INTEGRATED CARE
FOR IRELAND
IN AN INTERNATIONAL CONTEXT

CHALLENGES FOR POLICY, INSTITUTIONS AND SPECIFIC SERVICE USER NEEDS

Edited by

Tom O'Connor

D1477132

Published by OAK TREE PRESS, 19 Rutland Street, Cork, Ireland

www.oaktreepress.com

© 2013 Tom O'Connor

A catalogue record of this book is available from the British Library.

ISBN 978 1 78119 104 0 (hardback)
ISBN 978 1 78119 080 7 (paperback)
ISBN 978 1 78119 081 4 (ePub)
ISBN 978 1 78119 082 1 (Kindle)

Cover design: Kieran O'Connor Design
Cover illustration: bryljaev / 123RF Stock Photos

Printed in Ireland by SPRINT-print

CONTENTS

SECTION I: ECONOMIC AND PUBLIC POLICY INSIGHTS FROM IRELAND AND ABROAD

SECTION II: THE BIOMEDICAL AND SOCIAL INTERFACE OF INTEGRATED CARE: THEORY, POLICY AND SERVICE USERS' NEEDS

SECTION V: INTEGRATED CARE FOR MENTAL HEALTH AND DISABILITY SERVICE USERS

FIGURES

TABLES

ACKNOWLEDGEMENTS

The publication of this book was made possible by a wide variety of people. First, I'd like to thank all those who contributed to the book and served up what is a series of excellent chapters with scholarship in abundance. The expertise across the various fields is staggering. Thank you all very much.

I would like to thank the National Academy for the Integration of Research, Teaching and Learning for the financial support that has made this publication possible. In particular, my thanks to Jennifer Murphy, who strongly encouraged the endeavour from the outset. My thanks also to Damien Courtney, Margaret Linehan and Jim Walsh for their enthusiastic support for the book and to my colleagues, Ona McGrath and Moira Jenkins, who contributed chapters.

I would like to express my sincere gratitude to Brian O'Kane from Oak Tree Press, who displayed patience, diligence and camaraderie in equal measure in working with me throughout the project. Brian, you are one of the genuine 'nice guys'!

A big thank you to my partner, Déirdre, for her continuous support and enthusiasm throughout the time, and to Kathleen, my late mother, who loved me to share my work interests with her.

DEDICATION

I dedicate this book to my partner, Déirdre, who supports me every day in everything I do, and to Kathleen, my mother (recently deceased), for the gift of life and all the time we spent together.

CONTRIBUTORS

BENGT AHGREN earned his PhD at the Nordic School of Public Health and was later awarded an Associate Professor (Docent) position. He currently holds a professor chair in Public Health Management at the same institution. Nordic School of Public Health is a Nordic institution located in Gothenburg, Sweden.

RUNO AXELSSON was appointed Professor of Public Management at Uppsala University in 1984. In 2003, he was appointed Professor of Public Health Management at the Nordic School of Public Health in Gothenburg, Sweden. He is currently employed as Senior Adviser at the Sahlgrenska Academy, the medical faculty of Gothenburg University.

SUZANNE CAHILL is an Associate Professor of Social Policy and Ageing at Trinity College Dublin, where she teaches an undergraduate course on Ageing and Dementia and supervises several post-graduate students. She has worked as a social worker, researcher and educator and has served on many committees (in Ireland and Australia), campaigning for the rights of people with dementia. In 2011, she chaired the National Dementia Strategy Advisory Committee, which guided the evidence-based research review underpinning Ireland's forthcoming Dementia Strategy. She is currently Chairperson of Alzheimer's Café Ireland (Ireland's first Alzheimer's Café). Her research interests include (i) quality of life and dementia, (ii) social policy and family caregiving, and (iii) general practitioners and dementia. She has published widely nationally and internationally on ageing and dementia-related topics.

JIM CAMPBELL is Professor of Social Work, Goldsmiths College, University of London.

CLAIRE COLLINS is Director of Research at the Irish College of General Practitioners (ICGP). Claire has over 20 years' experience conducting and teaching qualitative and quantitative research in the academic, statutory and private sectors and has been the ICGP Director of Research since 2004, with responsibility for the promotion, development and implementation of research in general practice and representing the ICGP on various national and international committees. She is a Fellow of the

Royal Academy of Medicine in Ireland and is the Irish representative to the European General Practice Research Network.

CATHERINE DARKER is the Adelaide Professor in Health Services Research within the Department of Public Health & Primary Care, Trinity College Dublin. Dr Darker's research focuses on three areas: health policy and health services research; problem substance use and addiction; and primary care. Dr Darker has published widely across these diverse areas.

GAVIN DAVIDSON is Lecturer in Social Work, School of Sociology, Social Policy and Social Work, Queen's University Belfast.

LAURA DESMOND is a graduate of Cork Institute of Technology, BA Honours Social Care, and has been working in the area of drug addiction for the past number of years. Currently she is employed as a community-based drugs worker in a project in the north side of Cork City funded by the Health Service Executive, where she is administering the assessments (initial and comprehensive) developed by the National Drugs Rehabilitation Implementation Committee, which were piloted extensively across 44 services in Cork and Kerry. As a community-based drugs worker, Laura is involved in individual support, group work, onward referral to the relevant services, delivering drug awareness programmes for schools/groups and parents and also implementing programmes such a brief intervention programme and strengthening family programme.

MICHAEL DONNELLY is Reader in Health and Social Care Research in the School of Medicine, Queen's University Belfast (QUB), and Principal Investigator in the Northern Ireland Centre of Excellence for Public Health, QUB.

EITHNE FITZGERALD is Head of Policy and Research at the National Disability Authority, the independent statutory advisory body to the Government on disability policy and practice. Eithne is an economist. Her previous roles included working in the Department of Finance, with housing charity Threshold, as an independent researcher, serving in public life as Minister of State, and as a university lecturer.

MARK FLEMING is a Registered Mental Health Nurse who works in NHS Ayrshire and Arran in Scotland. He is also seconded part-time to Healthcare Improvement Scotland as National Integrated Care Pathways co-ordinator for mental health. Mark's work in Ayrshire is focussed on the development and implementation of integrated care pathways and their application within their electronic patient record. Mark's e-health work has expanded across many services; he loves to explore how technology can support clinical practice and is keen to try out new devices with clinicians to try to improve care.

VANESSA HETHERINGTON is Senior Policy Executive at the Irish Medical Organisation (IMO) since April 2008. She has a Master's degree in International Relations, a degree in European Business Studies, and a Diploma in Journalism and Media Studies. Prior to joining the IMO, Vanessa worked as research assistant on a number of media content analysis projects.

KATE IRVING joined Dublin City University in 2006 from University College Dublin, where she worked on Ireland's first Health Research Board-funded project in nursing decision-making. Kate's PhD was completed in Curtin University of Technology, Western Australia (2001: *Case Studies in the Use of Restraints*). Kate co-ordinates the Dementia Champion Module with the Health Service Executive and the North Dublin Alzheimer's Café, and is Clinical Lead in the Memory Works Clinic.

DEIRDRE JACOB is a social worker who holds qualifications to Master's degree level in Applied Social Research from Trinity College Dublin. She has worked in primary care as a member of two multidisciplinary teams in Dublin South West for approximately four years. She is currently Chairperson of the Irish Association of Social Workers Special Interest Group for Primary Care Social Workers and of the more recently-established Tallaght Roma Integration Project. She has a keen interest in combining community development approaches and primary health care approaches as a means of achieving better health outcomes in communities.

MOIRA JENKINS is an academic lawyer teaching on the social care and early childhood education degrees at Cork Institute of Technology. She practised as a barrister in Victoria, Australia, before lecturing on constitutional law and legal skills and analysis at University College Cork. She is admitted as a solicitor in the Supreme Court of England and Wales. Her current research interests focus on advocacy as a right, the participation rights of the vulnerable older person and the future role of the social care professional.

MARGARET MacADAM is president of The Age Advantage Inc., which provides consulting and strategic planning in policy and service delivery issues for the elderly. She is Associate Professor (Adjunct) at the

University of Toronto, Faculty of Social Work and teaches in the Health Studies Program of University College, University of Toronto.

LISA McGARRIGLE is a PhD candidate at Dublin City University currently researching cognitive protective and risk factors in dementia as part of Irish-led FP7-funded project, INMINDD. She holds a Bachelor of Social Science degree and a Master's degree in Sociology from University College Dublin, and a Higher Diploma in Psychology from Trinity College Dublin.

GRÁINNE McGETTRICK is the Policy and Research Manager for The Alzheimer Society of Ireland. This role includes commissioning research projects and policy papers, building strategic partnerships, engaging in policy analysis, securing funding and representing the organisation at various national and international fora. She holds a Bachelor of Social Science degree from University College Dublin and a Master's degree in Social Policy from NUI Maynooth.

ONA McGRATH is a lecturer in the Department of Social and General Studies, Cork Institute of Technology. She has an MSc in Adapted Physical Activity from the Katholieke University Leuven. Her interest areas are wellbeing, health promotion and adapted activities for persons with disabilities and chronic illnesses.

SHEENA McHUGH is a Health Services Researcher and Health Research Board Interdisciplinary Capacity Enhancement (ICE) Post-doctoral Research Fellow at the Department of Epidemiology and Public Health, University College Cork. Her research interests are health service delivery and organisation, quality of care and chronic disease management.

LINDA McKECHNIE has a professional background in mental health nursing, having qualified as a registered mental nurse (RMN) in 1985. Following completion of her RMN training at South West Scotland College of Nursing & Midwifery, she gained a Post Graduate Diploma in Community Care Studies from Glasgow University in 1995 and a Post Graduate Certificate in Project Management from Lancaster University Management School in 2006. She is currently undertaking an MSc in Dementia Studies at the University of Stirling. Linda has progressed her career in various clinical and managerial roles, and currently works as the Service Development Manager for the Mental Health, Psychology and Learning Disabilities Directorate in NHS Dumfries and Galloway. Her portfolio of responsibilities incorporates a wide range of strategic service improvement programmes. In addition to this role, Linda is the Deputy Chair of the Scottish Pathways Association. For five years, she worked part-time with Healthcare Improvement Scotland as a national co-ordinator for integrated care pathways (ICPs) and was involved in the development of the national standards for ICPs for mental health. She has co-authored publications on care pathways in the *International Journal of Care Pathways* and the *International Journal of Health and Social Care in the Community.*

JOE MORAN is a general practitioner, practicing in Fermoy, and a part-time lecturer in the Department of General Practice, University College Cork. He has worked in clinical and academic general practice in Ireland, Canada and the UK. His areas of special interest include case-reporting in general practice, doctor-patient communication, chronic disease management and medical education. He is a founding member and director of DiGP (Diabetes in General Practice) and a director and current chairman of the board of SouthDoc (out-of-hours family doctor service for Cork and Kerry).

MAURICE O'CONNELL took up the post of CEO of the Alzheimer Society of Ireland in 1999 and plays a central role in driving and growing the organisation. He is a non-executive director and former Chairman of Alzheimer Europe. Maurice currently participates in the Irish Joint Programming on Neurodegenerative Diseases hosted by the Health Research Board. He holds an MA in Applied Psychology.

TOM O'CONNOR is a College Lecturer in Economics/Health & Social Care Policy at Cork Institute of Technology. In 2006, he edited (with Mike Murphy) a book, *Social Care in Ireland*, and has published research reports and articles in the field of health and social care. He also has written widely on Irish economic policies in recent years and has been a frequent contributor to the national media.

DESMOND (DES) O'NEILL, a specialist in geriatric and stroke medicine, is also a writer and commentator in national media. Based in Tallaght Hospital and Trinity College Dublin, his practice and research are focussed on ageing and the neurosciences, and how they interact with the humanities. His particular interest in the longevity dividend – the many ways in which we have gained from our increase in life span – has contributed to national and international initiatives in many aspects of ageing. In Ireland, this includes developments in stroke, dementia and elder abuse: in 2010, he was awarded the All Ireland Inspirational Life Award for his work on behalf of older people.

MARGARET O'RIORDAN has been a general practitioner for the past 23 years. She holds an MBA in Leadership, Strategy & Renewal from Dublin City University, a BA in Adult Education & Training from NUI Galway, membership of the Irish College of General Practitioners and is a Fellow of the Royal College of General Practitioners. Dr O'Riordan has published research in the areas of medical education and quality improvement. Dr O'Riordan is the current Medical Director of the Irish College of General Practitioners. A senior management position operating at a strategic level within the College, the Medical Director has a key role in promoting general practice and shaping health policy through interaction with government, the public and the health sector. As head of professional competence, she supports GPs to attain and maintain excellence in clinical practice and patient safety and collaborates with external agencies to provide high quality general practice to agreed standards.

IVAN PERRY is Professor of Public Health and Head of the Department of Epidemiology and Public Health at University College Cork. He is a graduate of NUI Galway and the University of London. Professor Perry is the Foundation Director of Ireland's National Self Harm Registry. He is Principal Investigator (PI) on the Health Research Board (HRB) Centre for Health and Diet Research established in 2008 and a co-PI on the HRB-funded PhD Scholar Programme in Health Services Research. He was also co-PI on SLAN-07, Ireland's national health and lifestyle survey.

DIARMUID QUINLAN has an honours degree in physiology from University College Cork (UCC). Following an internship in Cork, he went to Kent, England to undertake a GP training scheme. He then worked in Australia for a year before returning to Ireland, where he started practice in Glanmire. He is chairman of the HSE South Diabetes Service Implementation Group and the Diabetes in General practice group and a member of the National Diabetes working group. He is an accredited clinical risk assessor in primary care with the Medical Protection Society – the only such assessor in the Republic of Ireland – and a tutor for undergraduate medial students at UCC.

WILLIAM REDDY is a Programme Manager at the Health Service Executive. He works in the Special Projects Unit of the Special Delivery Unit on ICT innovation and process improvement projects and also works with a number of acute hospitals on improving unscheduled and scheduled care performance.

JOHN SAUNDERS is the Director of Shine. He was a member of the 2003 Expert Group reviewing and updating mental health service policy, resulting in *Vision for Change*, and was Chair of the Second Independent Monitoring Group to oversee and report on its implementation. John was a member of the Second Mental Health Commission and is Chair of the current Commission. He has qualifications in nursing, a degree in Economics and a diploma in Public Administration.

FAISAL SHAIKH is a consultant at Tallaght Hospital and at the Royal College of Surgeons in Ireland.

STEVE THOMAS is an Assistant Professor in the Centre for Health Policy and Management, Trinity College Dublin. He leads research into the viability of universal health insurance in Ireland and the resilience of the Irish health system in austerity. He has a wealth of international experience in policy-oriented research.

DAVID THOMSON started his nursing career in 1992, specialising in mental health. When qualifying as a Registered Mental Health Nurse, he achieved the first-ever Distinction in Scotland at Diploma of Higher Education following nurse training being revised to promote higher levels of academia in the profession. He was awarded a Bachelor of Science in Health Studies in 1997 from the Caledonian University, Glasgow. He has worked in various health care settings, leading to secondment to Quality Improvement Scotland (now Healthcare Improvement Scotland) in 2008 as the National Programmes Manager for Mental Health attached to Scottish Government. He was responsible for leading and authoring the review of Best Practice Statement: Admissions to Adult Mental Health Inpatient Services, developing the national database of positive practice (**www.piramhids.com**), advisor/national trainer for the Releasing Time to Care programme and a member of two national programme boards: the National Prisoner Healthcare Group and the Scottish Patient Safety Programme Group. Currently, David is the National Co-ordinator for Integrated Care Pathways and an Inspector with Her Majesty's Inspectorate of Prisons. He is the Chairman of the Scottish Pathways Association and a member of the European Pathway Association International Committee. He has published in *International Journal of Care Pathways* and the *International Journal of Health and Social Care in the Community* and has presented his work both nationally and internationally.

SEAN TIERNEY is a Consultant Vascular Surgeon in Tallaght Hospital, Dublin and Dean of Professional Development and Practice in the Royal

College of Surgeons in Ireland. He was President of the Irish Medical Organisation in 2010-2011.

FOREWORD

Who could be against better integration of services? And yet one of the most common complaints of service users across many aspects of modern life is that integration that should be occurring is not taking place, that the various parts of the system are not 'talking' to each other.

A failure to integrate services is not just a matter of inconvenience: it has been shown repeatedly that outcomes, both personal and societal, are consistently better with more integrated services. In addition, a lack of integration inevitably means all the inefficiencies that duplication (or even triplication or worse) that ensue: this profligacy of human and organisational capital is unsustainable, particularly at a time of significant economic difficulties for the nation.

The picture is not uniformly bleak, and in some areas of care, interdisciplinary working in Ireland has developed considerably: examples include major improvements that have occurred in cancer care over the last decade, or the development of substance abuse programmes. However, it is not always obvious, even within health and social care services, as to which are the areas where we are integrating well, and which are the areas where we clearly are not.

Integrated Care for Ireland in an International Context therefore is particularly timely, and fills a gap in our knowledge of both what seems to work and also of areas where there is a patent failure to integrate services appropriately. Drawing on experience from a range of areas is a particular strength of the book, which includes overviews of mental health, services for older people and primary care, as well international perspectives.

The intensity and complexity of modern care provision is such that those in any one area usually have little opportunity to acquaint themselves with solutions in other areas of practice, and it is very likely that some elements of successful integrated care in one arena of care can provide insight and inspiration for improvement in care in others.

A broad perspective is helpful also in understanding the barriers and disincentives to integrated care. It is facile, and generally unhelpful, to lay all of the blame for the arrested development of integrated care on the government or the 'system', although clearly both are important aspects.

Some of the barriers come from within, whether from the dynamics of an Illichian regression of institutions and services from their primary goal of providing service to one of self-preservation or due to a lack of flexibility among various professional groupings to move beyond traditional practices of care.

Indeed, the rhetoric of most professions appears on the surface to embrace interdisciplinarity and integrated care: exercising this in practice is not a passive exercise but rather requires active engagement, often a degree of training, time and effort. This book provides insights that may facilitate this progress.

But perhaps the most important reason for producing this text is to remind us of the importance of moral and professional agency for those of us working in health and social care, and to provide an intellectual underpinning for advocacy that, at times, may be uncomfortable in its implication for our professional lives.

Sustained advocacy has made a difference in recent decades for a number of areas of care in Ireland, such as in care for stroke, and it is important that we develop synergies of purpose and method from this range of experiences. A hallmark of professionalism is a cautious optimism that the application of science and best practice will improve care. This must be no different for integrated care, a concept that is increasingly recognised as a professional and societal imperative. We might not just yet be at the point Victor Hugo described when he wrote that *"mightier than the tread of marching armies is the power of an idea whose time has come"*, but *Integrated Care for Ireland in an International Context* provides a welcome step forward for both action and debate.

Desmond O'Neill MA MD FRCPI AGSF FRCP(Glasg) FRCP
Dublin
June 2013

INTRODUCTION

This book has been produced to benchmark the use of integrated care systems in Ireland. Its starting point is examining policy in the overall sense on integrated care: **Chapter 1** traces the development of integrated care in an *ad hoc* way in public policy over the past 25 years or so, to a time when it started to unfold as an institutional model in the *Primary Care Strategy* of 2001, and in the clear parameters and model as laid out by the Health Service Executive (HSE) at the end of the 'noughties' and into the second decade of the 21st century. The chapter examines progress to date, with a particular focus on primary care, which is seen as the linchpin of integrated care. It takes as given that patients and clients need to be discharged to an integrated care environment within their community that has the appropriate configuration of primary care and community health and social care networks, in order to allow a patient to make a recovery, but also to allow them to remain in their own community into the future. In this context, a detailed discharge care plan, outlining these services at the level of primary/community care, is described in **Chapter 3** from a manager's perspective by William Reddy, a programme manager within the HSE. Of course, a suitable model for the financing of health care is a *sine qua non* for the successful development of integrated care going forward. Should we use a general taxation model, be more oriented to private funding models or use universal social insurance? These are the important questions dealt with by Steven Thomas and Catherine Darker in their detailed chapter on choosing the right model for health funding (**Chapter 4**).

Policy in Ireland can be compared to other countries within the Organisation for Economic Co-operation and Development (OECD) that have been developing integrated care for a lot longer than Ireland. For example, in **Chapter 5**, Bengt Ahgren and Runo Axelsson show that the development of integrated care in practice is more advanced in Sweden than in Ireland, though similar political and institutional blockages have developed. Similarly, Margaret MacAdam delimits the 'uneven journey' towards integrated care for the elderly in Canada (**Chapter 13**), depending on which region of the country a patient resides in and the varying level of commitment to integrated care by different stakeholders in different places.

Indeed, older people are probably the most significant sub-population group in Ireland for which integrated care is required. With a dramatic increase in the older population to about 1.25 million by 2030, and a sadly undeveloped system of home care and community care, integrated care for older people is urgent at this point. The urgency of this need, and the lack of sufficient progress to date, is described by Des O'Neill, whose chapter leaves the rolling out of integrated care for the elderly going forward as an open-ended question, 'perhaps jam tomorrow' (**Chapter 15**). Similarly, Suzanne Cahill decries the lack of progress to date for those who suffer with dementia, their families and their carers, asking if the promise of integrated care for those with dementia is indeed a 'dream or reality' (**Chapter 14**). In the same vein, in **Chapter 16**, Kate Irving, Lisa McGarrigle, Grainne McGettrick and Maurice O'Connell assess the strengths and weaknesses of the forthcoming National Dementia Strategy in delivering integrated care pathways.

Integrated Care in Ireland in an International Context clearly has an international focus: we already have seen references to Sweden and Canada. We also have an opportunity to examine progress within the United Kingdom, in Scotland and in Northern Ireland. Progress towards integrated care in Northern Ireland can be compared to that in the south of the country (**Chapter 2**), through the inclusion of a wide-ranging chapter by Jim Campbell, Gavin Davidson and Michael Donnelly. Scotland has been a leading exponent of technology transfer in the wider health and social care services in recent years. The experience of NHS Trusts and the development of integrated care for mental health service users is the focus of the work of Mark Fleming, Linda McKechnie and David Thomson in **Chapter 18**, which offers salutary lessons for the stalled Irish experience in implementing *Vision for Change*. The socially-regressive nature of this failure since 2006 is described by John Saunders in **Chapter 17**, whereby successive governments have been unwilling to fund and roll out *Vision for Change*, to the detriment of service users. This unwillingness has stopped the development of integrated mental health care in its tracks.

We can see that the book makes international comparisons on progress in developing integrated care in Ireland by comparing its progress internationally. But, there is a second focus on specific service user groups in urgent need of integrated care: the elderly and the mentally ill are cases in point. **Chapter 1** outlines the wider integrated care service model that is meant to deal with both the general population and all of the various sub-populations, including mental health and disability. The practicalities involved in providing supports for disabled people within the drive towards integrated care are the focus of **Chapter 20** by Eithne Fitzgerald of the National Disability Authority. This chapter brings us up-to-date on the various strands of government policy towards disability, including the *Disability Act, 2005* and the National Disability Strategy, going beyond the policy to examine what the practical benefits have been and where the shortfalls are in moving away from institutional living patterns towards integrated care in the community. Another increasing important sub-population in need of integrated care, in the context of rising rates of liver disease and suicide within young cohorts of the population, are those who are addicted. Laura Desmond and I provide evaluatory evidence, based on primary research with 'policy-makers' and 'policy-implementers', on the promising National Drug Rehabilitation Implementation Committee (NDRIC) (2010) integrated care framework for those in need of addiction services (**Chapter 7**). In a different vein, we are increasingly aware of the potential health time bomb that is diabetes, when examined from a population health perspective in Ireland. The gargantuan challenge that diabetes will provide, necessitating both integrated care treatment and health promotion urgently, is the subject of a deeply-analytical chapter by Sheena McHugh and Ivan Perry (**Chapter 6**), where the authors see the significant challenge of integrated care 'meaning different things to different people'. Reverting back to disability, the law has been a useful tool in pushing for the rights of disabled people in the past. In **Chapter 19**, Moira Jenkins explores the use of the law, by way of Ireland's ratification of the *United Nations Convention on the Rights of Persons with Disabilities*, to further progress towards achieving real social rights for disabled people in the move towards more independent living and appropriate integrated services, based on these rights. She argues that the establishment of a statutorily-defined social care advocate would greatly expand this agenda.

In addition to this three-fold approach to Irish policy, international and service user foci within the book, the fourth and final ingredient entails examining the future of integrated care in Ireland for the most significant professional groupings that are involved in rolling it out. This requires a greater level of understanding of other professional projects and much higher quantums of patience and forbearance to work in a multidisciplinary way. Some international evidence on the best way to achieve this is provided from Finland in the chapter by Ona McGrath on interprofessional working (**Chapter 10**). Of course, it is all very well for the

Irish Department of Health to publish policies towards integrated care and for the HSE to publish models for its administration and delivery but the practical implementation of such policies needs to be examined. In this regard, two Cork general practitioners, Diarmuid Quinlan and Joe Moran, offer a sobering assessment in **Chapter 9** of the current state of primary care as it has developed here to date, calling for the increasing incentivisation of evidence-based treatments in diabetes and other areas, as part of a series of necessary reforms of the general practice system, as we move towards integrated care. Similarly, Margaret O'Riordan and Claire Collins of the Irish College of General Practitioners explore the evidence-base for interdisciplinary working within primary care teams internationally and apply these lessons to the Irish experience in **Chapter 12**. Staying within the medical profession, in **Chapter 8** Vanessa Hetherington, Faisal Shaikh and Sean Tierney of the Irish Medical Organisation, consider the future for medicine across the different interfaces between primary, secondary and tertiary care, if integrated care in Ireland is to be successful. In a wide-ranging, structurally-oriented chapter, Deirdre Jacob of the Irish Association of Social Workers explores the deep-seated linkages between primary care and social work, two of the most pivotal professions in providing integrated care pathways 'as a new way of delivering services' (**Chapter 11**).

Integrated Care in Ireland in an International Context aims to bring the debate on the future of integrated care in Ireland to a wider audience than heretofore. It is intended to guide the thinking of policy-makers and the whole panoply of different health and social care professions that are stakeholders in the process. Equally important, it is hoped that groups representing the needs of the general population, those with disability, mental illness, older people with specific needs and others also will benefit from the text. The whole project is to improve the overall health and wellbeing of all who live in Ireland.

It is hoped also that this publication will be a spur to the further development of research and teaching in the area of integrated care, as well as being a catalyst for the resourcing and implementation of improved public policy in the area. As such, this book will be important to students and lecturers across the disciplines of medicine, social work, social care, gerontology, addiction, health management, lawyers in health and human rights areas, mental health therapists and other sister professions that are not included here, such as occupational and speech/language/auditory therapies.

On a personal level, I would like to sincerely thank all the contributors who have served up an outstanding array of chapters for this book. It has been a pleasure to read and edit your work and to work with you on this project. The depth and compass of this book has surpassed even the highest expectations I had when commissioning chapters at the outset. The chapters display an outstandingly high level of scholarship and attention to detail for which I will be eternally grateful.

I wish the readers of this book a fulfilling voyage in their study of integrated care in all its facets and with reference to the various patient/client groups, professions and international case studies, on offer in the book.

Bon appétit!

Tom O'Connor
Cork
May 2013

1: INTEGRATED CARE IN IRELAND: PROGRESS FROM POLICY TO PRACTICE TO DATE

Tom O'Connor

This chapter seeks to examine the extent to which integrated care has progressed in Ireland from the 1980s up to the present day.

The first section uses a historically-sequential structure to trace the development of a working public policy for integrated care in Ireland from the 1980s up to 2000. The second section covers the period from 2001 to the present, where real organisational models for the development of integrated care came to the fore. In both sections, there is an examination of the perceived practical benefits of integrated care with reference to various building block documents and covering different patient/client groups. The third section compares the organisational model for integrated care and varying policy prescriptions from 2001 to the present to the actual practical delivery of integrated care currently, commenting on the successes/failures in the translation of public policy to practical integrated care delivery, particularly on how far the actual health and social care infrastructure has followed the developments in public policy. This section also examines three main areas: the development of primary care teams (PCTs) and primary care centres (PCCs); mental health services; and disability services. The chapter ends with conclusions and comments on the future for integrated care in Ireland.

1980s TO 2000

The rudiments of integrated care were present in a variety of health policy documents going back nearly 30 years in Ireland. The mental health policy blueprint, *Planning for the Future*, advocated a de-institutionalised approach to mental health services delivery with a greater emphasis on care in the community-based mental health centres

(Department of Health (DoH), 1984). However, at that stage, the move to de-institutionalisation and community care was itself an innovative idea, and although in hindsight a significant pre-cursor to integrated care, it was not immersed in any wider and deeper model of integrated care, with the term itself not having been formally conceived of at the time.

Ten years later, *Shaping a Healthier Future* (DoH, 1994), a wide-ranging and comprehensive policy document that covered the whole spectrum of health and social care, demonstrated that public policy was moving towards a progressive realisation of incorporating integrated care into the health and social care landscape. For example, the belief that services needed to become integrated, and that both thinking and practice needed to be joined-up, seems clear in an opening salvo that called for:

> ... re-orientation of services with an increased emphasis on the provision of the most appropriate care, which in turn requires the improvement of the linkages between services (DoH, 1994: 14).

Integrated care requires that, for the person as a whole, services need to move beyond a singular focus on medical disease. Good health has wider dimensions that go beyond the absence of a medical condition and must incorporate social aspects: positive social interaction is crucially important to good mental health; healthy lifestyles are strongly influenced by exercise, diet, good nutrition and issues concerning a healthy work-life balance are all important, along with many others. These factors contribute to improved quality of life, a term that had only begun to be used in the policy discourse in the early 1990s. The recognition in *Shaping a Healthier Future* of health and quality of life was exemplified in its introduction of two new terms: 'health gain' and 'social gain', the former referring to the necessary health improvements that could be achieved using medicine, and the latter referring to the wider social dimensions that crucially impact on one's health. A further critical impetus to introduce social gain as a key public policy goal was the need to have due recognition that a significant proportion of the overall demand for services was accounted for by groups that were in need of interventions primarily based on social/psychological interventions, in particular those possessing intellectual disabilities or mental illness and other groups such as older people and children who needed what were previously called 'personal and social services', but which are now termed 'social care'.

A major breakthrough in moving towards integrated care was the introduction in *Shaping a Healthier Future* of the population health approach to health and social care (DoH, 1994). The document contained an emphasis on improving the epidemiological data on which critical population health decisions (the term 'health' in this chapter is used in the widest sense, incorporating the medical and social elements as discussed) were made. To bolster this approach, there was a strong emphasis on the two key elements of health promotion and disease prevention. Even more significantly for integrated care, *Shaping a Healthier Future* introduced an emphasis on 'care in appropriate setting' (DoH, 1994: 22). It also proposed the increased use of epidemiological and public health functions alongside health technology, research and evaluation and specific population groups.

Though the full conceptualisation and development of integrated care as a working concept, let alone clearly delineated models to deliver same, were not worked out at that stage, further building blocks were clearly committed to within the document. Key in this regard were 'service development linkages' (DoH, 1994: 22) between GPs, community-based services and acute hospitals. In a clear statement of what was to be done, and where integration was actually mentioned for the first time, the document stated:

> The system is too compartmentalised to achieve the objective of providing care in an appropriate setting, it is essential that there are effective linkages between the services. Hospitals, general practitioners and other community services should operate as elements of an integrated system within which patients can move freely as their needs dictate. At present, the system is too compartmentalised to permit this flexibility (DoH, 1994: 26).

This clear objective of an integrated system firmly rested on the role of the General Practitioner (GP). However, the remit for the GP was vast and to a large extent unrealistic, notwithstanding the critical role of the GPs who deal with close to 90% of medical needs (Brennan, 2003). This pivotal centrality of GPs, however, did not equip them to deal with the vast array of needs that the document posited, with the document making claims that in future GPs would have:

> ... a wider and more integrated role in the health system ... a holistic approach to the care of patients, taking full account of psychological, social and environmental factors influencing patients (DoH, 1994: 52).

One such chosen area to deliver integration was mental health, where the role of the GP in integrating with existing secondary mental services was set as a clear goal:

> To integrate mental health and primary health services and in particular to strengthen the role of general practitioners in the care of the mentally ill (DoH, 1994: 70).

The document did refer to the fact that, at the time, most GPs operated in single GP practices, which made this objective all the more daunting. However, it proposed that group practices should become the norm in the medium term, though these hardly equipped GPs for the wider role as envisioned.

In common with the development of integrated services in many other countries, the role of voluntary and community providers was seen as integral. Ireland had relied since the foundation of the State on voluntary service providers, mainly by way of the Catholic Church organisations. A litany of shameful events and the destruction of many lives occurred within this predominantly institutional approach, such as industrial schools, the Magdalene laundries and services for the intellectually disabled (see, for example, Rafferty and O'Sullivan, 1999; Doyle, 1989; Galvin, 2002; Goulding, 2005). Since the publication of reports such as Kennedy (1970) and the belated start of an emphasis on child protection, most notably in the *Child Care Act, 1991*, the near monopoly of the Catholic Church on social services has been eroded. In this context, *Shaping a Healthier Future* (DoH, 1994) envisaged an increasing role for a heterogeneous variety of voluntary and community service providers to liaise with GPs and other elements within the wider health system to start the process of providing integrated care for vulnerable groups such as the disabled, older people, mentally ill, children at risk and others. In this context, the document emphasises de-institutionalisation, which involves home and community care in which integrated care is sited:

> The continuing care services are in a process of rapid development. In particular, community-based services are being provided both as an alternative to institutional care where appropriate and to address previously unmet needs for support for vulnerable groups (DoH, 1994: 24).

It is salient to note in the extract below the reference to the seminal document, *Years Ahead: A Policy for the Elderly* (DoH, 1988), which also emphasised the importance of home and community care, in this case for the older population, though public policy to a large extent moved backwards towards nursing home care in the years that followed, which only served to hamper efforts to provide integrated care for the growing elderly population. The correct objectives, however, were laid down in the 1990s:

The objectives of health and personal social services for older people which currently guide the development of services were recommended in the Report of the Working Party on Services for the Elderly, *Years Ahead: A Policy for the Elderly*. They are: to maintain older people in dignity and independence at home, in accordance with the wishes of older people as expressed in many research studies; to encourage and support the care of older people in their own community by family, neighbours and voluntary bodies in every way possible (DoH, 1994: 66).

We will observe below that PCTs of health and social care professions, in liaison with a wider network of social service providers, became a policy blueprint for integrated care in the 2000s. However, with regard to the older population, the early stages of this policy began with the delineation of an emerging model of co-operation between GPs and others working in the health and social services at the level of home and community. The emphasis here was on allowing the vast majority of older people to be cared for at home. The aim was:

To restore to independence at home those older people who become ill or dependent. Strengthening the role of the general practitioner, the public health nurse, the home help and other primary care professionals in supporting older people and their carers who live at home. The target will be to ensure that not less than 90 per cent of those over 75 years of age continue to live at home (DoH, 1994: 67).

Consequently, the clear objective of developing an integrated system between hospitals, GPs and community services – the essence of integrated care – became a stated public policy goal as far back as 1994. It was not clearly worked out, however; in particular, it took years for the concept of a 'discharge planning system', whereby acute hospitals could discharge patients to enhanced integrated primary/community care services, even to become a suggestion. Furthermore, this period (and indeed until 2008, as shown below) is characterised by a piecemeal 'working up' to integrated care. Policy-makers and practitioners began working from a practical knowledge of what constitutes integrated care organically, rather than having a clear working definition or key underlying aims and objectives at the outset.

2001 TO DATE

Probably the most significant impetus towards the recognition of integrated care as the pre-eminent approach for the future delivery of health and social care services came with the publication of *Quality and*

Fairness (Department of Health and Children (DoHC), 2001a) and the accompanying *Primary Care Strategy* (DoHC, 2001b). These two documents set out the model for integrated care, yet there is no actual definition of what constitutes integrated care. In fact, there is no definition of integrated care in any of the core policy documents informing its development in Ireland, although these documents delineated a clear model for the future organisation, planning and delivery of services into the future.

Similar to the previous strategy, and in line with international best practice, primary care became the central focus for future development. The vision was to prevent patients and clients from having to seek the services of acute hospitals or residential care. The programme was driven by the high cost of admissions to acute hospitals, the long waiting lists for hospital beds and the fact that waiting on hospital trolleys had started to become a permanent feature of the Irish secondary health care system. Concomitantly, the fact that Ireland, with one of the youngest population demographics and people of working age in the EU, would become a reversed demographic by 2030, when at least 1.2 million people would be aged over the age of 65, added to the urgency. Numerous reports dealing with older people highlighted that the vast majority wished to receive health and social care services in their community and their own homes (National Council on Aging and Older People (NCAOP), 2002). This seamless integration of health and social care needs, though not yet specifically termed 'integrated care', was considered to be the gold standard (DoHC, 2001a), and added further impetus. Strong advocacy towards this imperative came from organisations such as Age Action and NCAOP. The National Disability Authority (NDA) and Inclusion Ireland also called for the de-institutionalisation of the Irish social care system, strengthening the call to deliver on integrated care.

Although *Quality and Fairness* (DoHC, 2001a) did not define specifically what was meant by the term 'integrated care', nonetheless it displayed an understanding of integrated care and planned for it in practical terms. Integrated care meant a co-ordinated system where the hospital system stay became a last resort; if there was recourse to hospital, then time would be minimised there; there would be a clear and seamless strategy integrating the acute hospital system with primary and community care services through the use of a discharge plan for patients, allowing them to receive the full configuration of health and social care that they needed once discharged. So, even though successful integrated care would have a strong emphasis on care in the primary and community care systems, integration would involve the acute hospital system also or indeed any system that 'warehouses' people to the point where they would need to be transferred to their community, in line with established policy. This included low to medium dependency disabled clients also, and other population groups where it was more appropriate to leave a hospital, a mental institution, a residential care home or nursing home. Consequently, the *Primary Care Strategy* (DoHC, 2001b) used a population health approach that applied to the health of the general population but also provided separate health/care strategies for specific sub-populations: those with chronic illnesses; the disabled; older people; mentally ill patients; and others.

Application of the Current Definition

It has been noted that, historically in Ireland, it took considerable time to develop a practical understanding of the application of integrated care, let alone define it. It is clear that the concept itself has proved to be unwieldy and can mean different things to different professions, depending on the context in which it is being applied. Even in this book, we see different definitions of integrated care, each emphasising a different aspect of the whole. There are many definitions in the international literature, and they differ significantly. This lack of agreement on a universal definition, the search for which could hamper the development of integration within the Irish health and social care services, probably informed the decision of Irish policy-makers to only loosely define its meaning, which itself only happened *circa* 2007 (Health Service Executive (HSE), 2007). This occurred a considerable time after the concept and its application had begun to slowly develop, and gradually melded into public health thinking almost through a process of osmosis.

Integrated care has two main foci, each operating in opposite directions:

- Preventing patients from entering acute hospitals or institutions through the provision of enhanced primary and community care;
- Enabling patients/clients to leave acute hospitals or institutions with a suitable discharge health (patients) social care plan (clients) into primary / community care services.

In both cases, a thoroughly revamped primary care system became necessary. In this context, one of the most positive innovations in the *Primary Care Strategy* (DoHC, 2001b) was the commitment to create up to 531 PCTs throughout the country. These had already been set up in many other countries years before (Kokko, 2009). The professional configuration of each team in the Irish context is shown in **Table 1.1**.

Table 1.1: Configuration of Primary Care Teams

Profession	Number of staff planned
General Practitioner	4.0
Health Care Assistant	3.0
Home Helps	3.0
Nurse/Midwife	5.0
Occupational Therapist	0.5 – 1.0
Physiotherapist	0.5 – 1.0
Social Worker	0.5 – 1.0
Receptionist/Clerical Officer	4.0
Administrator	1.0

Source: DoHC, 2001b: 24.

Note: For the purpose of calculations, the average population size served by the PCT is taken as 5,000. Eight additional whole-time equivalents (WTEs) would be required to provide extended hours care by the PCT and 24-hour GP and nursing/midwifery services.

The key feature of integrated care in this context was to integrate the health and social care needs of any patient/client in a holistic and relatively seamless way, thereby preventing admissions to acute hospitals or residential care. Of course, this could not succeed without the necessary ability of PCTs to refer members of the population to a full array of wider health and social care interventions within the hinterland that the PCT was to serve. The combination of both sets of services was needed to deliver full integration within one holistic entity. This integration was to be achieved by the established system linkages between the PCTs and what was then called Primary Care Networks (PCNs) (later subsumed into Health and Social Care Networks (HSCNs)) and wider specialist services. A PCN consisted of the professionals shown in **Table 1.2**.

Table 1.2: Configuration of Primary Care Networks

Chiropodist	Community Pharmacist
Community Welfare Officer	Dentist
Dietician	Psychologist
Speech and Language Therapist	

Source: DoHC, 2001b: 24.

The most significant level of integration would occur between the PCTs and the wider specialist services and professionals in those services, encompassing the full range of health and social care professionals:

> The primary care team will integrate with these .community-based specialist teams in ways similar to how the primary care team will integrate with the <u>specialist</u> institutional services, e.g. acute hospitals. The benefit of this from the perspective of users is that they are facilitated, through a single point of contact, in accessing whatever specialist services they require. Examples of specialist teams based in the community include:

- Palliative care;
- Mental health;
- Child care;
- Disability (intellectual and physical/sensory);
- Special client groups (e.g. homeless, Travellers);
- Community services for the elderly (DoHC, 2001c).

Figure 1.1: Integrating the Primary Care Team within the Health System

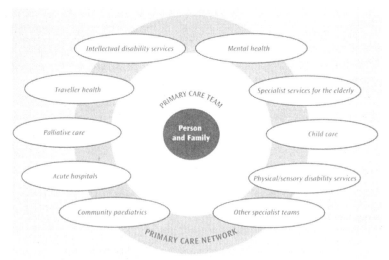

Source: DoHC, 2001b: 28.

Professionals in social work, social care, speech and language therapy and occupational therapy – the wider 'social professionals' – would work in many of the areas outlined in **Figure 1.1**: intellectual disability, Traveller health, services for the elderly, palliative care and physical/sensory disabilities. However, they would share information and expertise with health professionals and other social professionals in the PCT and PCN. This integrates medical and social care at the level of primary care, which itself occurs in the community. Hence there is integration between primary and community care. The primary and community care focus surrounds the person and his/her family in the community. Prevention of people being admitted to hospital or residential care in many cases would be achieved. Also, those patients in hospitals or in residential care (if in low to medium dependency and with sufficient supports) could be discharged into well-resourced primary and community care services that would be fully integrated with each other, delivering integrated care.

This is still the model for integrated care delivery in Ireland. However, there has been a change in nomenclature and emphasis: the PCN and the array of specialist services now form part of a HSCN (see **Table 1.4** later in this chapter and the HSE *National Service Plans*), alongside their collaboration with PCTs. These would work together in a mutually advantageous way and serve local populations of up to 5,000 people. The panoply of voluntary social care providers form part of this network, while aiding the proposed strengthening of working relationships between professionals working in a voluntary social care organisation (for example, disability) and GPs, nurses, counsellors, podiatrists or others in the PCT. Again, health and social care practice meet and a variety of providers, be they private, voluntary or public, across a variety of specialisms, work in close co-operation with PCT members, mostly focused on areas of medical expertise, to deal holistically with the total health and social care needs of the patient/client. Other services in community, such as support groups, that could improve the quality of life of the patient/client, are also included:

> It is intended that most of the primary and social care needs are met by locally based PCTs – the members of the PCT will be aligned to locally assessed needs and resources:
> - Teams have common goals based on health care outcomes and shared values. They also have shared standards and operating processes;
> - An average of five PCTs will make up a Health and Social Care Network (HSCN) serving a wider, but related, population of 30,000 to 50,000 people;
> - HSCNs will include a pool of specialised resources that serve PCT communities;

- PCTs and HSCNs will be integrated with hospitals, multi-agencies, private providers, voluntary agencies, and with support groups (HSE, 2010a: 9).

The way it would work is envisaged in a hypothetical (my own) case study of an older person:

> If an older woman had multi-system health/social care needs, she would be dealt with in a PCT (level 1 in the integrated services model), ideally situated in a PCC. Here, her GP would treat for her these conditions, prescribing medicine where necessary and other appropriate medical interventions. Follow-up health checks, the taking of blood samples and other important functions could be provided by the practice nurse. The social worker could organise additional care services from within the HSCN (level 2), which might include day care services, home help, speech and language therapy (for example, if the patient had been a stroke victim) or other necessary community care services (for example, home help or home care). Physiotherapy also might be necessary or the patient might be referred for sessions of counselling. These services would be provided after all the various professions involved had met as a team and had formulated an over-arching health and social care plan for the woman. A dedicated care plan, formulated to include all these necessary inputs for the woman, would be seamless and holistic and allow her to live at home without the necessity of being moved to hospital or a residential care facility. Subsequently, team meetings would be held to monitor the progress of the patient and to make any necessary modifications to her care plan. Any minor injuries could be referred to an urgent care centre in the community (level 3). If this woman developed severe renal problems, for example, she would be referred to a large acute hospital Centre of Excellence (level 4), situated in regional centres and where an enhanced ambulance service would be available at immediate notice to urgently speed this transition. A strong integrated and managed communication system would allow speedy assessment at all levels and the sharing of information in an integrated way across the four levels of this integrated services model.

Clearly, the model for this comprehensive delivery of integrated care had been put in place for the first time in the *Primary Care Strategy* (DoHC, 2001b). However, the progress towards showcasing new models of integrated care was delivered in a most impressive way *via* the publication of the *Vision for Change* (Mental Health Commission (MHC), 2006) mental health services blueprint. This offered a clear and structured programme for the delivery of integrated care services in the area of mental health. The term 'integrated care' became understood as the integration of medical care and other social interventions that were necessary for a person's holistic mental health. Fully-provided-for integrated care reflected the seamless aggregation of the medical and social into this new entity.

Vision for Change (MHC, 2006) almost immediately became accepted as government policy. It posited for the first time the view that any mental health problem was to be understood as an integrated problem through the use of a 'biopsychosocial model' of assessment, which itself required integrated solutions. This biopsychosocial model of mental ill-health meant that genetic predisposition, brain chemistry abnormalities and the development of psychological problems as a result of these and/or other faulty learning-induced psychological conditions, were treated alongside social everyday-life mental ill-health risk factors, such as alcohol misuse, work-related stress, bereavement and other factors.

These policy proposals required an integrated response to an integrated problem: the established PCTs would deal with the patient suffering from mental ill-health. A series of interventions would be designed by the team that might include drug therapy, home help or other services. The PCT then would refer the patient to a Community Mental Health Team (CMHT), a direct proposal in *Vision for Change*. Appropriate services, which might include cognitive behaviour therapy or other inputs, could be added. Ongoing liaison would occur regularly between the CMHT and the PCT. Also, the professional make-up of each CMHT would differ, depending on which segment of the population it was designed to work for: specific mental health services would be delivered to different population groups such as children, older people, those with intellectual disabilities, ex-prisoners or those from the general population. Services for these sub-populations would be designed and tailored for delivery within population catchment areas of specific size.

Other significant policy developments followed *Vision for Change*, so that by the end of the 2000s, integrated care had become the pre-eminent policy model for the delivery of all health and social care services across the various categories of the population in need of care. This required further plans for the re-structuring and organisational management of the health and social care systems. The re-structuring of the health services began with the introduction of the HSE, which included a further strong emphasis on more developed management models. As a result, the HSE published its *Transformation Programme for 2007-2010* (HSE, 2006) and subsequently its annual *National Service Plans* in the years thereafter. Planning for integrated care delivery and auditing the required resources became the linchpins of these programmes, alongside a strong commitment to a population health approach.

With the establishment of the HSE still in its early years, and with promises of a new era for the Irish health care services under its CEO, Dr. Brendan Drumm, the HSE's *Transformation Programme* (2006) made clear promises on the delivery of integrated care by 2010, which were included within six established priorities. **Table 1.3** quotes some of these specifically:

Table 1.3: Health Transformation Priorities

Priority one: 'Develop integrated services across all stages of the health journey'.

Priority two: 'Configure primary, community and continuing care services so that they deliver optimal and cost effective results'.

Priority four: 'Implement a model for the prevention and management of chronic illness'

Priority six: 'Ensure all staff engage in transforming health and social care in Ireland' (HSE, 2006: 11)

The programme set clear targets to be achieved by 2010 under each priority. Each priority was established as an action point and the programme guaranteed specific changes by way of 'where we will be by 2010'. The transformation towards achieving these priorities would mean that:

"My journey into, through and out of the health and social care system will be easy to navigate." (Priority one)

"I will be able to easily access a broad spectrum of care services through my local primary care team, i.e. conveniently and close to my home". (Priority two)

"I can expect high quality care and results from comprehensive and integrated care programmes which will involve my community and designated care centres." (Priority four)

With regard to staff: "My work will have a direct impact on delivering high quality care and contribute to overall transformation of health and social services." (Priority six) (HSE, 2006: 11).

Though there is a clear commitment to integrated care, the HSE, following the *Primary Care Strategy* (DoHC, 2001b), still recognises the pitfalls in using a rigid and highly specific definition of integrated care. Remember, at this point, the term 'integrated care' had been used since *Shaping a Healthier Future* (DoH, 1994). However, in 2008, the HSE offered the following loose working definition of integrated care:

An Integrated Health System is based on a way of delivering health care, i.e. a particular integrated model of care. In health systems that support the integrated model of care, patients can get in, through and out of the health service more quickly. They spend less time in hospital and more time being cared for in their communities or in their own homes. They are more likely to receive the type and quality of care they need, when they need it, in the most appropriate setting and from the most appropriate health care professional (HSE, 2008: 5).

The HSE *National Service Plans* in 2009 (and annually thereafter) evidenced clear examples of the use of information and 'technology transfer' (Cooper, 2011) to inform the development of integrated care services. They also included a strong focus on 'new public management' (Pollitt, 2003; Clarke and Newman, 1997). At this point, the use of high quality information, informed through a population health approach, resulted in a clear and well-designed model of integrated care for the whole country. The best and most impressive model using this approach up to that point had been *Vision for Change* (MHC, 2006).

The National Director for Integrated Care of the HSE described the model to a conference in 2010 (McCallion, 2010). In that presentation, he acknowledged that this highly-developed model included insights from previous policy documents such as: the *Primary Care Strategy* (DoHC, 2001b); *Vision for Change* (MHC, 2006); the *HSE Corporate Plan 2008-2011* (2008a); *Towards an Integrated Health Service or More of the Same?* (HSE, 2008b); section 33.2 of the *National Disability Strategy* (Department of Justice and Equality, 2004); *Towards 2016* (Department of the Taoiseach, 2006); *An Evaluation of Cancer Services in Ireland: A National Strategy* (DoH, 1996) and a report by PA Consulting, entitled *Inspiring Confidence in Children and Family Services: Putting Children First and Meaning It* (HSE, 2009a). More importantly, his presentation indicates that this new integrated care model could be used for all the health and social care services planned for in these policy documents. This model thus represents the 'gold standard' organisational, financial and human resource management system at the macro level, on which all services for the general population, as well as specific patient and client groups within the wider population, now rest.

Taking the focus of the 2001 primary care model, the variety of health and social care services documentation as described above, the HSE *Code of Practice for Integrated Discharge Planning* (2008c) and the service delivery model (included in HSE *National Service Plans* (2009b; 2010a; 2011a) below into consideration, it is clear that integrated care works in two directions:

- Hospital discharge planning/discharges from residential care by the HSE to enhanced primary and community care systems – that is, health/care in the appropriate setting, including home care;
- Enhanced illness prevention, health promotion and health/care treatment within primary and community care to prevent primary admission to acute hospital or residential care, in the context of the general population and various sub-populations, such as older people, the mentally ill, disabled, dementia sufferers, those with chronic diabetes, drug abusers and others.

Figure 1.2: The Health Service Executive's Service Delivery Model

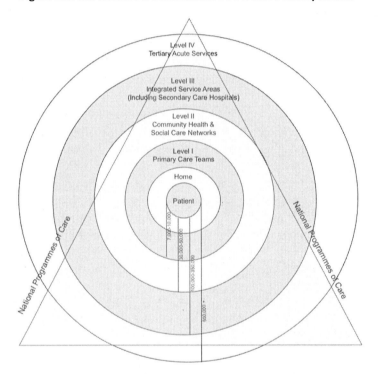

Source: HSE, 2011a: 14.

The model takes into consideration: an increase in the general population; the ageing demographic; and the projected increased incidence in numbers of people suffering from asthma, heart disease, cancer and diabetes (McCallion, 2010). In addition, McCallion pointed out that, in 2010, 531 PCTs (abbreviated from Primary Care Health Teams (PCHTs)) had been mapped out for the whole country to cater for these and other health care needs (level 1). Indeed, the following year, the HSE *National Service Plan* (2011a) confirmed that these had been formed and were in place. However, the HSCNs (level 2) were still work in progress in 2010. Given that patients require a discharge plan before they can be safely allowed to return home, as part of the new hospital configuration programme, hospital populations were to be synchronised to where integrated services were being rolled out. Integration was to happen by transferring 'non-complex acute services to local hospitals and/or PCTs' (McCallion, 2010: 11). These smaller local hospitals would work in close co-operation with PCTs and would have 'co-terminous populations'. These non-complex hospitals are situated at level 3 of the integrated services model. The PCTs would be designated into eight integrated service areas (ISAs) nationwide but would represent 'the building blocks for an integrated service area' (McCallion, 2010: 12). A large proportion of the secondary care needs of the population would be handled by these specifically designated acute secondary care hospitals. This is completely new: for the first time, primary care and secondary care would be virtually melded together in close co-operation between smaller local hospitals and primary care teams, all happening under a wider ISA within the integrated service delivery model but where integrated care is delivered across levels 1, 2 and 3 and 4 within the overall ISA:

> The new HSE Integrated Care model will deliver services across Integrated Service Areas (ISAs), where one person will be responsible for all hospital and community services ... The new HSE service delivery model puts the patient at the centre of the process – with Primary Care Teams (PCTs) at Level I, Community Health & Social Care Networks at Level II, Integrated Services Areas (including secondary care hospitals) at Level III and Tertiary acute services at Level IV ... The policy objective was to transfer non-complex acute services to local hospitals and/or PCTs. To support this concept, PCTs and related secondary care acute hospitals should have co-terminous populations (McCallion, 2013: 1).

The progress on level 3 of the ISAs within the overall service delivery model is quite slow. There is a lack of clarity about which acute hospitals will become the local hospitals performing non-complex acute services. In fact, there is not a large amount of clear confirmation within HSE policy documentation that smaller acute non-complex hospitals will always be located at level 3 of the integrated services model, though this can be deduced from some of the documentation – for example: HSE (2011a) and HSE South (2011a) but particularly in McCallion (2010; 2013). The HSE South (2011b) hospital reconfiguration plan (the *Higgins Report*) does not make it clear which hospitals currently delivering the full-range of acute services (complex and non-complex) will be expected in the future to handle non-acute cases, in the context of the transfer of complex acute cases to level 4 centres of excellence and the expanded role for local non-complex acute secondary hospitals in delivering integrated care within the ISAs across levels 1 to 3, and whereby tertiary care at level 4 will happen only at larger centres with high technology and specialised teams dealing with the most complex health care needs. There is a strong degree of local opposition to what has been perceived as a 'downgrading' (which is not necessarily the case) of acute hospitals in the south, such as Bantry General Hospital, South Infirmary Victoria University Hospital (SIVUH) and Mallow General Hospital. This extends to the whole country: including other hospitals in Munster, from Nenagh to Ennis to the debate on future hospital services in Waterford. However, the evidence suggests that, if acute hospitals in towns and cities previously offering the full range of services were now restricted to becoming local non-complex acute secondary hospitals (McCallion, 2013) at level 3, then this becomes a key element within the health and social care infrastructure and part of a logical plan to enhance integrated care at the level of primary/community care, improved by integration with local hospitals (level 3) also, and speedy ambulance services to tertiary hospitals at level 4 if required, thereby integrating services within the local area closest to the client. This is a key objective of integrated care delivery.

This also fits in to the re-organisation of the secondary acute hospital system by using only a smaller number of larger, more specialised 'centres of excellence' at tertiary care level, as previously suggested by the *Hanly Report* (DoHC, 2003a), the *Brennan Report* (DoHC, 2003b), the *Prospectus Report* (DoHC, 2003c) and others in the 2000s. These bigger centres of excellence then form level 4 of the model, as outlined.

The organisational model for integrated care as represented above then would need to be applied to specific health and social care services to cater for the whole population and to patients/clients with specific needs. In this context, McCallion (2010: 13) pointed out that over 20 'programmes of care' were to be rolled out by 2011 but that there was a 'separate project underway in child care and some gaps in other personal and social services'. Some of these areas have already been addressed in policy – for example, in the areas of disability (see HSE, 2011b), which in 2013 could most likely be viewed retrospectively as further additions to the programmes of care outlined by the HSE in 2010 (McCallion, 2010). These are listed in **Table 1.4** below as the 'national programmes for integrated care'.

Table 1.4: National Programmes of Integrated Care

Primary Care	Care of the elderly	Palliative Care	Radiology
Obstetrics and Gynaecology	Obstetrics and Gynaecology (Deputy)	Joint Stroke (Geriatrician)	Joint Stroke (Neurology)
Acute Coronary Syndrome	Heart Failure	Diabetes	COPD
Asthma	Mental Health	Epilepsy	Dermatology
Neurology out patients	Rheumatology	Joint Acute Medicine	Joint Acute Medicine
Emergency Medicine	Critical Care	Surgery	

Source: McCallion, 2010: 13.

At the time of writing (March 2013), detailed hospital re-configuration plans have been completed. It must be emphasised that these are 'plans' and not outcomes at this stage. Some configuration plans have been drawn up to cover more than one ISA – for example, in the case of Cork and Kerry, where the plan covers two separate ISAs (HSE South, 2011b). This plan puts smaller hospitals, such as Mallow General and others, on a re-configuration list. It is likely that hospitals, such as Mallow and other smaller ones in Cork and Kerry, and indeed Ennis in Co. Clare, represent the type of hospital that fits into the smaller non-complex, acute service hospitals in level 3 that are envisaged in the national HSE model for integrated care as put forward by McCallion (2010). However, reminiscent of the style of Irish policy-writing and mindful of local political sensitivities, the wording of the re-configuration document on Cork and Kerry does not state this with any degree of clarity. However, subsequent comments from the Minister for Health make it clear that Mallow (and presumably other county/smaller hospitals of this type) will be re-configured to level 3 non-complex acute hospitals but even this does not mean that all will survive. The Minister's comments following the furore over a negative Health Information and Quality Authority report on standards of health care at Mallow General Hospital in 2011 make the point clear:

> Local hospitals should be a vibrant element of local health services, providing treatment and care at the appropriate level of complexity to the patients in their area. Patients should only have to travel to the larger hospitals for more complex services (HSE, 2011c).

Clearly, this comment accentuates the positive in terms of closing down or downgrading local hospitals. Nonetheless, there is a clear logic and evidence-base for what has been planned. However, it is still understandable that local communities would be opposed to surrendering a local hospital either in totality or for a downgrade in return for the promise of the reform of the total health and social care services across the country. Services that exist are tangible; promises are not.

The actual decisions on which hospitals will be 'downgraded' to level 3 non-complex acute or to urgent day care centres is not set out to any great extent in documentation available from the HSE. Rather, the final decision is left to the Minister's discretion. But even in this context, there is an emerging type of downgrading: the closure of an acute hospital's A&E services with the introduction of a compensatory urgent treatment centre and/or the downgrading of a hospital to a non-complex one, but where it still retains its acute hospital designation. In the HSE South, an example of the former case has been the closure of A&E services at SIVUH in July 2012, with the introduction of the Mercy Urgent Care Centre, situated on the site of St. Mary's Orthopaedic Hospital, which had been closed previously. Mallow General Hospital combines both types of 'downgrading', involving A&E closure and the move to non-complex acute procedures. In late February 2013, the A&E in Mallow General Hospital was replaced by a new Urgent Care Centre, as was the unit in Bantry General Hospital. The wider vision is still a closely guarded secret, with all these moves emanating from the "Smaller Hospital Framework, a document that has yet to be published by the Government" (RTÉ News, 2013). Mallow and Bantry also are part of a network of hospitals in the South of the country that will be expected to carry out only non-complex acute procedures (HSE South, 2011b).

PROGRESS IN TRANSLATING INTEGRATED CARE POLICY INTO PRACTICAL DELIVERY FROM 2012 ONWARDS

This third section compares the organisational model and service plans for integrated care that have been delivered up to 2012 to the actual practical delivery of integrated care in Ireland at present and comments on the successes/failures in the translation of these public policy goals into practical integrated care delivery that touches peoples' lives.

This section will assess also the shortfalls in delivering what is being perceived as a seamless holistic 'integrated care delivery for the whole person', which attempts to integrate medical and social care, but which is endeavouring to do so in the face of far-deeper-seated challenges to population health that are 'structural' in nature (O'Connor and Murphy, 2006; O'Connor, 2008; 2009a; 2009b; 2011).

In this section, the key areas of health and social care provision are examined to evaluate the progress towards achieving integrated care to date: clearly, it would be impossible to do this for all 23 areas identified by the HSE (McCallion, 2010). With this in mind, this section focuses on progress within three key areas: first, given that PCTs are the most essential building block for integrated care and the logic of having accompanying PCCs, the progress to date in this regard will be examined. The city and county of Cork will be taken as a geographical microcosm for detailed examination. As the second largest city in the Republic of Ireland, Cork is strongly indicative of the progress that has been achieved nationally. The second is the area of mental health, chosen because an integrated care blueprint (MHC, 2006) has existed in government policy since 2006 and because of the current urgency in the context of rising incidence of mental ill-health and suicide in Ireland, alongside the over-reliance on pharmaceuticals as a single tier of treatment. The third area is that of disability. This was not included within the original 23 areas but, in the past three years, it has clearly been established by the HSE as a key area for integrated care in the context of de-institutionalisation and moving towards a community care model (HSE, 2011b).

Primary Care Teams and Centres

It is clear from the four-level model of integrated care that primary care is arguably the linchpin of the whole model, given that over 90% of all health care is delivered in primary care (Brennan, 2003). In this, the PCT is of critical importance. We have noted that the HSE originally pointed to 531 PCTs being mapped out nationally. The HSE *National Service Plan* (2011a) refers to 527 PCTs as the full national complement. The HSE also noted that it expected that the final figure for the number of PCTs holding clinical team meetings to be 394 in 2010. However, the report does not provide a figure for the number of patients receiving treatment from the teams. This is a curious omission and suggests that, while all these teams may have met at least once during the year, many may not have been delivering daily patient care, simply because PCT-based daily treatment of patients is far from a national reality in practice, irrespective of any team meetings that may have occurred. The HSE also planned to have 134 HSCNs operating by the end of 2011.

A PCT, previously known as a PCHT, is meant to be a one-stop-shop where patients in the locality can come to get an array of different professional interventions under one roof. This then requires a large, well-equipped PCC to house the different professionals involved and to provide the necessary equipment and facilities to carry out the whole range of professional interventions involved, in addition to providing space for meetings, information-sharing and health and technology transfer. Consequently, the absence of the various team members working within one facility in a single local area within a fit-for-purpose building renders the team effectively non-existent.

The HSE South *Regional Service Plan* (2011a) stated that, at the end of 2010, there were 47 PCTs in the region: 16 on the North Lee side of the city, 15 on the South Lee and eight each in both West Cork and North Cork. Yet, at the time of writing, there is still only one PCC in operation for the whole of Cork city, despite its now 30+ PCTs. The HSE South *Regional Service Plan* (2011a) accepts that members of the PCT may not be working in the same PCC, though co-location is the ideal:

> Ideally, all members of a Team are based in a single Primary Care Team building. Alternatively, Team members may be based in separate locations using ICT to facilitate team working. Co-location is not a pre-requisite for Team operation, and indeed may not be practical in certain situations where Teams span a large geographic area; however, meetings should be arranged in a suitable facility to allow all team members to attend (HSE South, 2011a: 26).

Notwithstanding the use of ICT and special meetings in a 'suitable facility' for different members of PCTs not working in the same PCC, the existence of only one PCC in Cork city does not sit well with the fact that there are 30+ PCTs supposedly meeting and working in tandem with each other to serve patients and clients. Realistically, the housing of PCTs under one roof within a PCC is a *sine qua non* for the operation of effective PCTs, which itself is a precondition in order to achieve excellent integrated care. Further, it is hard to imagine whether these 30+ PCTs are actually a daily reality at all in the delivery of social care in the first instance, apart from infrequent meetings, and the inclusion of these meetings on the pages of audit reports. Recourse to information on what is happening nationally suggests that many PCTs are not a reality in the daily functioning sense:

> So last year Minister for Health James Reilly and his Minister of State Róisín Shortall instructed the HSE to carry out an accommodation needs assessment for primary care teams around the country. The idea was to identify areas where gaps in provision existed and to suggest

what approach could be taken to plug these gaps. This assessment, completed in October 2011, found that only 55 primary care teams were in place, while 415 teams needed accommodation in 297 centres (some centres would house more than one team) (*The Irish Times*, 2012).

This data is clearly at variance with the HSE *National Service Plan* (2011a), which stated that 527 primary care teams were in place almost a year earlier.

Despite the 30+ PCTs identified as being in existence in Cork city north and south, only one PCC currently exists (January 2013), situated at Blackrock Hall on the south side. The PCCs potentially encompass several PCTs, as envisaged by the *Primary Care Strategy* (DoHC, 2001b) and many other HSE documents since then. The professional configuration within Blackrock Hall, a state-of-the-art PCC in Cork city, includes GPs (10 in total) and other professionals such as a physiotherapist, podiatrist, nutritionist, counsellor, pharmacist, speech and language therapist, home carers and others (Touchstone, 2013).

The wide array of health and social care professionals within Blackrock Hall is in keeping or even an extension of those set out in the *Primary Care Strategy* (DoHC, 2001b). **Table 1.4** above illustrates the DoHC (2001b) vision for a PCT that includes 23 members drawn from: social workers, home helps, health care assistants, physiotherapists, occupational therapists, five nurses/midwives, four GPs and five in administration. This requires a large building with highly developed facilities on a par with those in Blackrock Hall. Also, since 2001, the Blackrock Hall professional configuration and international evidence (Clifton *et al.*, 2006), suggests that several other health/care professionals also now need to be part of teams, including podiatrists, cognitive behavioural therapists and others.

Blackrock Hall is an exception. It was built not by the design of the HSE; it happened because a pharmacist, not a GP, who also was an entrepreneur, decided to develop it. So, this state-of-the-art PCC in Blackrock happened almost serendipitously due to a private entrepreneur, rather like the Blackrock Clinic did in Dublin in the 1980s (see Wren, 2003) and many of the other private hospitals that have followed suit, under the aegis of Dr. James Sheehan and the Beacon Group. The website that advertises Blackrock Hall makes the point clearly:

> The Touchstone Practice is owned by Fergus and Orna Hoban together with all of the practitioners who work here – in areas like pharmacy, dentistry, orthodontics, audiology, optics, physiotherapy, osteopathy,

home care, nutrition & dietetics, health food, occupational therapy, clinical fitness, speech & language therapy, podiatry & chiropody, diabetes, psychotherapy & counselling and smoking cessation. Fergus is one of the leading entrepreneurs in Ireland in the development of primary care services, is originally a pharmacist, and is Clinical Director of Touchstone (Touchstone, 2013).

Most PCCs identified as being a necessity within HSE *National and Regional Service Plans* in the past three years have yet to be built, with varying reasons being cited, all of which have to do with the property development process. In most cases, the building of PCCs is being carried out *via* Public Private Partnerships (PPPs).

Primary care in Ireland has been run by GPs, catering for the whole population, since the doing away of the dispensary system, the setting up of the health boards and the introduction of the General Medical Services system over 40 years ago (Wren, 2003; Curry, 2005). What now exists is a mix of fee-paying private patients and non-fee-paying public patients with medical cards within each GP practice. This private/public patient base, however, is owned and run completely as private practices by GPs or groups of GPs. The DoH/HSE contracts these private businesses to provide medical services to those with medical cards, whereby a capitation payment is received for each patient. The remaining patients, who are fee-paying, pay a set fee per visit out-of-pocket. Despite operating as private practices, many of which own the premises they operate from, GPs are not property entrepreneurs. As a result, the scale and excellence of the Blackrock Hall facility – a PCC that closely resembles the gold standard envisaged by the DoH and HSE – has not been replicated anywhere in Cork city or county to date (March 2013).

Given that PCCs will replace established group GP practices, the State needs to procure, plan and deliver the infrastructure of these centres itself. It cannot be left to private interests, including or excluding GPs or other consortia, to deliver the infrastructure. It is unwise to expect private capital *via* PPPs to develop these centres, as the New Zealand experience tells us (Crampton and Starfield, 2004). This model is not beneficial and clearly the State needs to lead the development and ownership of PCCs itself (Crampton and Starfield, 2004): the centres need to be procured and staffed through the public purse and contractual arrangements, such as leasehold, would need to be negotiated with GP practices wishing to be re-deployed in such centres. Thus, the ownership of primary care, at least in terms of the public infrastructure of PCCs needs to rest with the State, irrespective of the private contractual relationship between health providers and GPs or other health/care providers. The evidence internationally clearly points to far greater benefits than costs in delivering primary care with as much public ownership as possible (Crampton and Starfield, 2004; Pollock, 2005). If private finance initiatives are used to finance such centres (Cullen, 2012), this is likely to lead to poor value for money for the Irish State in the long run (Pollock, 2005).

In the current model, GPs obviously would need to be part of the consortia, alongside DoH and HSE in a PPP that would raise the significant capital required for the PCC, as well as the equipment and the costs of salaries for teams of people. Doctors and other health professionals may need to become large-scale business entrepreneurs to fulfil the task.

However, the rolling out of primary care in the context of private businesses and the necessity of GPs or consortia of GPs or others (as in Blackrock Hall) to purchase land and buildings is totally unsatisfactory as a way of rolling out a fully-developed national complement of PCCs. Furthermore, the whole process is subject to speculation and other motives that do not serve the needs of patients well, as is obvious in the case of Cork and the country as a whole:

> The last government favoured developing centres by leasing sites from the private sector, but the assessment found that many submissions made by developers were highly speculative. The economic downturn was also blamed for delays, plus the fact that many GPs had invested significantly in their premises in recent years and were unable to dispose of them (Cullen, 2012).

The progress to date in the areas where detailed information has been available from HSE South (2011a; 2012; 2013) has been slow and tortuous. Taking the 18 PCCs outlined in **Table 1.5**, only Ballineen, Macroom and Mahon are up and running, with two centres in Carrigtwohill and Schull due to be operationalised by the end of 2013. To this can be added one further PCC in Mitchelstown, which is not detailed in the HSE *Regional Service Plans* on which **Table 1.5** is based. Even so, were all six operational by the end of 2013, only one-third of the 18 PCCs will have been developed and made operational in the three years from 2011 to 2013. These centres are being developed through PPPs, which clearly are not delivering to any great extent at this point in time.

Furthermore, there are now 30+ PCTs in operation in the North and South Lee areas (HSE South, 2012). Yet there is only one PCC (Mahon) in Cork city, accounting for four PCTs in total. There is not a single PCC operating in the North Lee area, which contains the greatest areas of deprivation (Cork City Council, 2012). Judging by **Table 1.5**, a median of two PCTs per PCC is the optimum. Given that four teams are served by the two PCCs in Mahon and Macroom, 36 PCTs are left, which would need approximately 18 new PCCs to accommodate them.

Table 1.5: Primary Care Centre Development in HSE South

	Number of PCTs HSE RSP (2011)	Status HSE South RSP (2011)	Update HSE RSP (2012)	Update HSE RSP (2013)
Kinsale	2	Plans being prepared	No update	Work in progress
Ballineen	1	Negotiations underway	Proposal subject to HSE approval	Operational (not noted in HSE)
Cobh	1	New draft plan awaited	Agreement for lease signed Completion Q1 2014	Work in progress
Newmarket	1	Site location agreed Plans to be developed	Agreement for lease signed Q1 2014	Work in progress
Clonakilty	1	Potential site identified	No update	Work in progress
Fermoy	2	Negotiations ongoing	Negotiations ongoing	
Mayfield	1	Discussions ongoing	Discussions ongoing	Work in progress
Bishopstown	3	Location to be determined	No update	No update
Glanmire	2	Progressing	No update	No update
Castletownbere	1	Letter of intent issue Negotiations ongoing	No update	No update
Carrigaline	2-3	Going to HSE Board February 2011 for approval on rental details	Proposal subject to HSE approval	No update
Charleville	1	Layout plans being drafted	Agreement for lease signed Completion Q1 2014	Work in progress
Schull	1	Planning sought	Construction commenced	Operational 2013(e)

	Number of PCTs HSE RSP (2011)	Status HSE South RSP (2011)	Update HSE RSP (2012)	Update HSE RSP (2013)
Togher (inc. Greenmount & Lough)	3	Site to be determined	City Council to offer site for sale inc PCC site	No update
Macroom	1	Lease agreement close to completion	Due to open	Operational (not noted on HSE)
Mahon	2	Lease agreement close to completion	Up and running	Operational
Carrigtwohill	1	Layout plans finalising	No update	Operational 2013 (e)
Ballincollig	3	Layouts agreed Two sites	No update	No update

The HSE South 2013 *Regional Service Plan* (2013) promises an improvement in the city and county environs on delivering PCCs, outlining its commitment to:

- "Progress development of a Primary Care Centre in Cork City (Ballyphehane, Togher);
- Progress the development of a Primary Care Centre for Cork City NW (Knocknaheeny, Fairhill and Gurranebraher), in St. Mary's Health Campus by direct build;
- Work with Estates in progressing development of Primary Care Centres in Cork City NE (Mayfield, Montenotte), Charleville, Kinsale, Clonakilty, Newmarket and Cobh;
- Continue to explore provision of accommodation in Glanmire, Bantry, Carrigaline, Beara, Fermoy and Youghal" (HSE South, 2013: 30).

The lack of accommodation in Cork city for its PCTs is striking, considering the HSE (2011d) list of PCTs on the North Lee and South Lee areas as evidenced in **Table 1.6**.

There is clearly a blockage in building and developing PCCs in Cork. This is also the case on a national basis in Ireland and, unless there is a drastic improvement, it will be many years before the HSE's proposed integrated service model will become a reality.

Table 1.6: Primary Care Teams, Areas, Population: Cork City North, September 2011

North Lee 20 PCTs		South Lee 19 PCTs	
Area	Population	Area	Population
Riverstown / Glanmire 1	17,130	Kinsale x 2	30,544
Riverstown / Glanmire 2		Bandon 1	
Blackpool	5,123	Bandon 2	
Fairhill / Farranree	8,000	Mahon 1	25,539
Gurranebraher	6,487	Blackrock 1	
Dillons Cross/St. Lukes	6,651	Blackrock 2	
Knocknaheeny	4,574	Ballincollig / Bishopstown 1	42,217
Blackpool 2	3,143	Ballincollig / Bishopstown 3	
Mayfield East	7,828	Ballincollig / Bishopstown 3	
Macroom 1	12,796	Ballincollig / Bishopstown 4	
Macroom 2		Ballincollig / Bishopstown 5	
Youghal	10,603	Ballincollig / Bishopstown 6	
Blarney 1	14,000	Douglas / Frankfield / Grange 1	23,627
Blarney 2		Douglas / Frankfield / Grange 3	
City Centre	7,470	Douglas / Frankfield / Grange 3	
Midleton 1	12,440	Greenmount / The Lough 1	26,790
Midleton 2	6,007	Ballyphehane / Togher (x2)	
Midleton 3	4,623		
Carrigtwohill (Midleton 4)	6,007		
Mayfield West	8,406		

Source: HSE, 2011d.

The national replication of the problem is highlighted by Paul Cullen of *The Irish Times,* who points out that the unsatisfactory nature of progress in the planning and development process for PCCs, and the severe lack of progress in building them across the whole country, was of concern to the former junior Minister for Health, Róisín Shortall, in 2012:

> In April, Shortall instructed the officials to rationalise the list down to 200 centres. She said the existing private leasing arrangements were moving too slowly and were failing to help target the areas of greatest need (Cullen, 2012).

This controversy at the end of 2012 between the Minister for Health, Dr. James Reilly, and his junior minister, Róisín Shortall, over her perception that the Minister had added PCCs of his own choosing to a priority list, and which subsequently resulted in her resignation, illustrates a further danger. The location of PCCs in the future may be influenced by party politics at the expense of careful planning.

An investigation by *The Irish Times* journalist, Paul Cullen, based on statements from the HSE and reports of meetings that took place in 2011 and 2012, reveals that, as of 2011, 297 PCCs needed to be sited and provided to house 415 PCTs (Cullen, 2012). A smaller priority list of 200 was put forward by Róisín Shortall in April 2012, based on extra weighting being given to areas of social deprivation. A final priority list of 30 was finalised later in 2012. The controversy between Ms. Shortall and Minister Reilly arose when she perceived that five extra centres were added by him in July of that year, of which she was unaware and where the correct criteria to justify their addition to the list was absent. This list of 35 was released to the press. It included Balbriggan and Swords. The public controversy that erupted resulted in the resignation of Ms. Shortall amid allegations that Minister O'Reilly had pulled a 'stroke':

> Opposition parties are calling on the Health Minister James Reilly to resign after former Junior Minister Róisín Shortall accused him of "stroke politics" and said he had blocked attempts to reform the health service (*Irish Examiner*, 2012).

The whole planning of PCCs based on private property development bids and immersed in political intrigue is clearly an anathema to the development of integrated care in Ireland.

Disability

Organisational Model
At the end of 2007, Ger Reaney (2007), Health Manager of HSE South, outlined the vision for disability services nationally to the Disability Federation of Ireland. The model of integrated care for those with disabilities is within the broad framework as outlined previously. Within the best practice principles for community care (Means *et al.*, 2008), the health and social care needs of disabled people are to be more effectively dealt with by PCTs (level 1) and specialist providers within the wider HSCN (level 2). This is consistent with a subsequent commitment in 2010 by the HSE (as noted earlier) that "HSCNs will include a pool of specialised resources that serve PCT communities" (HSE, 2010b: 9), referring to the wider community HSCN, which is consistent with the *Primary Care Strategy* (DoHC, 2001b) and McCallion (2010). The rationale is that more disabled people, previously housed in residential facilities,

can be transferred to independent community living, either at home or in independent units, once there is this suitable four-level integrated service model and infrastructure to cater for their needs. It also seems clear that, although certain disabled sub-populations may need to remain in residential care, this service will form part of level 3 services within the integrated services model but at a far reduced level. Critically complex care will be delivered at level 4 for disabled populations, as it will be for all other members of the general population. The benefits of integration in the area of disability, according to Reaney, are:

Primary Care Teams:
- Opportunity for engagement with local community;
- Contribution of voluntary sector to shaping of transformation programme;
- Need to maintain quality, specialist knowledge and expertise in transition to new system (Reaney, 2007: 9).

Working together – in the future:
- Opportunities for increased levels of collaboration;
- Transformation programme;
- Need to provide PCTs with specialist information, expertise and support (Reaney, 2007: 16).

Reaney's vision includes a strong commitment also to user involvement and partnership arrangements with voluntary providers through various collaborative fora.

While the vision is a good one, in examining the *Primary Care Strategy* (DoHC, 2001b), HSE *National Service Plans* (2007; 2010a), McCallion (2010), HSE South *Regional Service Plan* (2011a) and Reaney (2007), there is still some ambiguity about the interface between levels 2 and 3 with regard to those in need of specialist health and social care services. It is clear that non-complex acute hospitals and urgent day care centres will be in level 3. We are left to assume from rather broad policy statements what the configuration of level 3 will look like regarding disability services, the most helpful of which has been noted earlier as:

PCTs and HSCNs will be integrated with hospitals, multi-agencies, private providers, voluntary agencies, and with support groups (HSE, 2010a: 9).

Taking this assertion in the context of McCallion (2010) and HSE South (2011a; 2012; 2013), it seems that residential care services for those with disabilities will be in level 3 within the ISA spanning levels 1 to 4, as will nursing homes. This is implicit from the documentation, but it needs to be confirmed and elaborated more clearly and precisely. As it stands, level 3 seems to include: larger campus-type accommodation in health and social care; nursing homes; acute hospitals that are non-tertiary, many of which would be non-complex; and various other residential care campuses or addiction centres. Nonetheless, with the slow transformation of Irish social care services for disability away from residential care, in the future it would be expected that a large proportion of the disabled population currently in residential care would move to home and community living and consequently that most of the services for the disabled would occur at levels 1 and 2 of the integrated services delivery model as put forward by the HSE.

Disability Priorities

The various HSE *National Service Plans* since 2011 have delivered a strong emphasis on disability services. For example, in 2011, the HSE's priorities included the following:

Children's disability therapy services:
- Reconfiguration of existing therapy resources to geographic-based teams progressed and monitored (0-18 Yrs).

Adult residential services:
- Engagement with service providers and cross-sectoral agencies on reconfiguration objectives;
- Development of outline implementation plan in line with VFM and Policy Review.

Adult day services:
- Engagement with service providers and cross-sectoral agencies on reconfiguration objectives;
- Development of outline implementation plan in line with VFM and Policy Review (HSE, 2011a: 41-44).

The reconfiguration objectives are those related to de-institutionalisation, as confirmed by the subsequent report on congregated settings (HSE, 2011b) as discussed below. At the moment, there are supposed to be 134 HSCNs (*Irish Medical Times*, 2011) established to integrate with the PCTs and further on to levels 3 and 4. However, apart from a change in nomenclature, there is little evidence of the actual existence of these HSCNs, presumably because most of the PCCs are not available (as detailed above) to house the PCTs that would be integrated with these 134 HSCNs. This seems to be a significant challenge going forward.

Similarly, though not listed separately as one of the 23 national programmes of care in **Table 1.4**, the HSE in its report on congregated settings (HSE, 2011b) sets out disability services as a national priority for integrated care. Its plan is to end what is perceived as a glaring human rights issue in having large numbers of disabled people living in institutional/residential/congregated care settings of more than 10 people. HSE is proposing to enable the majority of the 4,000 disabled people in these settings to live independently in their own homes or in shared units of no more than four people in normal local communities.

In doing so, the report sets out 31 recommendations for public policy. Yet by early 2013, progress has been exceptionally slow (Inclusion Ireland, 2013). There may be a reluctance among existing institutional providers to forego block grants for residential care in favour of a system of independent home care grants/supports that would follow the client as an individual (NDA, 2011). Also, the same under-developed integrated care infrastructure on the ground will hamper any acceleration of plans in this area, given that:

> HSE Primary Care Teams should be the first point of access for all medical and social care including public health nursing, home help services, meals on wheels, social work, psychological interventions, with a clear pathway to secondary specialist disability-specific teams when required (HSE, 2011a: 9).

These support services have been ravaged by public expenditure cutbacks since 2008: for example, cuts of up to 1 million home help hours were introduced by the HSE in 2012 (Wall, 2012) and there has been an embargo on public service recruitment, which includes social workers. Even social work services in child protection have witnessed dramatic increases in caseloads to the point where they have "Big caseloads being juggled with little support" (*Irish Independent*, 2012). These cuts are typical of those running across the infrastructure that is being planned for the delivery of integrated care, making it difficult to see how the plans can be translated into reality in the short-to medium term.

Mental Health

Mental health services are located in same organisational priority as disability services, whereby government policy is committed to most services being provided by PCTs and the wider team of specialist providers within the HSCN working in close co-operation, within the integrated care service delivery model (McCallion, 2010). Mental health services are also one of the 23 'programmes of integrated care' identified in **Table 1.4**. Obviously, consistent with the implementation of *Vision for Change* (MHC, 2006), a small proportion of mentally ill patients, at least temporarily, at different points in time, would continue to require specialist residential care at level 3 of the integrated services model.

The urgency for the introduction of this integrated care model for mental illness, which strongly emphasises primary, community health and social care delivery, is long overdue in Ireland. The promotion of positive mental health and the treatment of mental ill-health have had a poor history in Ireland (MHC, 2006). Historically, even as recently as the 1960s, patients were treated with heavy doses of insulin, putting them in to a dangerously vegetative state, from which they might somehow benefit once recovered, and gratuitous use of electro-convulsive therapy happened, often without anaesthetic (*The Irish Times*, 2013). The heavy use of institutions in an almost Dickensian model of care was the norm (*The Irish Times*, 2013). Sub-populations – some with addiction problems, women suffering post-natal depression, children and those with severe mental health conditions – were all placed in large institutions that were pejoratively termed 'the mad house' or 'the loony bin' by members of the general public. This stigma was reinforced by the popular media, using terms such as 'nutter' and 'loony' in the popular press (Prior, 2013).

Saunders (2007) points out that mental health has been treated always as a residual issue for Irish health policy and that there is a widespread level of ignorance on the subject by many politicians. The residual status of mental health, despite the fact that mental ill-health will affect 25% of the population at any given time, is strongly indicated by the fact that the mental health spending normally absorbs around 7% of total health spending (Saunders, 2007; MHC, 2006). *Vision for Change* strongly showcased an integrated care approach to mental health:

> Most mental health problems are dealt with in primary care without referral on to specialist services. Primary care is therefore the main supplier of mental health care for the majority of the population ... The GP in primary care is also the main access point to specialist mental health care for most of the population (MHC, 2006: 23).

Vision for Change demonstrated a clearly integrated model for mental health services delivery that involved both primary care and secondary care. The PCT would be fully staffed with mental health professionals, who would refer patients to an array of appropriate mental health services in community care. In the case of more serious or protracted mental health problems, the PCT would refer the patient to the newly-established CMHTs, which like the PCTs would themselves be multidisciplinary in nature. These teams would then provide and refer patients to a full range of dedicated mental health services, also which would be based in the community.

The CMHTs would be part of a clearly defined structure working from national to local: the Mental Health Services Directorate would be mediated by Mental Health Catchment Area Teams (MHCATs) covering 300,000 people, to which CMHTs would be accountable. The HSE *Transformation Programme 2007-2010* (HSE, 2006), as mentioned above, similarly proposes ISAs, which are broadly similar, in terms of their place in the management structure and the populations they are designed to service, as the MHACTs in *Vision for Change* (MHC, 2006). CMHTs would have a management structure that included a team leader, a team co-ordinator and a practice manager. Each team would be designed to deal with specific population sub-groups with a full complement of professionals, including specialist services for children and adolescents, and be designed to cover specific population catchment areas offering home-based mental health services delivery. The composition of the various teams would vary depending on the sub-population group, although the underlying configuration of any team is set out in recommendation 9.1:

> **9.1**: To provide an effective community-based service, CMHTs should offer multidisciplinary home-based treatment and assertive outreach, and a comprehensive range of medical, psychological and social therapies relevant to the needs of service users and their families. Each multidisciplinary team should include the core skills of psychiatry, nursing, social work, clinical psychology and occupational therapy. The composition and skill mix of each CMHT should be appropriate to the needs and social circumstances of its sector population. (MHC, 2006: 79).

In terms of the new CMHT infrastructure, the report provided a detailed breakdown of what was needed across the population spectrum to include disability services also (MHC, 2006). The following 'Summary of new infrastructure requirement bases for Community Mental Health Teams' (MHC, 2006: 269) was considered necessary, as shown in **Table 1.7**.

The report estimated that the cost of revamping (let alone revolutionising) the Irish mental health systems into a thoroughly integrated service, where service users were integrated and where CMHTs were integrated into primary care, would be €21.5 million above current spending per year over seven years (in 2005) with a capital cost of €797 million, only a fraction of which could be defrayed through the sale of older institutional sites. Apart from regular maintenance and upgrading where necessary, this initial capital investment could be considered a once-off investment by the Irish State in the mental health services.

Table 1.7: Infrastructure for Community Mental Health Teams

Specialisms	No. of CMHTs
General Adult	78
Early Intervention	2
Adult Liaison	13
Rehabilitation and Recovery	39
Older People	39
Intellectual Disability	26
Child and Adolescent	63
Liaison Teams	7
Eating Disorder Teams	1
Intellectual Disability Teams	13
Substance Misuse	4
Homeless People	2
Forensic Adult	4
Forensic Child and Adolescent	1
Co-Morbid Mental Health & Substance Misuse	13
Adult Eating Disorders	4
Neuropsychiatry	2
Total	**311**

Source: MHC, 2006: 29.

The progress in achieving a new mental health service, integrated with primary care and using the strong evidence-base of a population health approach, essentially representing a state-of-the-art service, has been nothing short of abysmal. Relatively small amounts of extra resources in the tens of millions have been drip-fed into the mental health system at the discretion of the relevant minister at different stages since the adoption of *Vision for Change* (MHC, 2006) as Irish government policy. In 2008, the Mental Health Coalition, a campaigning coalition of mental health service user groups, using the Department of Health's own figures, showed that €24 million of the €51.2 million earmarked for the implementation of *Vision for Change* was diverted into other areas of HSE spending in 2006 and 2007 (Expert Group on Mental Health Policy, 2008).

In the same vein, an Amnesty International report on the mental health services in Ireland and particularly the *Mental Health Act, 2001*, states:

> Amnesty has stated that, as long as Ireland fails to implement *Vision for Change*, it will continue to fail to meet international standards and there will continue to be cases where people are deprived of their liberty under the Act, in situations which might not have arisen were adequate community-based services and supports available (Amnesty International, 2011: 26).

Finally, the report of the Independent Monitoring Group for *Vision for Change* (DoHC, 2011c) points to an exceptionally slow and tortuous approach to implementation, pointing to large staffing shortages, with austerity policies over-zealously choking off resources:

> Mental health services had taken a "proportionally much greater reduction in staff numbers" than other areas of the health service, submissions to the body had said. The public service recruitment embargo made it "extremely difficult" to change mental health services as per the plan, the report said ... There were some 1,500 vacant posts in community health teams which were "poorly populated", it said. There had been "very slow progress" in fully staffing community mental health teams, it found (*The Irish Times*, 2012).

Shockingly, the report found that mental health spending as a proportion of total health spending had not risen from the 6.8% at the time of publication of *Vision for Change* (MHC, 2006) to the 8.4% needed for implementation. This figure is consistent with the current 1,500 vacancies in CMHTs.

CONCLUSION

In overall terms, the evidence as discussed shows that the progress towards achieving fully-functioning PCTs and PCCs in Ireland has been slow and tortuous. There is far more left to do than has been done. There is evidence of over 500 teams having been formed and having met; but there is no evidence that these are in any way embedded in the day-to-day treatment of patients, which still seems predominantly the preserve of individual GPs at this point in the HSE South Region and indeed nationally. The failure to develop PCCs seems to be the biggest impediment towards rolling out properly and full functioning PCTs. This is a *sine qua non* for enhanced primary care, which itself is a prerequisite for integrated care. This failure to develop PCCs and to house teams that actually work and integrate together, rather than existing only in published reports without any verifiable delivery of care quantums, prevents the move to develop integrated care for the whole range of the 23 national care programmes as identified by the HSE in 2010 and the others that have come onstream since then. This affects diverse population health and social care groups, from those who are in need of critical care to those with disabilities or poor levels of mental health.

Furthermore, the involvement of private investment in an integrated care system is causing tremendous delays. International evidence does not support PPPs as the most desirable way to fund primary care. It is clear that a major rethink on how best to finance PCCs and other integrated care infrastructure, particularly at levels 1 and 2 of the integrated care service delivery model, needs to happen. Waiting for private consortia and investors or developers to come on board to develop urgent policy-based integrated care services is serving the population health needs of Irish society very badly.

Finally, there is still a high level of uncertainty on what acute hospitals, residential care or other services will be specifically designated as a level 3 service. The expectations on this, as articulated in this chapter, are based on piecing together a large variety of HSE documentation, which even still does not display the level of certainty one might expect in clarifying the services configuration at level 3.

The tertiary services at level 4 are also a somewhat moveable feast at the moment, but it seems clear that the largest and most well-equipped hospitals that deal with the highest health speciality areas presently, and are located in the major cities, will be retained as the new tertiary centres of excellence, with the vast majority of other acute hospitals dealing with less complex needs being reconfigured as non-complex acute hospitals or urgent care centres at level 3 of the model.

What is also an open question is the management of integrated care across the four levels. This is not yet worked out, it would seem. It seems apparent that a new professional grade entitled something like 'integrated care co-ordinator' will need to be employed at the interface between each of the four levels across all 531 PCT catchment areas in the country. Thus, 2,000 health personnel specialising in managing the interfaces between the different levels, with specialised integrated knowledge spanning a variety of disciplines, will likely need to be employed. Such personnel would need to be trained in both health and social care and have strong management skills sets also. The provision of key personnel in this area seems to be a further pre-requisite for delivering successful integrated care in the future and would represent strong value for money in the long run. We still await the arrival of real integrated care in Ireland at this point, however.

REFERENCES

Amnesty International (2011). Mental Health Act 2001: A Review, Dublin: Amnesty International.

Brennan, R. (2003). 'Primary Care: New Directions' in Kinsella, R. (ed.), *Acute Health Care in Transition*, Cork: Oak Tree Press.

Clarke, J. and Newman, J. (1997). *The Managerial State*, London: Sage.

Clifton, M., Dale, C. and Bradshaw, C. (2006). *The Impact and Effectiveness of Interprofessional Education in Primary Care*, London: Royal College of Nursing.

Cooper, T. (2011). *Driving Quality Improvements in Social Care*, presentation, CIT Visiting Speaker series, 6 May.

Cork City Council (2012). *Building Co-ordination around Communities and Local Needs: The Future of a More Inclusive Europe*, Cork: Cork City Council.

Crampton, P. and Starfield, B. (2004). 'A Case for Government Ownership of Primary Care Services in New Zealand: Weighing the Arguments', *International Journal of Health Services*, 34 (4), 709-727.

Cullen, P. (2012). 'Care centres list grew to 35 locations after reviews', *The Irish Times*, 21 September.

Curry, J. (2005). *The Irish Social Services*, Dublin: Institute of Public Administration.

Department of Health (DoH) (1984). *Planning for the Future: Report of the Study Group on the Development of the Psychiatric Services*, Dublin: Stationery Office.

Department of Health (DoH) (1988). *Years Ahead: A Policy for the Elderly: Report of the Working Party on Services for the Elderly*, Dublin: Stationery Office.

Department of Health (DoH) (1994). *Shaping a Healthier Future: A Strategy for Effective Healthcare in the 1990s*, Dublin: Stationery Office.

Department of Health (DoH) (1996). *An Evaluation of Cancer Services in Ireland: A National Strategy*, report prepared by Deloitte, Dublin: Stationery Office.

Department of Health and Children (DoHC) (2001a). *Quality and Fairness: A Health Strategy for You*, Dublin: Stationery Office.

Department of Health and Children (DoHC) (2001b). *Primary Care, A New Direction: Quality and Fairness - A Health System for You Health Strategy*, Dublin: Stationery Office.

Department of Health and Children (DoHC) (2001c). *Primary Care: A Description*, available http://www.dohc.ie/publications/fulltext/primary_care_new_direction/ part_two.html.

Department of Health and Children (DoHC) (2003a). *Report of the National Task Force on Medical Staffing (The Hanly Report)*, Dublin: Stationery Office.

Department of Health and Children (DoHC) (2003b). *Commission on Financial Management and Control Systems in the Health System (The Brennan Report)*, Dublin: Stationery Office.

Department of Health and Children (DoHC) (2003c). *Audit of Structures and Functions in the Health System (The Prospectus Report)*, Dublin: Stationery Office.

Department of Health and Children (DoHC) (2006). *A Vision for Change: Report of the Expert Group on Mental Health Policy*, Dublin: Stationery Office.

Department of Health and Children (DoHC) (2011c). *Report of the Independent Monitoring Group for* Vision for Change, Dublin: Stationery Office.

Department of Justice and Equality (2004). *National Disability Strategy*, Dublin: Stationery Office.

Department of the Taoiseach (2006). *Towards 2016: Ten-Year Framework Social Partnership Agreement 2006-2015,* Dublin: Stationery Office.

Doyle, P. (1989). *The God Squad*, London: Corgi.

Expert Group on Mental Health Policy (2008). *Second Report on Implementation of Vision for Change*, Dublin: Stationery Office.

Galvin, P. (2002). *The Raggy Boy Trilogy*, Dublin: New Island.

Goulding, G. (2005). *The Light in the Window*, London: Ebury.

Health Service Executive (HSE) (2006). *Transformation Programme 2007-2010*, Dublin: HSE.

Health Service Executive (HSE) (2007). *National Service Plan*, Dublin: HSE.

Health Service Executive (HSE) (2008a). *Corporate Plan 2008-2011*, Dublin: HSE.

Health Service Executive (HSE) (2008b). *Towards an Integrated Health Service or More of the Same?*, Dublin: HSE.

Health Service Executive (HSE) (2008c). *Code of Practice for Integrated Discharge Planning*, Dublin: HSE.

Health Service Executive (HSE) (2009a). *Inspiring Confidence in Children and Family Services: Putting Children First and Meaning It, Strategic Review of the Delivery and Management of Children and Family Services*, prepared by PA Consulting, Dublin: HSE.

Health Service Executive (HSE) (2009b). *National Service Plan*, Dublin: HSE.

Health Service Executive (HSE) (2010a). *National Service Plan*, Dublin: HSE.

Health Service Executive (HSE) (2010b). *Improving Team Working: A Guidance Document*, Dublin: HSE.

Health Service Executive (HSE) (2011a). *National Service Plan*, Dublin: HSE.

Health Service Executive (HSE) (2011b). *Time to Move on from Congregated Settings: A Strategy for Community Inclusion, Report of the Working Group on Congregated Settings*, Dublin: HSE.

Health Service Executive (HSE) (2011c). 'HSE South Reassures the Public on Safety of Services at Mallow General Hospital and Future Role of the Hospital', Press release, 19 April, Dublin: HSE.

Health Service Executive (HSE) (2011d). *List of Primary Care Teams*, Dublin: HSE.

Health Service Executive (HSE) South (2011a). *Regional Service Plan*, Dublin: HSE.

Health Service Executive (HSE) South (2011b). *A Roadmap to Create an Integrated University Hospital Network: Reconfiguration of Acute Hospital Services Cork and Kerry Region, Report of the Director of Reconfiguration Professor John R. Higgins*, Dublin: HSE.

Health Service Executive (HSE) South (2012). *Regional Service Plan*, Dublin: HSE.

Health Service Executive (HSE) South (2013). *Regional Service Plan*, Dublin: HSE.

Inclusion Ireland (2013). *Implementing the National Disability Strategy*, Position Paper, Dublin: Inclusion Ireland.

Irish Examiner (2012). 'Pressure on Reilly as Shortall backs "stroke politics" claim', 29 September.

Irish Independent (2012). 'Big caseloads being juggled with little support', 21 June.

Irish Medical Times (2011). 'Briefing Notes on Health', 21 February.

Kennedy, E. (1970). *Reformatory and Industrial Schools System Report*, Dublin:
    Stationery Office.
Kokko, S. (2009). 'Integrated Primary Health Care: Finnish solutions and
    experiences', *International Journal of Integrated Care*, Apr-Jun; 9: e86.
McCallion, D. (2010), *Integrated Services Programme – Integrating Hospital and
    Community Services: An Overview*, IPHA conference presentation, September.
McCallion, D. (2013). 'How the ISAs Will Work', *Health Manager*, March.
Means, R., Richards, S. and Smith, R. (2008). *Community Care: Policy and Practice*,
    London: Palgrave Macmillan.
Mental Health Commission (MHC) (2006). *Vision for Change*, Dublin: MHC.
National Council on Aging and Older People (NCAOP) (2002). *Towards Care
    Management in Ireland: Conference Proceedings*, Dublin: NCAOP.
National Disability Authority (NDA) (2011). *The Introduction of Individual Budgets
    as a Resource Allocation System for Disability Services in Ireland*, Dublin: NDA.
O'Connor, T. (2008). 'Towards the Development of a Learning Model that
    Integrates the Social Structural Causes Of Clients' Needs in to Social Care
    Practice, paper to *National Academy for the Integration of Research, Teaching and
    Learning Annual Conference*, November, Waterford Institute of Technology.
O'Connor, T. (2009a). *The Need for an Integrated Social Care Profession* in Share, P.
    and Lalor, K. (eds.), *Applied Social Care*, Dublin: Gill & Macmillan.
O'Connor, T. (2009b). 'Using Research to Develop Plans for Holistic Social Care:
    Professional Responses to Societal Failure of Clients in Social Care', paper to
    ENSACT European Conference, Dubrovnik, April.
O'Connor, T. (2011), *An Investigation in to the Health and Social Care Needs of Ageing
    Positive Action Clients in the Medium-term*, Dublin: Positive Action.
O'Connor, T. and Murphy, M. (eds.), (2006). *Social Care in Ireland: Theory, Policy
    and Practice*, Cork: CIT Press.
Pollitt, C. (2003). 'Public Management Reform: Reliable Knowledge and
    International Experience', *OECD Journal on Budgeting*, 3(3), 121-136.
Pollock, A. (2005). *NHS Plc: The Privatisation of our Health Care*, London: Verso.
Prior, P. (2013). *Asylums, Mental Health and the Irish 1800-2010*, Dublin: Irish
    Academic Press.
Rafferty, M. and O'Sullivan, E. (1999). *Suffer the Little Children: The Inside Story of
    Ireland's Industrial Schools*, Dublin: New Island.
Reaney, G. (2007). 'Working Together for the Future', presentation to Disability
    Federation of Ireland, 21 November.
RTÉ News (2013). 'Mallow hospital's emergency department to close, replaced
    with urgent care centre', 28 February.
Saunders, J. (2007). 'Mental Health Care Services: Policy, Politics and
    Prescriptions', presentation, CIT Visiting Speaker Series, 16 October.
The Irish Times (2012). 'Delivery of mental health plan slow and inconsistent', 18 July.
The Irish Times (2013).'Misery in Ireland's "massive mausoleums of madness", 2
    February.
Touchstone (2013). 'The Best Primary Care in Cork', touchstone.ie/blackrockhall.
Wall, M. (2012). 'HSE to implement home help cuts', *The Irish Times*, 5 October.
Wren, M.-A. (2003). *Unhealthy State: Anatomy of a Sick Society*, Dublin: New Island.

SECTION 1: ECONOMIC AND PUBLIC POLICY INSIGHTS FROM IRELAND AND ABROAD

2: THE INTEGRATED SERVICE IN NORTHERN IRELAND

Jim Campbell, Gavin Davidson and Michael Donnelly

INTRODUCTION

Successive UK governments have struggled to deliver health and social care policies equitably and efficiently. Amongst the many problems identified by policy-makers and practitioners has been the disjointed nature of services, despite the attempts to deal with this issue (Johnson *et al.*, 2003). One of the solutions, it has been argued, is to construct and develop a more integrated approach to service delivery, though the concept of 'integration' is often contested. In their review of the literature on this subject, Reed *et al.* (2005) summarise the key policy and practice developments with particular attention given to the needs of older people. They found that attempts to make systems of health and social welfare in the UK more integrated have tended to be incremental, involving bridging and increasing connectivity between disparate organisations and professional groupings. It appears that 'whole system change', despite the experience of other European countries, has either not been considered or has been thought to be too complex for the UK. Glendinning (2003, cited in Heenan and Birrell, 2009) suggests that integrated services are characterised by: a single point of access for service users; continuity of care; single management arrangements; holistic approaches to meeting need; agreed set of aims and objectives; common information systems; and co-location of services.

This chapter, on the Northern Irish experience of integration, reflects some of these debates. As we describe below, the integrated service in Northern Ireland offers many positive opportunities for the delivery of more coherent health and care services than is possible in the rest of the UK. On the other hand, nearly 40 years after its introduction, the extent to which the policy has delivered on such promises is not clear.

The chapter begins with an historical overview of the origins and development of the service. It is argued that, in the case of Northern Ireland, policy-making was shaped as much by the particular circumstances of political conflict as by conventional rationalities about how governments should address health and social care need. Next, we discuss the available evidence that supports or contradicts the view that the specific model of integrated services in Northern Ireland has been successful. The relative paucity of this evidence-base implies that our assessment of the achievements of the integrated service can be tentative only in nature. The discussion focuses on findings from selected research in four areas: older people; mental health; comparative studies; and victims and survivors of the conflict in Northern Ireland. This literature reports on two key areas: how services appear to be delivered, mostly in terms of professionals' views; and comparisons that are made between the Northern Irish experience of health and social welfare services and the experience in other parts of the UK. We conclude with an overview of the key messages that can be drawn from this literature and suggest that a more expansive understanding of integration is required in order to meet in a holistic way the needs of citizens in Ireland, the UK and elsewhere.

THE DEVELOPMENT OF AN INTEGRATED SERVICE IN NORTHERN IRELAND

This section explores the origins and development of what is commonly described as the 'integrated service' in Northern Ireland. There are a number of aspects of this service that makes it unusual when compared to health and social care organisations in the other devolved regions of the UK. Tentative proposals for an integrated service were debated in a *Green Paper* published by the Northern Ireland Government in 1969, where it was suggested that "nothing short of a fully integrated administrative system can provide an adequate framework for comprehensive care" (Northern Ireland Government, 1969: para.24). These ideas occurred at a time when Northern Ireland was entering a period of prolonged conflict, euphemistically described as 'the Troubles'. When the Westminster Government revoked the powers of the Northern Ireland Government a few years later, a system of Direct Rule was used to introduce new types of State bureaucracies to deliver government across many departmental areas. It has been argued that these mechanisms of Direct Rule had much to do with policy responses by the State to manage the ongoing political conflict. The creation of these welfare bureaucracies implied a loss of local political and community accountability in systems of governance and resource allocation; the policy assumption was that the devolved administration had failed to deal with the discrimination that had led to the Troubles. There was, however, a consequential increase in the influence of professional decision-making processes (Ditch and Morrissey, 1992; Pinkerton and Campbell, 2002). *The Health and Personal Social Services (NI) Order, 1972* established an organisational structure in which most statutory health and social care professionals were employed by one of four Health and Social Services Boards. In the House of Lords debate on the *Order*, Lord Windlesham suggested that:

> In many fields the health of a community and its social needs are interrelated. The elderly, the handicapped and the mentally ill, for example, are particularly vulnerable groups in need of both medical and social care. The combined administrative structure will enable the health and social services for these groups to be fully co-ordinated. I should add that certain safeguards will be included in the administrative structure to protect the professional autonomy of both services (Hansard, HL Deb 27 July 1972, volume 333, cc1542-53).

The service was administered by a hierarchy of professional groups, including medical staff, nurses, professionals allied to medicine, administrators and social workers, with each profession having separate line management structures. Under the *1972 Order*, the four Boards had access to considerable financial resources and substantial decision-making authority to plan and provide for services. A positive consequence was that the new service avoided the problematic separation of functions that historically existed between local authorities and health authorities in the rest of the UK (Heenan and Birrell, 2006). This was not, however, a fully integrated system. The delivery of education and housing services, which are delivered in integrated ways in Britain, were separated into freestanding bureaucracies (Education and Library Boards and the Northern Ireland Housing Executive respectively). Discourses about the integrated service also tend to focus on the role of statutory agencies and professionals and not on the extensive range of community, voluntary and private sector organisations that increasingly contribute to the health and social wellbeing of the population (Acheson, 2010; Heenan, 2004). This problematic of a 'partial' integrated service is an issue that we will return to later in the chapter.

The perception that the integrated service was something of an experiment by the central State was reinforced by subsequent changes in policy and law that shaped the organisation and delivery of organisations

(Campbell and McLaughlin, 2000). Substantial modifications to the service continued throughout the 1990s, beginning with the publication of *People First* (Department of Health and Social Services (Northern Ireland) (DHSS (NI)), 1990). As in the rest of the UK, a cornerstone of community care policy was the imperative to de-institutionalise, part of a wider attempt to achieve the '3 Es' of economy, efficiency and effectiveness (Means and Smith, 1994) through the marketisation of health and social care provision. What was not able to be achieved in the rest of the UK was possible in the Northern Ireland. A radical experiment in the administration of health and social welfare was taking place, in which the decentralisation of statutory services and devolution of budgets was achieved. *The Health and Personal Social Services (NI) Order, 1993* confirmed these new relationships by re-organising the service into four commissioning Health and Social Services Boards and over 20 community and hospital trusts. What was radical, some might say irrational, was that the creation of so many organisational units took place in such a small geographical area and a population of around 1.5 million people. Nearly two decades later, new sets of administrative changes have led to what appear to be more coherent structures, involving one commissioning authority, five provider trusts and a streamlined system of acute and other hospital service provision (Northern Ireland Executive, 2006; Heenan and Birrell, 2009). The most recent review of these arrangements, however, indicates how much further needs to be done to achieve optimum levels of integration. Compton (2011: 23) has suggested that, despite this history:

> Our system often does not deal with multiple conditions in an integrated way, which for the individual can mean having to engage with multiple clinicians and services which are not well joined up. The consequent personal experience is often very frustrating.

Therefore, the review has proposed that 17 Integrated Care Partnerships should be created to facilitate the further integration of the planning and delivery of health and social care services in Northern Ireland.

What is often missing in analyses of this history is the impact of political violence on this society and consequences for health and social care services. Despite the fact there appears to be deep layers of unmet psychological and social need (Ferry *et al.*, 2010), health and social care professionals historically have been reluctant to explore how the services they provide can help victims and survivors of the conflict (Office of the First Minister and Deputy First Minister (OFMDFM), 2009), nor how the conflict has impacted upon their practice (Pinkerton and Campbell, 2002).

When the problems faced by citizens with higher levels of health and social care need (Hillyard *et al.*, 2003; Tomlinson, 2007) also are considered, we can better understand the challenges that the integrated service faces.

HOW WELL DOES THE INTEGRATED SERVICE WORK?

The policies that have evolved in Northern Ireland offer a number of potential benefits. For the last 40 years, health and statutory social care professionals have been employed by the same types of authorities (although as we explained above, the way that these have been planned and arranged over the years led to some degree of disruption and, ironically, disorganisation). All statutory provision, across primary, secondary and tertiary medical care and community-based social care services, to a lesser or greater extent, are characterised by some form of interdisciplinary working. It has been argued that these features of the service enabled more efficient planning, particularly around the vexed interface areas between hospital and community, and forms of multi-disciplinary working.

Managers' Views

The only study that has been designed to test these ideas with managers of the service was initiated by Heenan and Birrell (2006). They carried out interviews with strategic managers (n=24) and group interviews with operational managers (n=16). One of the strengths of the study was that participants were drawn from the range of managers across different health and social care trusts. Perhaps not surprisingly (given that they were key stakeholders in the service that they managed), they tended to view the service positively.

Four key themes emerged from the data. Respondents were strongly of the opinion that the structuring services around programmes of care enabled good multi-disciplinary working to take place and ensured that holistic forms of assessment and interventions could take place. A second theme focused on systems of professional management and accountability. In the Northern Irish system, following the introduction of general management in the 1980s (McCoy, 1993), the old hierarchical, single professional line of accountability was broken. The result has been that, in operational terms, any professional can manage any other. Professional line management issues now are dealt with through different arrangements, usually single professional *fora* and named individuals who are allocated this responsibility. Although there was some unevenness in these arrangements, the respondents in the study were generally positive about how these forms of multi-disciplinary management systems worked. There were, however, some concerns that professional silos remained, particularly because cross-disciplinary education was the exception at both qualifying and post-qualifying training. A third theme that emerged from the interviews was the perception that the integrated service has been relatively successful in dealing with the complex processes associated with de-institutionalisation and community care. The problems caused by the separation of health and social care functions in the rest of the UK (mentioned earlier in this chapter) were viewed to be more easily resolved in the Northern Irish system because of the unified system of planning and delivery of services across this continuum. Systems of care management, alongside other community care reforms, supported these policy changes. The final theme, described by Heenan and Birrell (2006) as the 'hegemony of health', reveals some tensions between staff, particularly those who were concerned that health care priorities dominated the system in terms of resourcing and planning. Nonetheless, most respondents were optimistic that these inequalities and preferences could be overcome.

The authors conclude by arguing that, on this evidence, the integrated service is more successful than systems elsewhere in the UK, but that much hinges on the attitudes of professionals and a willingness to break down interdisciplinary barriers if the service is to fulfil its vision.

We now turn our attention to studies that relate to the activities of professionals involved in specific parts of the integrated service.

Services for Older People

The twin goals of de-institutionalisation and community care continue to inform the organisation and delivery of health and social care services in Northern Ireland, as they do in the rest of the UK. Most studies that have tested these ideas focus on the needs of adults, in particular older people. For example, initiatives such as home-from-hospital services have been designed to enable quicker, appropriate discharge from general hospitals through the use of community-based supports. In an early evaluation of one initiative led by a hospital-based social services team in collaboration with the voluntary sector, Donnelly and Dempster (1999) found that the service was beneficial, particularly in terms of increased levels of independence and satisfaction with services. Medical, nursing and social work staff estimated that patients probably would have remained in hospital for an extra 10 to 13 days on average in the absence of the service. Similar findings have been reported for other patient and client groups, including patients with complex needs (Scott and Donnelly, 2008). For example, Donnelly *et al.* (2004) found that a community-based team of health and social care professionals led by a community care manager (with access to consultant medical staff, if required) provided cost-effective rehabilitation in the homes of stroke patients who, in the absence of the service, would have had longer hospital stays and lower quality of life. Other services for older people and their carers operate at the 'front' end of the integrated service, such as a nurse/social worker-provided service that connects into primary and community services to raise awareness of cognitive problems and to identify early signs of dementia (Scott and Donnelly, 2005). The success of these community care services is dependent on factors related to integration, such as organisation, funding and communication. Of particular importance is the quality and retention of sufficient community-based staff to deliver high quality care. Fleming and Taylor (2007) surveyed home care workers in a health and social care trust service for older people that was designed to prevent hospital admissions and facilitate earlier discharge. Staff were committed to delivering this form of community care, despite facing increasing pressures – for example, in terms of the complex needs of clients and the demands of policies around governance and risk management. The authors conclude by recommending improved training and management in order to ensure the continuing success of the service.

Discourses on integration often assume that closer working arrangements between health and social care professionals will result in the better management of risk and delivery of improved services for older people. The literature suggests that the evidence is mixed in this respect. In a study designed to explore how professionals assessed and managed elder abuse, McLaughlin and Lavery (2000) found that there were high levels of physical, psychological, financial and sexual abuse, as well as care-giver neglect of people aged 65 and over, in caseloads. One of the key findings of the study was the lack of direction and cohesion in some aspects of multi-disciplinary working in this important area of adult care. Taylor (2006) used a grounded theory approach to explore the issue of risk to older people, as perceived by staff, across a range of disciplines (social workers, care managers, consultant geriatricians, general medical practitioners, community nurses, occupational therapists, home care managers and hospital discharge support staff). The author suggests ways in which the findings from the study can be translated into practice. In a similar vein, Killick and Taylor (2011) examined factors in professional decision-making in relation to identifying and reporting abuse of older people. A systematic review and a panel of expert practitioners were used to identify factors that might influence professional recognition and reporting of elder abuse by social workers and other professionals Although some progress has been made in this area, the views and needs of carers often are neglected, particularly at key points of transition between community and institutional systems of care (McCann *et al.*, 2011).

Mental Health Services

At an important moment in the history of mental health service in Northern Ireland, the DHSS (NI) used a three-year period of bridging finance to facilitate discharge from mental health and learning disability hospitals. In the only large-scale research into this process, Donnelly *et al.* (1994) found that there was no substantial change in the quality of life for patients who had been discharged in the period 1990-1992, although there was variation in the benefits of community supports provided by the private, voluntary and statutory care sectors. Interestingly, the authors also found that the packages of care offered to these clients were cheaper, on average, than was the case in other similar British studies.

A number of other studies have identified forms of interdisciplinary practice in the way mental health social workers carried out their statutory functions. Manktelow (2002), in a cross-sectional survey of Approved Social Workers (ASWs), revealed some difficulties in the relationships between GPs and ASWs at times of assessment for compulsory admission to psychiatric hospitals. In a later study, Davidson and Campbell (2010) also found difficulties in interdisciplinary working between social workers, GPs and the police service. These were mainly related to practical difficulties of communicating and co-ordinating assessments and interventions at times of crisis.

The final study we wish to mention is in the area of mental health services for children (Teggart and Menary, 2005). Of the 64 children in substitute care who were assessed using a behavioural screening instrument, the authors found over half of the children were likely to have a diagnosable disorder. They conclude by arguing that more developed mental health services for this group of children and young people are necessary. The introduction of a single assessment framework for children in need (Martin, 2007, cited in Heenan and Birrell, 2009) should improve multidisciplinary approaches to helping children and young people in this field.

Comparative Studies

A number of researchers have attempted to investigate the integrated service using a comparative framework. For example, in a series of studies on care management with older people (Challis *et al.*, 2006), and people with mental health problems (Reilly *et al.*, 2007), the integrated service in Northern Ireland was compared with the separate organisational arrangements that pertain in England (where local authorities have lead responsibility for community care and care management). The Northern Irish system of care management was characterised by: a greater level of involvement by health care staff; more multidisciplinary working; a shared, joined-up approach to assessment and care planning processes; a more differentiated approach to care management, including better targeting of resources; and closer links between care management and specialist provision. Structurally, the organisation of health and social services in Northern Ireland was found to be more conducive towards, although insufficient to secure, integrated working. The nature, type of services and ways of working appeared to be broadly similar in both jurisdictions, thereby implying that greater structural integration *per se* may not lead to better service outcomes. Reilly *et al.* (2003) reported broadly similar findings in a comparative study of the views of consultants in old age psychiatry in England and Northern Ireland, as did Clarkson *et al.* (2009, 2010) in a comparative analysis of performance measurement systems regarding care for older people. Whilst the comparative analytical approach used in these studies provides important insights about the operation and delivery of the integrated service, there is need for research that investigates and assesses the benefits for service users and their families.

The Integrated Service and the Troubles

We began this chapter by highlighting the unusual and political circumstances that led to the establishment of the integrated service in Northern Ireland. In 1972, the worst years of the Troubles, over 500 people lost their lives and many more were physically and psychologically traumatised. Surprisingly, there are few written accounts of this period. Darby and Williamson (1978) describe how health and care professionals struggled to practice in the midst of violence and the collapse of civil authority. We also mentioned earlier that decisions taken by the Direct Rule Government led to the creation of a State populated by health and social care professionals employed by unified organisations. The political parties at the time were largely excluded from the management and governance of these organisations. This loss of political accountability proved to be a double-edged sword. The State viewed the moment as an opportunity to deal with various forms of discrimination and alleged discrimination that had occurred since the foundation of the Northern Irish State in 1921; what emerged, on the other hand, was what was described later as a 'democratic deficit' where health and social care agencies became increasingly detached from the communities they were employed to serve. Therefore, we can view the integrated service as relatively successful in its first decade in terms of an increasingly well-qualified workforce, bridging a variety of competently trained and educated disciplines. It has been argued also, however, that this sense of bureaucratic detachment often left practitioners unable, or unwilling, to deal with the effects of ongoing social and political conflict (Pinkerton and Campbell, 2002).

As with other aspects of the integrated service, we have only limited evidence to test these assumptions. Early studies of psychiatric *sequelae*, perhaps surprisingly, suggested that patients who had experienced the effects of violence were more likely to recover than expected (Lyons, 1971, 1972). Some researchers have speculated that the apparent absence of symptomology might be explained by psychosocial coping mechanisms that occur when traumatic events occur (Cairns and Wilson, 1984). Increasingly, however, others have identified increasing levels of post-traumatic stress disorder (PTSD) amongst different populations. Bell *et al.* (1988) and Loughrey *et al.* (1988) reported that 23% of patients who had experienced incidents of political violence reached threshold levels of PTSD. It may be that particular groups are more likely to experience PTSD, especially individuals and communities that experienced single incident traumas – for example, following Bloody Sunday and the Enniskillen and Omagh bombs (Curren *et al.*, 1990; Duffy *et al.*, 2007; Hayes and Campbell, 2000; Shevlin and McGuigan, 2003; McGuigan and Shevlin, 2010). Despite this increasing awareness of unmet psychological and other needs, it is less than clear how well the integrated service in Northern Ireland has dealt with the aftermath of such traumatic incidents. There is a perception, which is understandable given the intensity of the conflict in the early years of the Troubles, that professionals struggled to come to terms with these events and the implications for patients and clients (Darby and Williamson, 1978; Hayes and Campbell, 2000). However, one would expect that the integrated nature of services and the importance placed on professional management would have lead to more adequate responses to meet this need. This may not have been possible for a number of reasons. However able professional groups were technocratically (Gibson and Iwaniec, 2003), generally they were drawn from the society that was experiencing the conflict and its sectarian manifestations. Silence and fear, it has been argued, characterised everyday practice (Pinkerton and Campbell, 2002). In the years since the signing of the Belfast Agreement in 1998, however, gradual shifts in politics and society have allowed piecemeal efforts by professionals and health and social care agencies to deal with the legacy of conflict (OFMDFM, 2009). Although many legacy issues continue to affect professionals (Smyth *et al.*, 2001), like their clients, there is a willingness to develop more appropriate responses (Campbell and McCrystal, 2005; Duffy *et al.*, 2007). It also may be the case that the voluntary and community sectors are more likely to embrace new ways of dealing with trauma (Manktelow, 2007; Dillenburger *et al.*, 2008).

CONCLUSION

We started this chapter by arguing that the experience of the integrated service in Northern Ireland suggests a better system of health and social care than exists elsewhere in the UK. These arguments are well rehearsed by Heenan and Birrell (2009). Appropriately-designed partnerships tend to deliver better targeted services to clients and to ensure that the interface between community and hospital services is managed efficiently. Other advantages include common systems of information, resource and personnel management and multi-disciplinary education and training opportunities. Limitations in the Northern Irish integrated health and social care service include the piecemeal nature of its coverage across different client groups and concerns about the excessive influence of medical discourses regarding service planning and delivery.

Much of our understanding about the integrated service in Northern Ireland tends to be based on speculative views and practice wisdom; the evidence-base is partial and weak. Most of the studies focus on the views of professionals and have not given sufficient attention to other key stakeholders, such as service users, carers and communities. Also, in order to gain a more thorough understanding of the integrated service, there is a need to examine the important, but often poorly recognised, roles that the private, voluntary and community sectors play, alongside statutory organisations, particularly in a policy context that advocates a mixed economy of care.

In our review of this evidence, we highlighted findings from studies in a number of key areas: services for older people, mental health services, comparisons between Northern Ireland and the rest of the UK, and how the service has responded to political conflict. It appears that, in some situations, the joint working between health and social care professionals enables the problematic interface between hospital and community to be managed and controlled. This output is facilitated *via* a number of mechanisms, including good systems of communication and interprofessional working and training. Also, in an increasingly risk-averse world, locating professionals under the same roof and shared working space enables more comprehensive assessments of vulnerable adults and children to be undertaken. It is probable that, following the lead from politicians, health and social care professionals will become more skilled in dealing with the needs of victims and survivors of the conflict in Northern Ireland.

Finally, progress towards achieving a holistic approach to the planning and delivery of health and social care will occur more quickly in relation to the degree to which services across all health and welfare are joined up – and should include housing and education, because these contexts have an important, often unrecognised, impact upon population health and wellbeing. There are also factors transcending any type of care system that influence the degree of integration and decision-making about the balance of hospital and community care. These include important issues such as community safety and attitudes to risk and its management (Taylor and Donnelly, 2006a; 2006b). An ideal integrated care system crosses disciplines and sectors, but this ideal requires policy-makers, service planners and practitioners to take account of important social contexts that contribute to health and wellbeing; and, arguably, to design service responses that focus on wellness and welfare rather than on illness and crises.

REFERENCES

Acheson, N. (2010). 'Welfare State Reform, Compacts and Restructuring Relations between the State and the Voluntary Sector: Reflections on Northern Ireland's Experience', *Voluntary Sector Review*, 1(2): 175-192.

Bell, P., Kee, M., Loughrey, G.C., Roddy, R.J. and Curran, P.S. (1988). 'Post-traumatic Stress in Northern Ireland', *Acta Psychiatrica Scandinavica*, 77(2): 166.

Cairns, E. and Wilson, R. (1984). 'The Impact of Political Violence on Mild Psychiatric Morbidity in Northern Ireland', *British Journal of Psychiatry*, 145: 631-635.

Campbell, J. and McCrystal, P. (2005). 'Mental Health Social Work and the Troubles in Northern Ireland: A Study of Practitioner Experiences', *Journal of Social Work*, 5(2): 173-90.

Campbell, J. and McLaughlin, J. (2000). 'The 'Joined up' Management of Adult Health and Social Care Services in Northern Ireland: Lessons for the Rest of the UK?', *Managing Community Care*, 8(5): 6-13.

Challis, D., Stewart, K., Donnelly, M., Weiner, K. and Hughes, J. (2006). 'Care Management for Older People: Does Integration Make a Difference?', *Journal of Interprofessional Care*, 20(4): 335-348.

Clarkson, P., Challis, D., Davies, S., Donnelly, M. and Beech, R. (2009). 'Has Social Care Performance in England Improved?', *Policy Studies*, 30: 1-20.

Clarkson, P., Challis, D., Davies, S., Donnelly, M., Beech, R. and Takayuki, H. (2010). 'Comparing How to Compare: An Evaluation of Alternative Performance Measurement Systems in the Field of Social Care', *Evaluation: The International Journal of Theory, Practice and Research*, 16: 59-79.

Compton, J. (2011). *Transforming Your Care: A Review of Health and Social Care in Northern Ireland*, Belfast: Department of Health, Social Services and Public Safety.

Curran, P.S., Bell, P., Murray, A., Loughrey, G., Roddy, R. and Rocke, L.G. (1990). 'Psychological Consequences of the Enniskillen Bombing', *British Journal of Psychiatry*, 156(4): 479.

Darby, J. and Williamson, A. (1978). *Violence and the Social Services in Northern Ireland*, London: Heinemann.

Davidson, G. and Campbell, J. (2010). 'An Audit of Assessment and Reporting by Approved Social Workers (ASWs)', *British Journal Social Work*, 40(5): 1609-1627.

Department of Health and Social Services (Northern Ireland) (DHSS (NI)) (1990). *People First: Community Care in Northern Ireland for the 1990s*, Belfast: DHSS (NI).

Dillenburger, K., Fargas, M. and Akhonzada, R. (2008). 'Evidence-based Practice: An Exploration of the Effectiveness of Voluntary Sector Services for Victims of Community Violence', *British Journal of Social Work*, 38(8): 1630.

Ditch, J.S. and Morrissey, M.J. (1992). 'Northern Ireland: Review and Prospects for Social Policy', *Social Policy and Administration*, 26: 18-39.

Donnelly, M. and Dempster, M. (1999). 'A Home from Hospital Service for Older People', *Ulster Medical Journal*, 68: 79-83.

Donnelly, M., McGilloway, S., Mays, N., Perry, S., Knapp, M. and Kavanagh, S. (1994). *Opening New Doors: An Evaluation of Community Care for People Discharged from Psychiatric and Mental Handicap Hospitals*, London: HMSO.

Donnelly, M., Power, M., Russell, M. and Fullerton, K. (2004). 'Randomised Controlled Trial of an Early Discharge Rehabilitation Service: The Belfast Community Stroke Trial', *Stroke*, 35: 127-133.

Duffy, M., Gillespie, K. and Clark, D.M. (2007). 'Post-traumatic Stress Disorder in the Context of Terrorism and other Civil Conflict in Northern Ireland: Randomised Controlled Trial', *British Medical Journal*, 334: 147-150.

Ferry, F., Bolton, D., Bunting, B., O'Neill, S. and Murphy, S. (2010). 'The Experience and Psychological Impact of "Troubles"-related Trauma in Northern Ireland: A Review', *Irish Journal of Psychology*, 31: 95-110.

Fleming, G. and Taylor, B.J. (2007). 'Battle on the Home Care Front: Perceptions of Home Care Workers of Factors Influencing Staff Retention', *Health and Social Care in the Community*, 15(1): 67-76.

Gibson, M. and Iwaniec, D. (2003) 'An Empirical Study into the Psychosocial Reactions of Staff Working as Helpers to those Affected in the Aftermath of Two Traumatic Incidents', *British Journal of Social Work*, 33(7): 851-870.

Hayes, P. and Campbell, J. (2000). 'Dealing with Post-traumatic Stress Disorder: The Psychological *Sequelae* of Bloody Sunday and the Response of State Services', *Research on Social Work Practice,* 10: 705-720.

Heenan, D. (2004). 'Learning Lessons from the Past or Re-Visiting Old Mistakes: Social Work and Community Development in Northern Ireland', *British Journal of Social Work,* 34(6): 793-809.

Heenan, D. and Birrell, D. (2006). 'The Integration of Health and Social: The Lessons from Northern Ireland', *Social Policy and Administration,* 40(1): 47-66.

Heenan, D. and Birrell, D. (2009). 'Organisational Integration in Health and Social Care: Some Reflections on the Northern Ireland Experience', *Journal of Integrated Care,* 17(5): 3-12.

Hillyard, P., Kelly, G., McLaughlin, E., Patsios, D. and Tomlinson, M. (2003). *Bare Necessities: Poverty and Social Exclusion in Northern Ireland – Key Findings,* Belfast: Democratic Dialogue.

Johnson, P., Wistow, G., Schulz, R. and Hardy, B. (2003). 'Interagency and Interprofessional Collaboration in Community Care: The Interdependence of Structures and Values', *Journal of Interprofessional Care,* 17(1): 70-83.

Killick, C. and Taylor, B.J. (2011). 'Judgments of Social Care Professionals on Elder Abuse Referrals: A Factorial Survey', *British Journal of Social Work,* Advance Access: doi:10.1093/bjsw/bcr109.

Loughrey, G.C., Bell, P., Kee, M., Roddy, R.J. and Curran, P.S. (1988). 'Post-traumatic Stress Disorder and Civil Violence in Northern Ireland', *British Journal of Psychiatry,* 153(4): 554.

Lyons, H.A. (1971). 'Psychiatric *Sequelae* of the Belfast Riots', *British Journal of Psychiatry,* 118: 265-273.

Lyons, H.A. (1972). 'Depressive Illness and Aggression in Belfast', *British Medical Journal,* 1: 342-344.

Manktelow, R. (2007). 'The Needs of Victims of the Troubles in Northern Ireland: The Social Work Contribution', *Journal of Social Work,* 7(1): 31-50.

Manktelow, R., Hughes, P., Britton, F., Campbell, J., Hamilton, B. and Wilson, G. (2002). 'The Experience and Practice of Approved Social Workers in Northern Ireland', *British Journal of Social Work,* 32: 443–61.

McCann, M., Donnelly, M. and O'Reilly, D. (2011). 'Living Arrangements, Relationship to People in Household and Admission to Care Homes for Older People', *Age and Ageing,* 40: 358-363.

McCoy, K. (1993). 'Integration: A Changing Scene in Social Services Inspectorate', in Social Services Inspectorate, *Personal Social Services in Northern Ireland: Perspectives on Integration,* Belfast: Department of Health and Social Services.

McGuigan, K. and Shevlin, M. (2010). 'Longitudinal Changes in Post-traumatic Stress in relation to Political Violence (Bloody Sunday)', *Traumatology,* 16(1): 1.

McLaughlin, J. and Lavery, H. (2000). 'Awareness of Elder Abuse among Community Health and Social Care Staff in Northern Ireland: An Exploratory Study', *Journal of Elder Abuse and Neglect,* 11(3): 53-72.

Means, R. and Smith, R. (1994). *Community Care: Policy and Practice,* London: Macmillan.

Northern Ireland Executive (2006). *Better Government for Northern Ireland – Final Decisions of the Review of Public Administration*, Belfast: Northern Ireland Executive.

Northern Ireland Government (1969). *The Administrative Structure of the Health and Personal Social Services in Northern Ireland* [*Green Paper*], Belfast: HMSO.

Office of the First Minister and Deputy First Minister (OFMDFM) (2009). *Strategy for Victims and Survivors*, Belfast: OFMDFM.

Pinkerton, J. and Campbell, J. (2002). 'Social Work and Social Justice in Northern Ireland: Towards a New Occupational Space', *British Journal of Social Work*, 32(6): 723-737.

Reed, J., Cook, G., Childs, S. and McCormack, B. (2005). 'A Literature Review to Explore Integrated Care for Older People', *International Journal of Integrated Care*, 5: 1-8.

Reilly, S., Challis, D., Donnelly, M., Stewart, K. and Hughes, J. (2007). 'Care Management in Mental Health Services in England and Northern Ireland: Do Integrated Organisations Promote Integrated Practice?', *Journal of Health Services Research and Policy*, 12(4): 236-241.

Reilly, S., Challis, D.J., Burns, A.S. and Hughes, J. (2003). 'Does Integration Really Make a Difference? A Comparison of Old Age Psychiatry Services in England and Northern Ireland', *International Journal of Geriatric Psychiatry*, 18(10): 887-893.

Scott, D. and Donnelly, M. (2005). 'Early Identification of Cognitive Impairment: A Stakeholder Evaluation of a "Dementia Awareness Service"', *Dementia*, 4: 207-232.

Scott, D. and Donnelly, M. (2008). 'Buying Time for Better Decision-making: The Impact of Home-based Rehabilitation on Frail Older People', *Rehabilitation Journal*, 1: 5-14.

Shevlin, M. and McGuigan, K. (2003). 'The Long-term Psychological Impact of Bloody Sunday on Families of the Victims as Measured by the Revised Impact of Event Scale', *British Journal of Clinical Psychology*, 42(4): 427-432.

Smyth, M., Morrissey, M. and Hamilton, J. (2001). *Caring through the Troubles: Health and Social Services in North and West Belfast*, Belfast: North and West Belfast Health and Social Services Trust.

Taylor, B.J. (2006). 'Risk Management Paradigms in Health and Social Services for Professional Decision-making on the Long-term Care of Older People', *British Journal of Social Work*, 36: 1411-1429.

Taylor, B.J. and Donnelly, M. (2006a). 'Professional Perspectives on Decision-making about the Long-term Care of Older People, *British Journal of Social Work*, 36: 807-826.

Taylor, B.J. and Donnelly, M. (2006b). 'Risks to Home Care Workers: Professional Perspectives', *Health, Risk and Society*, 8: 239-256.

Teggart, T. and Menary, J. (2005). 'An Investigation of the Mental Health Needs of Children Looked After by Craigavon and Banbridge Health and Social Services Trust', *Child Care in Practice*, 11: 39-49.

Tomlinson, M. (2007). *The Trouble with Suicide. Mental Health, Suicide and the Northern Ireland Conflict: A Review of the Evidence*, Belfast: Department of Health, Social Services and Public Safety.

3: INTEGRATED DISCHARGE PLANNING: A PROGRAMME MANAGER'S VIEW

William Reddy

INTRODUCTION

One of the key goals of most health services, including the Irish health service, is to deliver safe and efficient integrated care. The provision of enhanced clinical integration is perhaps the most challenging and ultimately by far the most important to the patient/client. It requires excellent co-ordination of care at all levels to ensure 'things don't fall between cracks'.

As patients move through the various components of the health care system, a number of obstacles prevent timely access to care. In particular, hospitals have struggled to reduce the delays faced by patients who have been assessed as needing acute care but cannot get access to an acute inpatient bed because all capacity is occupied. This has led to serious delays resulting in an acute access block, which typically manifests as patients suffering long 'trolley waits' in Emergency Departments.

Developing solutions to the problem of delays in access to emergency care is challenging because the causes of delay are not in the Emergency Department itself. Rather it is multi-factorial, complex and systemic in nature and requires system-wide solutions.

One of the most effective strategies for reducing total patient journey time is to focus on the bottlenecks in both the admission and the discharge process. A mismatch between variation in demand (admissions) and the variation in capacity (resulting from discharges) gives rise to queues and, in many cases, unnecessary waits, which can be resolved by bringing the two elements into alignment.

Hospitals usually experience far more variation in patterns of patient discharge than in patterns of admission. The main reason for this is the way we manage processes such as ward rounds, inpatient tests and communication with families and community services to deliver a planned and controlled patient journey. This leads to a highly variable and unpredictable length of stay (LOS), even among patients admitted with similar conditions. Generally, discharges peak on Fridays, with a trough over the weekend where the numbers admitted exceed the numbers discharged and thus reduce the capacity to meet the general patterns of increased attendances at the start of each week.

DISCHARGE PLANNING

Given the limited capacity that is an acute hospital bed, it is important that we get the most value from this resource. Reducing the length of stay releases capacity in the system but requires pro-active planning of the whole process of care, which involves what we can term 'integrated discharge planning'. In order to address these matters in a systematic manner, it is important that we focus on the fundamental routine practices, processes and procedures that facilitate integration across services and over time. Of particular importance are transition points across the health system. This can involve simple matters to promote handovers in the hospital system to other multidisciplinary teams or other health care professionals, streamlining the processes of assessment, diagnosis and treatment such that the patient receives appropriate and timely care. The transition that has received the most focus is the transfer from hospital care to the community. Effective discharge planning that integrates care pathways into the community is imperative to re-orienting practice from discrete and isolated interventions towards integrated and continuous care, which is a key goal of all health care reform. This can involve such obvious matters such as taking timely steps to arrange transport to home for a frail elderly patient, organising prescriptions or follow-up care or applying for nursing home support in time.

It is important to recognise that discharge from a hospital is a process, not an isolated event, involving the development and implementation of a plan to facilitate the transfer of an individual from hospital to an alternative setting where appropriate. Components of the system (individual, family, carers, hospitals, primary care providers, community services and social services) must work together to ensure an integrated person-centred approach and the best outcome for the individual. The discharge process is thus a lens through which we can focus our attention on the internal organisation factors within hospitals that influence lengths of stay, bed occupancy and bed utilisation and also draw clear attention to the nature, capacity and availability of community-based services to be pro-active and responsive in order to avoid unnecessary admissions to acute care and to facilitate earlier discharge.

Many hospitals across the world have found it helpful to focus on the time of day when discharges occur. Moving discharges to the morning before peak arrival times helps keep the flow through an organisation. The simple premise is that the sooner an acute bed is vacated by the person who has finished their acute care, the sooner the next person can be accommodated in it. That is why there is now a national focus on discharging patients as early as possible each day (before 11 am) to ensure bed capacity is available when it is most needed for those who are the most acutely ill. This requires that all the clinical team and family know when discharge is likely to happen and have adequate notice (at least 24 hours) so that things can be organised in advance – for example, the medical certificate, the prescription, the follow-up appointment and the transport. It also requires that discharging ward rounds are conducted early each day and on a seven-day basis.

Patient surveys have consistently highlighted that this is not the normal practice and confirm that many patients state that they were given very little notice of their discharge, with a significant minority only being told on the morning of their discharge. Even when this notice is given, there are still further waits: for GP letters, medical certificates for work, prescriptions, transport and follow-up appointments. In practice, the four most common waits in accessing emergency care relate to: waiting for assessment, waiting to see a specialist; waiting for a diagnostic test and waiting for a bed.

One of the trends that impacts on Emergency Departments is that the numbers of admissions over weekends and on Mondays greatly exceed the number of discharges, which then typically leads to capacity issues on Tuesdays and Wednesdays – consistently the worst days for Emergency Department overcrowding. There is a general recognition that a situation exists in our hospitals such that patients are admitted seven days a week but typically discharges occur on only five of these (Monday to Friday). These patterns have been highlighted in a number of published reports such as the *Emergency Department Task Force Report* (Health Service Executive (HSE), 2007). This mismatch is now the focus of increased attention, especially with regard to the implementation of new working practices around extended working days, working in teams and the delegation of discharging powers within clinical teams or to other disciplines such as nurses within controlled parameters. New contractual arrangements and the implementation of the 'Croke Park' agreement and care programmes are key enablers to addressing these matters.

The introduction of visual aids such as white boards on inpatient beds showing the expected day of discharge have been introduced in many places and are proving effective in facilitating better communication, planning and timely discharging of patients. The key emphasis is on having a plan for each patient and ensuring that this plan is pro-actively managed by a named person over an explicit timeline and that potential delays are anticipated and addressed.

From the point of view of improving overall bed availability, the development of a strategic approach to discharge planning has been advocated by many national reports and is advocated by a large body of international literature. These consistently highlight a number of blockages and obstacles that have held back improvements in the discharge process, which need to be addressed in a systematic and structured way if we are to improve. Some of these blockages and obstacles include:

- Clinical management plan does not include expected date of discharge (EDD) based on an anticipated length of stay (LOS) resulting in:
  o Discharges mainly happening in the afternoon;
  o Fewer discharges over the weekend and on public holidays;
  o Patients staying longer in hospital than clinically necessary;
- No framework to plan the discharge;
- Lack of clearly-defined roles and responsibilities amongst multidisciplinary team around management of discharge;
- Multidisciplinary team unclear about knowledge, skills and competencies needed to support discharge decisions;
- Feelings that nurse-initiated discharge is too 'risky' or concerns about patient safety.

THE NATIONAL CODE OF PRACTICE FOR INTEGRATED DISCHARGE PLANNING

In order to address the situation in a sustainable manner, the HSE developed a standards-based *National Code of Practice for Integrated Discharge Planning*, which was finalised in November 2008 (HSE, 2008). This Code provides an explicit and measurable means to ensure that patient care, in, through and out of hospital, is managed in a consistent, coherent and efficient manner. It provides a reference point against which we can measure how well we are doing and where everyone is clear about what is expected of them.

It comprises a suite of national standards, recommended practices, forms, toolkits, key metrics and audit tools covering the following areas:

- Communication and consultation;
- Organisational structure and accountability;
- Management and key personnel;
- Education and training;
- Operational policies and procedures for discharge planning;
- Discharge planning process;
- Audit and monitoring;
- Key performance indicators.

The key indicators focus on the following areas, which are deemed critical to enabling efficient and controlled patient flow:

- **Referral:** Receipt of referrals shall be documented on a integrated discharge planning tracking form in the patient's health care record **within 24 hours of receiving the referral**;
- **Nurse (or Health and Social Care Professional (HSCP)/Other):** Within **one hour of patient admission to the ward**, an appropriate and competent nurse (or HSCP/Other) shall be identified and assigned to actively manage the patient pathway of care;
- **Estimated length of stay:** Each patient shall have an estimated LOS, which will be:
  o Identified during pre-assessment, on the post-take ward round or within 24 hours of admission to hospital;
  o Discussed and agreed with the patient/family and carers;
  o Documented in the health care record;
- **Treatment plan:** Each patient shall have a treatment plan;
- **Discharge plan:** The discharge plan shall be documented in the patient's health care record and the hospital shall advise service providers, as appropriate, of the planned discharge date as soon as possible, and at least two days prior to patient discharge (for patients who are inpatients for five days or longer);
- **Transport arrangements:** Transport arrangements shall be confirmed 24 hours before discharge;

- **Time of discharge:** Each patient discharge shall be effected (hospital bed becomes available for patient use) by 12 noon on the day of discharge.

A programme of implementation was agreed nationally and locally through the formation of local Joint Implementation Groups (JIGs) consisting of clinicians and managers from across primary and secondary care services. Self-assessments against the standards by multidisciplinary audit teams using a structured audit tool were conducted, leading to the development of local improvement plans.

A number of education and learning programmes were developed to facilitate improved practice in patient journey management, including:

- E-learning programme and resource tools;
- Irish participation with international partners in developing and evaluating patient pathways and Lean Thinking.

It is recognised that nurses and the nursing profession have a pivotal role in supporting improvements in integrated discharge planning and more efficient and effective management of the patient journey. In order to empower the nursing profession in this regard, a *Guideline* was developed and issued in July 2009, which outlines core elements for nurse/midwife-facilitated discharge planning (HSE, 2009). The guideline is intended to support and formalise existing discharge planning practice, while providing a template for local guidelines to be developed and adopted. The guideline emphasises that discharge planning is an element of the domains of competency in the undergraduate nursing curriculum and nurses and midwives continue to develop this competency in daily practice.

The nurse/midwife role in the discharge planning process includes:

- Collaborative input into determining the patient's estimated length of stay (ELOS);
- Collaborative input to the discharge plan;
- Tracking the progress of the discharge plan against the ELOS;
- Inclusion of progress of the discharge plan at each handover; and
- Completion of relevant discharge documentation.

The guideline also promote the use of criterion-based patient discharge, which refers to patient discharge by a nurse or midwife when specific clinical criteria have been achieved – for example, no raised temperature for 24 hours, wound healed, mobilising safely or no evidence of respiratory distress. The consultant/medical team will have documented discharge criteria or targets in the patient's health care record. The patient's consultant/medical team agree that the patient is fit for discharge once the patient has achieved these discharge criteria. This will allow additional discharges to occur out-of-hours and at weekends.

CONCLUSION

The *Code of Practice* (HSE, 2008) and associated guidelines provide a framework within which efficient care and case management can be delivered, thus providing clarity around key roles, responsibilities and performance standards. They are key enablers in facilitating components of the system (individual, family, carers, hospitals, primary care providers, community services and social services) working together to deliver integrated, efficient and appropriate care. They provide an evidence-based and transparent mechanism for dialogue, audit and evaluation supporting the whole system changes that are necessary to improving the quality and safety of our care system. Fundamentally, they operate as a 'chassis' or integration engine for engagement and performance improvement in delivering clinically-led reform through the emerging care programmes where the right care is delivered in the right place at the right time by the right person.

REFERENCES

Health Service Executive (HSE) (2007). *Report of the Emergency Department Task Force*, Dublin: HSE.

Health Service Executive (HSE) (2008). *National Code of Practice for Integrated Discharge Planning*, Dublin: HSE.

Health Service Executive (HSE) (2009). *Guideline for Nurse/Midwife-facilitated Discharge Planning*, Dublin: HSE.

4: WHICH IS THE RIGHT MODEL OF UNIVERSAL HEALTH INSURANCE FOR IRELAND?

Steve Thomas and Catherine Darker

INTRODUCTION

The global health policy agenda is dominated by discussions about the need for health systems to achieve universal coverage (Garrett *et al.*, 2009; Murray, 2010; Orentlicher, 2009; Yamey, 2010). There are two key elements to the concept of universal coverage: providing financial protection from the costs of health care and ensuring access to needed health services for all. This implies that the underlying health care financing mechanism must enable income cross-subsidies (from the rich to the poor) and risk cross-subsidies (from the healthy to the ill), while raising sufficient revenue (McPake and Normand, 2008).

The *Programme for Government* entitled *Towards Recovery, Programme for a National Government 2011-2016* (Fine Gael/Labour, 2011) opened up a new and exciting chapter in health policy development for Ireland (Garrett *et al.*, 2009; Murray, 2010; Orentlicher, 2009; Yamey, 2010). For the first time since the foundation of the Irish State, a Government endorsed a vision for the health system that embraces universal coverage – that individuals will access care on the basis of need rather than ability to pay. The *Programme for Government* states:

> Under this system there will be no discrimination between patients on the grounds of income or insurance status. The two-tier system of unequal access to hospital care will end (Fine Gael/Labour, 2011: 32).

Furthermore, the vehicle to achieve this is universal health insurance (UHI). The aim of this chapter is to compare and contrast available models of universal health insurance in Ireland in 2012 and to consider the best option. It is critically important to design the optimum model for UHI. Much of the available evidence has been compiled and reviewed by the Expert Group on Resource Allocation and Financing (Ruane, 2010) and there is little point in repeating such analysis.[1] Consequently, the analysis is restricted to a comparison of two key models of UHI.

It is worth noting also that Ireland, along with the USA, tends to talk about UHI, rather than social health insurance (SHI) which, historically at least, is a Western European concept. This is partly because the term 'social' has negative connotations in more libertarian societies. UHI also is technically more accurate where it refers to all the population being covered by insurance rather than just those in formal sector employment. Nevertheless, in much of the international literature, SHI is used more frequently, but both terms can be seen and sometimes they are used interchangeably.

The structure of this chapter is as follows. First, the authors assess the general theoretical and empirical features of UHI, cognisant of the experience of different countries. Second, the chapter highlights in detail the two main options for UHI: the official policy outlined in the *Programme for Government* and that developed and championed by the Adelaide Hospital Society (AHS), which has commissioned several studies on UHI in Ireland and developed its own position paper (AHS, 2010). These models are then evaluated against key criteria related to:

- Technical merit and likely performance;
- Feasibility for implementation in relation to the changes required; and
- The likelihood of support from key stakeholders.

Conclusions are then developed for the way forward for UHI in Ireland.

THE THEORETICAL AND EMPIRICAL FEATURES OF UNIVERSAL HEALTH INSURANCE

Basic Features

The common underlying principles that define UHI are the provision of access to care on the basis of need, and the payment for insurance on the basis of income or ability to pay. This contrasts with private insurance, which relates payment for insurance to the risk of the individual falling ill and excludes those who have not paid the premium.

---

[1]   The three-volume report of the Expert Group is an excellent and valuable resource. However, it deliberately shies away from developing a recommended option for health financing. Instead, it endorses principles for achieving universalisation through whatever health financing system is chosen. The political input into, and guidance and composition of, the group may have made the selection of a preferred option impossible.

The key characteristics of the basic UHI model are:

- Insured persons pay a regular contribution based on income or wealth, and not on the cost of the services they are likely to use;
- Access to treatment and care is determined by clinical need and not ability to pay;
- Contributions to the social insurance fund (or funds) are kept separate from other government-mandated taxes and charges;
- The social insurance fund finances care on behalf of the insured persons, and care may be delivered by public and private health care providers.

UHI funds are formally separate from general taxation, and may be organised and managed by autonomous organisations. Since UHI is separate from taxation and other publicly-mandated systems, the income from contributions must cover the fees paid for the services to which members are entitled. However, it is common for UHI to be subsidised in two ways: from government subsidies directly to providers of care (such as grants for capital developments) and through government payment of the premiums for people unable to pay for themselves.

SHI/UHI *vs* Taxation-based Financing

No country has a health financing system that relies purely on one funding mechanism. Indeed, all European systems are financed through a mix of public and private contributions (Bentes *et al.*, 2004). Nevertheless, most high income countries tend to be characterised by their primary reliance on either taxation or social health insurance to fund their health system. Many universal health care systems are funded primarily by tax revenue (for example, Portugal, Spain, Denmark and Sweden). Some nations, such as Germany, France and Japan, employ a multi-payer system in which health care is funded by private and public contributions. However, much of the non-government funding is by contributions by employers and employees to regulated non-profit sickness funds. These contributions are compulsory and defined according to law. In Western Europe, private voluntary insurance and out-of-pocket payments exist in virtually all countries but are rarely a major contributor of funding.

In terms of contributions and entitlement to services, the basic model of UHI has much in common with tax finance. Nevertheless, despite the similarities, UHI has retained much of the tradition and rhetoric of insurance. In practice, the differences between SHI and tax-financed systems are more significant for several reasons. First, the separate structures for collecting and managing funds tend to give the system greater transparency. Second, the fact that members are insured, and that access to care is dependent on contributions to the fund, can give the patient the status of a customer. Third, in order to keep the system in balance, it is necessary to be more explicit about the range of services to which the contributor is entitled: the 'common basket' of services.

UHI systems tend to be more popular with their populations than taxation-based systems, possibly because they have less rationing and greater transparency and possibly because the money follows the patient. Also the two systems have recently tended to borrow features from each other, resulting in less distinction in performance (McPake and Normand, 2008). For instance, many insurance systems get substantial taxation-based subsidies. Most importantly, the term SHI covers a multitude of different options and often it is the specific design features adopted in a country and the prevailing context and values that determine performance. Hence, it is important to look closely at differences in the models proposed for Ireland as they might have quite different impacts on health system performance, including value-for-money and fairness.

International Prevalence of UHI

Any adoption of, and move towards, UHI in all probability would be relatively fast in Ireland (within five to 10 years) and therefore it is important to review countries that have adopted UHI over a shorter time period as well as high income country systems where UHI has evolved over decades.

Conventional wisdom on UHI used to be that it would take several decades to introduce, with the experience of Western European countries highlighted (Normand and Busse, 2002). The transition was achieved through waves of reforms rather than a single one-off transformation. Several high income countries in Western Europe (including Belgium, France, Germany, Austria and Luxembourg) have a significant SHI component in their health system financing. Some countries have recently adopted SHI quite quickly. In particular, in Central and Eastern Europe and Central Asia, after the collapse of the Soviet bloc, SHI has emerged as a dominant financing model (Waters, 2008; Wagstaff and Moreno-Senna, 2009). By 1995, seven countries had SHI systems with a share of total health financing over 50%; this rose to 14 countries by 2003 (Waters, 2008). In 2009, China launched the first phase towards achieving UHI by 2020 and an early appraisal of progress suggests that nearly 92% of the country is now covered by insurance (Yip *et al.*, 2012). This suggests, at least superficially, that a quick development of UHI with broad coverage is possible even without a previous history and culture of health insurance. Thus Ireland's attempted swift transformation is not without precedent.

The Diversity of UHI Design
Mobilising Funds
There are three main models for paying for UHI. By far the most popular approach is a payroll tax. Where there is little government subsidy, as in Germany and many Eastern European models, the premium needs to be quite high. Most high-income country models have quite substantial subsidies to SHI from general taxation. This risks making the system more complex and less transparent but may be more politically acceptable and involve less upheaval where taxation systems are firmly rooted.

The second approach, employed in Switzerland and in part in The Netherlands, is to have a uniform flat fee, regardless of income. The advantage of such an approach is simplicity. The disadvantage is that it is by itself very inequitable. To compensate, subsidies are needed from government so that the poor are not penalised. It is possible but complicated to develop a system of subsidies that preserves equity, though it requires effective government regulatory capacity.

The third approach to funding UHI is to use a variety of financing bases, as in the French system. Here premiums are based on all income sources and not just payroll payments. Furthermore, there are additional 'sin' taxes and corporation taxation to spread the financing burden. This can be complex but, where the burden cannot be absorbed by a payroll tax alone, it may be more acceptable. There is also a resonance with the population in relating sin taxes to health spending.

The World Health Organization's (WHO) report *Health Systems Financing: The Path to Universal Coverage*, (WHO, 2010), and the associated declaration of the World Health Assembly (WHA, 2011), reached the conclusion that mandatory prepayment (or public funding) has to be the core of any universal health system. Mandatory prepayment funds in universal systems are 'public' in the sense that they are used for the benefit of all; they can be used to purchase needed health care for the whole population from public and private providers. There is strong evidence that raising funds through compulsory prepayment provides the most efficient and equitable path towards universal coverage. The funds are also 'public' in the sense that they are pooled in such a way as to ensure that there are income and risk cross-subsidies. As indicated earlier, these cross-subsidies are central to universal coverage.

Sharing Risks

A key choice is evident between the Western European models and those in Central and Eastern Europe. In the former, there is universal coverage but they are typically more expensive than taxation-based systems. In the latter, there is often significantly less than universal coverage, often with quite high user fee payments. The latter systems are far less equitable, both in terms of access and financing, but cheaper to run. They may fail, however, to meet key policy objectives.

The dominant European model relies on competition between several funds. However, this encourages insurers to cherry-pick the younger and fitter populations and to engage in competition that is not helpful for the system as a whole. Risk-equalisation becomes more important in this context. Although some risk-equalisation schemes possess much better predictive power for morbidity risk than others, all risk-equalisation systems are imperfect. The alternative is a single-fund mechanism, which is more common in East Asia.

Equity

More than any other design issue, policy decisions about exemptions, ceilings on payments and the general progressivity of the system reflect a nation's values. Hence, even in Western Europe, there is a broad range of approaches to different target groups such as the unemployed, pensioners and households on low wages. From an equity perspective in financing – where paying for health care should be according to ability – the progressivity of a system requires that the rich pay not only more but also a larger proportion of their income. More specifically, a system that has exemptions or very low payment rates for those who cannot afford is better, as is any system that does not have ceilings on payment for the rich.

UHI will not remove entirely the demand for private insurance, as is clear from reviewing mature health care systems in Western Europe. Nevertheless, as long as private insurance does not allow the member an advantage in the waiting list, demand for private insurance will likely drop sharply. Consequently, it will not skew access towards those who can afford to pay.

While UHI is more easily implemented into a system where user fees exist, it often does better to replace user fees than to live alongside them. The reason is that user fees are often poor at promoting equity. They limit access to services, especially for those on lower incomes, and frequently do not generate significant funds for the system as a whole. Therefore, they can undermine the progressive features of UHI financing.

Competing Models for Ireland

Given the diversity of choice of design for systems based on SHI internationally, it is interesting to analyse and reflect on the choices made in the Irish context. To do this, it is important to restate briefly the main features of UHI design as stated in Government policy and in the AHS position paper.

UHI according to the Programme for Government
The current coalition Government favours universal health care through a system that draws on the model introduced in 2006 in The Netherlands. This is a system of compulsory[2] private for-profit insurance with strong government regulation (Enthoven and van de Ven, 2007). In the new Irish system, everyone will have a choice between competing insurers and Voluntary Health Insurance Healthcare (VHI) will be kept in public ownership to retain a public option in the UHI system.

While current details are incomplete, it appears that there will be two payments into the system:

- The first is a premium, paid by the consumer where they can afford it or paid or subsidised by the government depending on the income bracket of the consumer. The consumer indicates their choice of insurer through this premium payment. The government automatically chooses and pays the VHI for those who cannot afford the premium;

- The second payment is from general government taxation revenue to each insurer according to the revealed patient choices and taking into account risk-equalisation across the schemes. This second payment is likely to be the larger funding flow.

Competition between the insurance funds is used as a tool to increase efficiency and innovation in the health system (though there is little evidence to suggest that this has happened (Ryan *et al.*, 2009). Health insurers compete on the basis of premium, service and quality of care. All insurers must offer to everyone the same standardised basic benefit package (although they can compete on supplementary insurance packages). This system requires a sophisticated risk-equalisation mechanism to minimise cream-skimming of low-cost patients.

---

[2]   Citizens who have not enrolled face harsh penalties (Leu *et al.*, 2009).

The *Programme for Government* states that universal primary care 'insurance' will be phased in from 2012 to 2015 and that the Government will act speedily to reduce costs in the delivery of both public and private health care and in the administration of the health care system (Fine Gael/Labour, 2011). Nevertheless, it appears now that this will be achieved primarily in the context of public taxation funding rather than any special insurance arrangement.

Under UHI, public hospitals will be managed no longer by the Health Service Executive (HSE). They will be independent, not-for-profit trusts with managers accountable to their boards. Hospitals will be paid according to the care they deliver and will be incentivised to deliver more care in a 'money follows the patient' system.

The Adelaide Hospital Society Model
This model, which is based on a series of three commissioned reports, also supports universalisation of access to health care through a system of UHI. It differs from the *Programme for Government* policy, however, in several important regards:

- First, it emphasises that, in the initial phase, a *single non-for-profit* national SHI fund should be established: "International evidence is clear that extreme caution is required when considering introducing competition between SHI funds in a SHI system" (AHS, 2010: 6). However, it would be possible to have private firms compete to run the not-for-profit UHI fund and paid in accordance to their successes in meeting targets. It leaves open the possibility for competition between funds once the system beds down;

- Second, the common basket of care prescribed by this model includes not only access to primary care providers but also free prescription drugs for all. This is a substantial additional benefit to the *Programme for Government* model;

- Third, the model emphasises removing all user fees from the system and drawing on earmarked sin, carbon and/or property taxes to supplement taxation and to raise sufficient revenue for universalisation of care;

- Fourth, it emphasises a covenant approach, which gives entitlements and improves transparency and trust. This is exemplified by the use of a *carte vitale* for the whole population, which includes patients' medical records, facilitates electronic payments and simplifies administration.

EVALUATING THE MODELS

In evaluating the models, it must be said that neither policy option is fully fleshed out. Hence, the analysis can focus only on key features of design and timetables for implementation as set out in the public domain. Still, each model presents a distinctive flavour of values and an individual pathway for development of the policy of UHI. The evaluation framework set out by the authors draws heavily on the main justifications for introduction of UHI in any context (McPake and Normand, 2008) but also the key contextual challenges for implementation in the Irish health system (Thomas and Burke, 2012).

The criteria against which each policy is measured are as follows:

- Technical merits:
  - o Efficiency;
  - o Equity and fairness;
  - o Transparency;
  - o Effectiveness;
  - o Social solidarity;
- Capacity and implementation challenges:
  - o Evolving context of recession;
  - o Supply capacity;
  - o Architecture, relationships and legislation.

TECHNICAL MERITS

Efficiency

In single-payer systems, one organisation – typically the government – collects and pools revenues and purchases health services for the entire population, while in multi-payer systems several organisations carry out these roles for specific segments of the population. Single-payer systems include all citizens within a single risk pool, while multi-payer systems have pools at potentially different levels of health risk. Single-payer insurers have monopsony power in purchasing health services; multi-payer systems offer the possibility of consumer choice of insurer with associated competition. The Irish Government has rejected the notion of a single-fund insurance model (Fine Gael/Labour, 2011) and has chosen a complex model relying on competing private insurance firms and strong and effective governance through risk-equalisation to avoid cream-skimming and dumping.

Some countries, such as the Czech Republic, have opted to forego a single-payer insurance system in favour of a multi-payer system. This raises the formidable technical challenge of avoiding adverse selection among the insurance pools. An insurance company will not price individual health insurance at the average cost of covering the uninsured. If it did, the individuals who purchased the policy would be disproportionately those who knew they were likely to have high health care costs, and so the company would lose money. To address adverse selection risks, most insurers use medical underwriting and incorporate a risk premium into the actual price of coverage. One possibility for addressing this challenge is through risk adjustment. Sophisticated risk adjustment systems exist, designed to explain as much variation in utilisation as possible; however, these sophisticated systems are rarely used. One reason is that they require detailed data that are frequently not available to most health insurance systems. A second reason is that, even if the data were available, even the most sophisticated risk adjustment system cannot predict all of the variation in utilisation. Nonetheless, an investment in information technology is one approach countries could take to prevent adverse selection in a multi-payer system. Another option is to use regulation to avoid the effects of adverse selection. For example, insurance pools could be limited in the benefit packages that they may offer to beneficiaries. This approach, however, eliminates one of the main advantages that multi-payer systems offer: diverse benefit packages. Risk adjustment processes are considered complex and expensive, and administration costs are usually higher with multiple funds, and for competition to be useful, it must improve efficiency in the delivery of care (WHO, 2010).

There is evidence that a single main payer for care (a monopsony) lowers the costs of provision. It is important to understand that it is not UHI *per se* that affects efficiency so much as the structures of provision, the system of paying providers and the resulting incentives. The multiple funds model, therefore, may not necessarily realise the potential advantages of competition (Barnighausen and Sauerborn, 2002). The gains from competition are thus less clear (Ryan *et al.*, 2009).

The Swiss and Dutch reforms, both of which have multi-payer models, have led to rapidly rising costs:

> The introduction of selective contracting by health insurers has actually reduced patients' choice of provider in Switzerland and The Netherlands ... The expansion of private insurance led to increased risk selection in Switzerland and The Netherlands. Indeed, shifts toward decentralised private governance also increased the

administrative complexity and overhead costs in those countries (Okma and Crivelli, 2010).

In The Netherlands, health care expenditure continues to outpace inflation at an annual rate of 5% since 2006; at the same time, the total costs of health insurance for Dutch families, including premiums and deductibles, increased by 41%. In The Netherlands, mergers may have reduced competition as funds seek economies of scale and premiums rose sharply to cover initial losses. Further, older and sicker patients tend to be less mobile (van de Ven *et al.*, 2007) and so consumer choice of fund may not help boost efficiency. In 2010, The Netherlands spent 14.8% of its GDP on health care and welfare, including long-term care and other social services. Premiums for low-income families have proved expensive and cover more than 40% of Dutch families; it also required more than 600 extra staff in the national tax department to check incomes each month and to calculate the value of the vouchers (Okma *et al.*, 2011). The Irish Government's model of competing insurance funds will necessitate a sophisticated risk-equalisation mechanism at the heart of the new system. This will be a major and costly challenge, as even the best risk-equalisation system is not perfect (Brandt, 2008).

Single-payer health care insurance pays for all services through a 'single' insurance pool, typically run by the State. It can be financed from a pool to which many parties – employees, employers, and the State – have contributed. The term 'single-payer' thus only describes the funding mechanism – referring to health care financed by a single public body from a single fund. Although the fund holder is usually the State, some forms of single-payer systems use a mixed public-private system. In a single-payer system, all hospitals, doctors, and other health care providers would bill one entity for their services. This alone reduces administrative waste greatly.

It has been argued that market-based efficiencies are achievable with a single-payer system, which is transparent and accountable (Hsiao *et al.*, 2011). Recently, Professor Hsiao of Harvard School of Public Health has undertaken a major study for the State of Vermont to assist it in the transition to UHI. The Vermont experience shows an 8% saving of total health spending by moving to a single-payer system (through administrative simplification and consolidation) and another 5% by reducing fraud and abuse. It is estimated that it will reduce costs by 12% to 14% over time. The Vermont study found:

> ... that the system capable of producing the greatest potential savings and achieving universal coverage was a single-payer system – one

insurance fund that covers everyone with a standard package, paying uniform rates to all providers through a single payment mechanism and claims-processing system (Hsiao, 2011).

It recommended that the single-payer be a public-private partnership with an independent board with representation from both the major health care payers (employers, the State, and workers) and the major beneficiaries and recipients of payment (providers and consumers). The board would negotiate updates to the benefit package and payment rates. It also proposed contracting out claims administration through a competitive bid to create incentives to develop more efficient systems. The system proposed in the Vermont study reduces the rate of cost increases over time by insulating major decisions about health care spending from politics, as well as by paying providers through capitation rather than fees for services. It reduces the rate of cost increases also by promoting delivery system integration and reducing the practice of defensive medicine by implementing a no-fault medical malpractice system. All told, it estimated that Vermont could save 25% in health care expenditures over 10 years.

Examples of single-payer insurance systems include Australia's Medicare, Canada's Medicare and Taiwan's National Health Insurance. Taiwan is arguably the most successful example of the introduction of universal health care. Taiwan introduced UHI in 1995 for its 23 million people, providing a very comprehensive benefit package. In 2007, these broad benefits were available at a total national expenditure from all sources of 6.13% of GDP (Okma and Crivelli, 2009). The planning task force for Taiwanese National Health Insurance, relying on the experience of other industrialised countries and the expertise of consultants, recommended a single-payer health system, primarily for reasons of efficiency (Chiang, 1997). A single-payer system, with global budgets used to purchase care from private providers, was identified as the best way to control health care costs. More centralised systems:

> … have been more successful in realising the goal of cost containment because of uniform administration and the imposition of countrywide fees and tariffs (Okma and Crivelli, 2009: 206).

Single-payer systems may contract for health care services from private organisations (as is the case in Canada) or may own and employ health care resources and personnel (as is the case in the UK). The single-payer method is advocated by the AHS (2010).

Equity and Fairness

Multiple pools can make it difficult also to attain equal access to services. Ensuring an entire population has access to similar benefits generally requires the rich and poor to pay into, and be covered from, the same pool. Financial risk protection is enhanced also when people with different incomes and health risks pay into, and draw from, the same pool. It is possible to achieve equity and financial protection using multiple insurers competing for consumers if there is sufficient public funding and participation is compulsory: however, for such structures to work, it is necessary to ensure pooling across pools, effectively creating a virtual single pool through risk-equalisation, whereby funds are transferred from insurers that cover low-risk people to those that cover higher-risk people. This approach is administratively demanding, requiring an ability to monitor risks and to collect and transfer funds across pools. Competing insurance groups with a public option, the VHI, is the approach recommended within the *Programme for Government* (Fine Gael/Labour, 2011).

The choice of revenue collection mechanisms determines the degree to which insurance systems are financed regressively or progressively and, in turn, will impact on equity and fairness (Hussey and Anderson, 2003). Regressive financing is a system by which the poor contribute a greater proportion of their income than do the rich. Flat taxes represent the same proportion of income for all individuals regardless of income level. Upper limits on the amount that can be paid in flat tax systems can make them regressive. Premiums and out-of-pocket payments are the most regressive financing options, since each individual pays the same amount, regardless of income. This will represent a greater proportion of income for the poor than for the affluent. Progressive financing arrangements, such as income taxes, are those where the proportion of income contributed rises with income level, so that the affluent contribute a greater proportion of their income than do the poor by paying higher income tax rates. Through progressive financing arrangements, insurance systems can provide greater subsidisation of the costs of health care for low-income individuals.

Single-payer systems typically accomplish this through progressive taxation. Multi-payer systems are more likely to be financed more regressively through mechanisms such as a payroll tax, as in a social insurance system after the German model, or through premiums, as in the market-oriented system in the US. In Japan, interpool transfers are made to the insurance pool containing the elderly population. Each insurance pool contributes an equal amount per beneficiary to the elderly insurance pool; in addition, the central and local governments contribute 30% of the revenues of the elderly insurance pool (Ikegami, 1996).

Single-payer systems, therefore, usually have an advantage over multi-payer systems in the efficiency of collecting revenues, overall cost control, and the capacity to subsidise health care for low-income individuals, and thus stand a better chance of being more equitable and fair. Multi-payer systems may be better able to collect revenues in countries with a weak taxation system, and can limit the amount of government control over revenue collection.

Transparency

Transparency within a health care system can be thought of in terms of people's understanding of the benefits to which they are entitled and their obligations under the benefits package (and the understanding of health workers as well), along with the extent to which these benefits and obligations are realised in practice; and transparency in the health financing agencies (for example, reporting requirements, audits, and so on). In Switzerland, for example, it is the citizens who directly purchase health insurance, not the government or employers, and therefore control of purchase and transparency of costs are known to each individual citizen (Herzlinger and Parsa-Parsi, 2004).

Important challenges remain with regards to transparency in the transition to UHI, such as: patient information on price and quality should be continuously updated and made available; quality of health care has to be made visible and measurable; and transparent and uniform pricing systems are needed for the mandatory purchase of insurance. There is a need within Ireland for an extensive public campaign setting out costs, benefits and potential pitfalls during further implementation of UHI.

Effectiveness

Incentives to provide efficient, equitable and quality services are essential, whether service providers are publicly- or privately-owned (WHO, 2010). Preventive and promotion interventions can be cost-effective and can reduce the need for subsequent treatment. Effective governance is the key to improving efficiency and equity. The pace of reform should be monitored to establish whether there are subsequent improvements in the population's health. While it can be argued that not enough time has passed to determine whether the policy changes have made an impact of the population's health, we can still assess whether the concept of monitoring effectiveness was mentioned within either model. The *Programme for Government* established the Special Delivery Unit to assist in reducing waiting lists and to introduce a major upgrade in IT capabilities (Fine Gael/Labour, 2011).

Within the AHS policy paper (2010), a *carte vitale* system, similar to that in France, is proposed. The *carte vitale* contains a patient's entire medical record, is the size of a credit card and is used by every French citizen. This use of information technology creates major financial savings by reducing paper-based administrative overheads. It is a key part of a strategy to keep administrative costs low, while providing better and easier access to timely care for each patient. The AHS proposed that such a card be developed and used in Ireland. Other countries, such as Taiwan and Germany, also make use of a digital record for every citizen. If such a system was introduced, it would allow easy tracing of patients as they move through the system. This will become especially important within the Government's proposal of 'money following the patient'.

Social Solidarity

Social solidarity in health care involves social and political acceptance that all citizens should receive equal care and treatment on the basis of their health care needs rather than financial means. However, these values are by no means shared by all societies, giving rise to a broad array of national concepts of solidarity in the area of health care.

As described above, single-payer health insurance systems, as advocated by the AHS, tend to be financed more progressively than multi-payer systems. Sharing the burden of health care financing in this way may increase the solidarity between richer and poorer segments of the population. Single-payer systems are more likely to create a sense of national solidarity through national redistribution of resources and to foster citizens' trust in the ability of the government to protect their welfare. This solidarity could contribute to building 'social capital', such as trust in others and civic participation.

However, in some cases, multiple insurance pools might improve the political support of the government. For example, better-off individuals who feel that they are contributing more than their fair share towards insuring the health risks of others may oppose the health insurance system. Allowing them to opt out of a single-payer insurance system may provide greater social solidarity in a normative sense, by securing the political support of high-income earners for the public insurance system. Multi-payer insurers also could create a sense of solidarity among smaller groups of society – for example, middle class professionals – at the possible expense of national solidarity.

CAPACITY AND IMPLEMENTATION CHALLENGES

The Evolving Context of Recession

Ireland has experienced one of the worst recessions in Western Europe. After the boom of the 'Celtic Tiger' years, the economy contracted very sharply from 2008 to 2010 and was barely able to register positive economic growth positive growth in 2011 (Duffy *et al.*, 2012). More worryingly, the debt to GDP ratio is now well over 100% and unemployment has increased sharply to 14% and is only being mitigated by outward migration (Barrett *et al.*, 2011).

The consequent cutbacks in public health funding have been quite stark, with over €1 billion being taken from health in 2010 and a further €750 million in 2011, with the prospect of further cuts of around €450 million before 2015 (Department of Finance, 2011). There also will be transitional costs to any new system and competition for scarce funding from other several sectors, as well as debt servicing obligations. Typically, UHI systems tend to be more expensive than taxation-based systems, perhaps being less able to ration. Resources are going to be very scarce.

Still, perhaps surprisingly, the current recession is not all bad news for the Irish government in its bid to reform the health system. The crisis is driving down the cost base of the Irish health system. Salaries for public health staff have fallen by between 5% and 15%. In addition, specialists on contracts also have had their unit costs cut. Such efficiencies make UHI more affordable. Further, the recession has highlighted the need for change among stakeholders and reduced the amount of opposition to change. A recent stakeholder analysis has shown that virtually all stakeholders believe that the system should shift towards universal cover (O'Riordan and Thomas, 2011). All this may confirm the view that recessions make for good windows of opportunity for reform.

Additional Services

Typically, UHI systems provide more services than taxation-based systems (Normand and Thomas, 2009). However, switching financing systems does not guarantee an adequate supply of services and, by itself, will not alleviate capacity constraints in provision. As noted, in Ireland these largely relate to overcrowding problems with acute care and insufficient human resources in specialist positions. Therefore, UHI reform must be complemented by better management of acute facilities and redirection of care towards lower levels (Thomas *et al.*, 2006). While this will alleviate some of the significant overcrowding in hospitals, it is dependent also on an expansion' of GP and primary care. The government's push to build more primary health care facilities has fallen way short of targets and the need for additional GPs is immediate if Government is to ensure appropriate free access to care at the point of contact (Thomas *et al.*, 2006). A mixture of encouraging later retirement, substitutions of nurses and pharmacists for GPs, additional GP training places and greater use of temporary migrants will have to be exploited fully if GP numbers are to match those required by universal access to primary care (Teljeur *et al.*, 2010). Failure to resolve such issues will mean that access to services may be equalised but poor expectations will be thwarted and citizens' trust in government damaged.

The issue of what will be covered within the 'common basket' of services is still to be decided. The AHS advocates that prescribed medicines should be included, as well as access to GP care and acute hospital care and treatment. Within the *Programme for Government*, it states that the guaranteed UHI package relating to universal hospital care will be determined by the Minister for Health, but that it will not cover prescribed medicines in primary care (Fine Gael/Labour, 2011).

A key question for any country considering UHI is which benefits should be universally covered and which should be covered only for those who are willing and able to pay a supplement. The breadth of the services that will be covered within the common basket will have an effect on staff and services. Different countries have included different services within their common basket (Schreyögg *et al.*, 2005). For example, the SHI benefits package within Germany covers preventive services; inpatient and outpatient hospital care; physician services; mental health care; dental care; prescription drugs; medical aids; rehabilitation; sick leave compensation; and long-term care (Busse *et al.*, 2005). The French health insurance system – a mix of explicit and implicit regulations – offers wide-ranging reimbursement in the fields of preventive, curative, rehabilitative, and palliative care (Bellanger *et al.*, 2005). Alongside the issue of what will be in the common basket of services within this country is to consider whether we have the capacity to deliver on the basic tenets of UHI.

Architecture, Relationships and Legislation

Transitioning to UHI will require new and adapted institutions (in purchasing, regulation and provision) and new ways of relating (through contracting and information flows). Government will have a primary role in designing this UHI architecture, monitoring, defining a benefit package and legislating. In brief, UHI would entail a system of contracting service providers. To move to such a system design would mean that several funding institutions would purchase services from providers, whether public or private, according to set specifications. Providers will need to have the ability to manage their own deployment and use of resources. For many State hospitals, this would mean more autonomy in decision-making, which would require a shift in current public sector culture and legislation. Furthermore, the management of each hospital would have to be strengthened to negotiate and manage contracts from funding agencies for provision of services. The budgeting process for hospitals would have to change also to reflect the contracting approach and, in all likelihood, all funding to providers then would be based on case mix. Hence, additional skills and information systems will be needed in the system and a different configuration of relationships between institutions. In particular, UHI will place new demands on management and information and will require new legislation. Within the *Programme for Government*, there is reference to the legislation that will be required to introduce UHI (Fine Gael/Labour, 2011). The legislative basis for UHI will be established by a *Universal Health Insurance Act* by 2016. Likewise, the proposed universal primary care will be established under a *Universal Primary Care Act*.

Changing the composition of health payments and benefits for different segments of the population will create both support and opposition. Vested interest groups are liable to oppose reform. Such opposition can derail reforms as has been seen in other countries, such as the USA and Sweden (Thomas and Gilson, 2004). Nevertheless, the political landscape in Ireland has changed significantly since the progressive health reforms in the 1940s and 1950s were defeated by the Catholic church and the consultants (Wren, 2003; Barrington, 1987). Further, the managed competition solution actually may bring on board many private sector interests that would otherwise oppose a more 'socialised medicine' option. In addition, and as noted earlier, the recession may limit the expectations of stakeholders and help to subdue opposition.

CONCLUSION

There is no universal solution to the design of health insurance systems. Countries vary greatly in their priorities, populations, development, systems of government, and other factors. This variety has provided countries considering reforms with a number of experiences to consider.

Single-payer and multi-payer systems each have advantages, which may meet countries' priorities for their health insurance system. Single-payer systems usually are financed more progressively, and rely on existing taxation systems. Effectively, they distribute risks throughout one large risk pool, and offer governments a high degree of control over the total expenditure on health. Multi-payer systems sacrifice this control for a greater ability to meet the diverse preferences of beneficiaries. However, this diversity tends to result in the segmentation of risk groups unless adequate safeguards against adverse selection are used.

While less of an outright block to reform, failure to resolve design issues may delay implementation, cause problems for system performance and, ultimately, impair financial sustainability. Irrespective of the source of financing for the health system selected, equitable prepayment and pooling at population level, and the avoidance, at the point of delivery, of direct payments that result in financial catastrophe and impoverishment, are basic principles for achieving universal health coverage.

Reform is not a one-shot effort: it is a journey, but each step on the 'road map' should take us closer to the goal. These various experiences illustrate some of the approaches that countries have used to surmount the problems in design of a health insurance system. No country has the single answer for how to design an effective health insurance system. The plethora of experiences, however, provides countries such as Ireland that are considering reform with many lessons to consider.

REFERENCES

Adelaide Hospital Society (AHS) (2010). *Universal Health Insurance: The Way Forward for Irish Health Care*, available http://www.adelaide.ie/publications.php.

Barrett, A., Kearney, I., Conefrey, T. and O'Sullivan, C. (2011). *Quarterly Economic Commentary, Winter 2010*, Dublin: Economic and Social Research Institute.

Barnighausen, T. and Sauerborn, R. (2002). 'One Hundred and Eighteen Years of the German Health Insurance System: Are There Any Lessons for Middle- and Low-income Countries?', *Social Science and Medicine*, 54: 1559-87.

Barrington, R. (1987). *Healthcare, Medicine and Politics*, Dublin: Institute of Public Administration.

Bellanger, M.M., Cherilova, V. and Paris, V. (2005). 'The "Health Benefit Basket" in France', *The European Journal of Health Economics*, 6(Suppl 1): 24-29, doi:10.1007/s10198-005-0315-0.

Bentes, M., Dias, C., Sakellarides, C. and Bankauskaite, V. (2004). *Health Care Systems in Transitions: Portugal*, Brussels: European Observatory on Health Systems and Policies.

Brandt, N. (2008). *Moving Toward More Sustainable Healthcare Financing in Germany,* OECD Economics Department Working Papers, No.612, Paris: OECD Publishing.

Busse, R., Stargardt, T. and Schreyögg, J. (2005). 'Determining the "Health Benefit Basket" of the Statutory Health Insurance Scheme in Germany', *The European Journal of Health Economics,* 6(Suppl 1): 30-36, doi:10.1007/s10198-005-0316-z.

Chiang, T. (1997). 'Taiwan's 1995 Health Care Reform', *Health Policy,* 39(3): 225-239, doi:10.1016/S0168-8510(96)00877-9.

Department of Finance (2011). *The National Recovery Plan 2011-2014,* Dublin: Stationery Office.

Duffy, D., Durkan, J. and O'Sullivan, C. (2012). *Quarterly Economic Commentary, Winter 2011/Spring 2012,* Dublin: Economic and Social Research Institute.

Enthoven, A.C. and van de Ven, W. (2007). 'Going Dutch: Managed-Competition Health Insurance in The Netherlands', *New England Journal of Medicine,* 357(24): 2421-2423.

Fine Gael/Labour (2011). *Towards Recovery, Programme for a National Government 2011-2016,* retrieved from http://www.labour.ie/policy/listing/129943050328508293.html.

Garrett, L., Chowdhury, A.M.R. and Pablos-Méndez, A. (2009). 'All for Universal Health Coverage', *Lancet,* 374(9697): 1294-1299, doi:10.1016/S0140-6736(09)61503-8.

Herzlinger, R.E. and Parsa-Parsi, R. (2004). 'Consumer-driven Health Care: Lessons from Switzerland', *Journal of the American Medical Association,* 292(10): 1213-1220, doi:10.1001/jama.292.10.1213.

Hsiao, W.C. (2011). 'State-based Single-payer Health Care: A Solution for the United States?', *The New England Journal of Medicine,* 364(13): 1188-1190, doi:10.1056/NEJMp1100972.

Hsiao, W.C., Knight, A.G., Kappel, S. and Done, N. (2011). 'What Other States Can Learn from Vermont's Bold Experiment: Embracing a Single-payer Health Care Financing System', *Health Affairs (Project Hope),* 30(7): 1232-1241, doi:10.1377/hlthaff.2011.0515.

Hussey, P. and Anderson, G. (2003). 'A Comparison of Single- and Multi-payer Health Insurance Systems and Options for Reform', *Health Policy,* 66(3): 215-228, doi:10.1016/S0168-8510(03)00050-2.

Ikegami, N. (1996). 'Overview: Health Care in Japan', in Ikegami, N. and Campbell, J.C. (eds.), *Containing Health Care Costs in Japan,* Ann Arbor, MI: University of Michigan Press.

Leu, E., Rutten, F., Brouwer, W., Matter, P. and Rütschi, C. (2009). *The Swiss and Dutch Health Insurance Systems: Universal Coverage and Regulated Competitive Insurance Markets,* New York: Commonwealth Fund.

McPake, B. and Normand, C. (2008). *Health Economics: An International Perspective,* 2nd edition, London: Routledge.

Murray, T.H. (2010). 'American Values and Health Care Reform', *New England Journal of Medicine,* 362(4): 285-287, doi:10.1056/NEJMp0911116.

Normand, C. and Busse, R. (2002). 'Social Health Insurance Financing', in Mossialos, E. (ed.), *Funding Healthcare: Options for Europe,* London: Open University Press.

Normand, C. and Thomas, S. (2009). 'Health Care Financing and the Health System', in Carrin, G., Buse, K., Heggenhougen, K. and Quah, S.R. (eds.), *Health Systems Policy, Financing and Organization*, Oxford: Elsevier.

Okma, K. and Crivelli, L. (2009). *Six Countries, Six Reform Models: The Health Care Reform Experience of Israel, The Netherlands, New Zealand, Singapore, Switzerland and Taiwan - Health Care Reforms 'Under the Radar Screen'*, Singapore: World Scientific Publishing.

Okma, K. and Crivelli, L. (2010). *Six Countries, Six Reform Models: The Health Care Reform Experience of Israel, The Netherlands, New Zealand, Singapore, Switzerland and Taiwan*, Singapore: World Scientific Publishers.

Okma, K.G.H., Marmor, T.R. and Oberlander, J. (2011). 'Managed Competition for Medicare? Sobering Lessons from The Netherlands', *New England Journal of Medicine*, 365(4): 287-289, doi:10.1056/NEJMp1106090.

Orentlicher, D. (2009). 'Health Care Reform: Beyond Ideology', *Journal of the American Medical Association*, 301(17): 1816-1818, doi:10.1001/jama.2009.613.

O'Riordan, M. and Thomas, S. (2011). *Support for Policy Development of SHI in Ireland: A Review of Stakeholder Views and Values*, Dublin/Galway: Trinity College Dublin and NUI Galway.

Ruane, F. (2010). *Report of the Expert Group on Resource Allocation and Financing in the Health Sector*, Dublin: Department of Health and Children, retrieved from http://www.esri.ie/publications/search_for_a_publication/search_results/view/index.xml?id=3123.

Ryan, P., Thomas, S. and Normand, C. (2009). *Translating Dutch: Challenges and Opportunities in Reforming Health Financing in Ireland*, Irish Journal of Medical Science.

Schreyögg, J., Stargardt, T., Velasco-Garrido, M. and Busse, R. (2005). 'Defining the "Health Benefit Basket" in Nine European Countries', *European Journal of Health Economics*, 6(Suppl 1): 2-10, doi:10.1007/s10198-005-0312-3.

Teljeur, C., Thomas, S., O'Kelly, F.D. and O'Dowd, T. (2010). 'General Practitioner Workforce Planning: Assessment of Four Policy Directions', *BMC Health Services Research*, 10(148).

Thomas, S. and Burke, S. (2012). 'Coping with Austerity in the Irish Health System', *Eurohealth*, 18(1), 7-9.

Thomas, S. and Gilson, L. (2004). 'Actor Management in the Development of Health Financing Reform: Health Insurance in South Africa, 1994-1999', *Health Policy and Planning*, 19(5): 279-291.

Thomas, S., Normand, C. and Smith, S. (2006). *Social Health Insurance: Options for Ireland*, Dublin: Centre for Health Policy and Management, Trinity College Dublin.

van de Ven, W.P., Beck, K., Buchner, F., Chernichovsky, D., Gardiol, L., Holly, A., Lamers, L.M., Schokkaert, E., Shmueli, A., Spycher, S., Van de Voorde, C., van Vliet, R.C., Wasem, J. and Zmora, I. (2007). 'Risk Adjustment and Risk Selection on the Sickness Fund Insurance Market in Five European Countries', *Health Policy*, 83(3): 162-79.

Wagstaff, A. and Moreno-Serra, R. (2009). 'Europe and Central Asia's Great Post-Communist Social Health Insurance Experiment: Aggregate Impacts on Health Sector Outcomes', *Journal of Health Economics*, 28(2): 322-340.

Waters, H. (2008). 'Health Insurance Coverage in Central and Eastern Europe: Trends and Challenges', *Health Affairs*, 27(2).

World Health Assembly (WHA) (2011). *Sustainable Health Financing Structures and Universal Coverage: 64th World Health Assembly Agenda Item 13.4*, retrieved from http://www.sciencedirect.com/science?_ob=RedirectURLand_method=exter nObjLinkand_locator=urland_issn=01406736and_origin=articleand_zone=art _pageand_plusSign=%2Band_targetURL=http%253A%252F%252Fapps.who.i nt%252Fgb%252Febwha%252Fpdf_files%252FWHA64%252FA64_R9-en.pdf.

World Health Organization (WHO) (2010). *The World Health Report - Health Systems Financing: The Path to Universal Coverage*, Geneva, WHO, available http://www.who.int/whr/2010/en/index.html, accessed 18.06.2012.

Wren, M.-A. (2003). *Unhealthy State: Anatomy of a Sick Society*, Dublin: New Island.

Yamey, G. (2010). 'Obama's Giant Step towards Universal Health Insurance', *British Medical Journal (Clinical Research ed.)*, 340: c1674.

Yip, W.C.-M., Hsiao, W.C., Chen, W., Hu, S., Ma, J. and Maynard, A. (2012). 'Early Appraisal of China's Huge and Complex Health Care Reforms', *The Lancet*, 379(9818): 833-842, doi:10.1016/S0140-6736(11)61880-1.

5: INTEGRATED CARE: PATHFINDINGS FROM SWEDEN

Bengt Ahgren and Runo Axelsson

BACKGROUND

There are many similarities between the health systems of Ireland and Sweden, which means that Swedish experiences may be relevant in an Irish context. Both Ireland and Sweden have a 'Beveridge' type of health system, based on general taxation and universal access to health services. Moreover, in both countries, there has been an increasing differentiation of roles and responsibilities within the health system, which has generated a corresponding need for integration of health services (Kodner and Spreeuwenberg, 2002). Thus, integration has become a more and more important task for the health authorities.

By the end of the past millennium, however, the Swedish health authorities were increasingly drawing on external inspiration in their efforts to improve the performance of the system. Inspired by success stories from the private sector (Deming, 1986), the focus of organisational development shifted from a division of functions to an integration of multi-functional activities (Andreasson *et al.*, 1995). This new focus generated two main approaches for the integration of health care: improvement of intra-organisational processes and design of interorganisational structures (Ahgren, 2007). Before describing this development in more detail, it is necessary to provide a short background.

During the 1960s, there was an ambition in Sweden to create an integrated system of health care at regional level. Responsibility for primary health care and psychiatric care was decentralised from the national government to the county councils, which already were responsible for general hospitals. By 1967, the county councils were responsible for all the different branches of health care. They also were quite independent of the national government, since most of their activities were financed through county taxes. Thus, since the 1960s, the political as well as the financial power in the Swedish health system has rested at a regional level (Axelsson, 2000).

In the early 1990s, this decentralised health system was further decentralised when responsibility for the care of the elderly was transferred from the county councils to the municipalities. This was a national reform in order to improve the integration between the health services of the county councils and the social services of the municipalities, and also to improve the collaboration between health professionals and social workers (Adamiak and Karlberg, 2003). For the same reasons, there was another national reform a few years later, where responsibility for the care of the functionally-disabled and long-term psychiatric care was transferred also from the county councils to the municipalities (Danermark and Kullberg, 1999).[3]

After these reforms in the 1990s, the county councils are responsible for all health care except care delivered in nursing homes and other forms of housing for older people with somatic and psychiatric long-term diseases, and for mentally-retarded patients. These are the responsibility of the municipalities.

There are currently 21 county councils and 290 municipalities in Sweden. The role of central government is to establish principles and guidelines for care and to set the political agenda for health care. This is achieved by means of laws and ordinances. The National Board of Health and Welfare has an important role as the central government's expert and supervisory authority.

Although health care in Sweden is financed mainly from public sources, there has been a growing private sector involvement in the health system from the beginning of the 1990s. There have been an increasing number of private providers, mainly in primary health care and care of the elderly, which have been contracted through competitive procurement and financed by the county councils and the municipalities. This is similar to the financing of voluntary hospitals and the contract agreements with self-employed general practitioners in Ireland (McDaid *et al.*, 2009). In Sweden, the process of privatisation has increased the differentiation of the health system and today private providers account for almost 10% of the total health care expenditures (Baroni and Axelsson, 2011).

The increasing differentiation, reinforced by the increasing number of private providers, has run contrary to the integration of health and social

---

[3]   In order to avoid the conceptual confusion in the literature of integrated care, the term 'integration' will be used in this chapter mainly in interorganisational contexts, while 'collaboration' will be used in professional contexts. For a discussion of this terminology, see Axelsson and Bihari Axelsson (2006).

services in the county councils and municipalities. So also have the market-oriented models with purchaser-provider split that were introduced in about half of the county councils in the beginning of the 1990s. Both of these developments were inspired by the ideas of New Public Management, which meant an application of management principles from the private sector in the public sector (Hood, 1991; Pollitt, 1990). There were political as well as economic considerations behind these ideas, and they were promoting competition rather than collaboration in health care (Hallin and Siverbo, 2003).

By the end of the 1990s and the beginning of the 2000s, most county councils had abandoned their market-oriented models, since they were not delivering the efficiency that had been expected. One reason for this was the high transaction costs connected with these models (Siverbo, 2004). Partly as a reaction to the 'economism' of the market models, many county councils instead introduced different models of quality improvement and quality management in health care. Since most of these models are process-orientated, they also brought a renewed interest in integration and collaboration (Axelsson, 2000).

This chapter will explore further the recent history of integrated health care in Sweden. Tracing its origins back to the 1990s, the focus will be on the development of integration and collaboration in the Swedish health system during the first decade of the 2000s. In addition to the historical account, there will be some analytical reflections in connection with the different stages of the development. There also will be an analysis of the successes and setbacks with the wisdom of hindsight. Finally, some of the challenges of integrated health care for the present decade will be discussed and also partly reflected on in comparison with the Irish development.

THE BEGINNINGS IN THE 1990s

The first efforts to integrate health care in Sweden were inspired by the so-called 'producer model' from manufacturing industry (Anthony *et al.*, 1989). According to this model, the core processes within an organisation must be integrated in order to create predetermined outcomes in a cost-effective way. Furthermore, such processes should be repetitive, consist of sequential activities, and have a distinct start and end.

Many well-known methods of process development have been derived from the producer model – for instance, 'business process re-engineering' (Hammer and Champy, 1994) and 'business process improvement' (Harrington, 1991). The successful use of these methods in the private sector inspired health care organisations in Sweden to integrate their processes in the same way. In the beginning of the 1990s, methods of process development were used in settings similar to manufacturing – that is, when health care activities were repetitive, sequential and had predetermined outcomes. Elective surgery was one of the areas where Swedish health care was successful in developing integrated intra-organisational processes (Ahgren, 2007).

By the end of the 1990s, when more and more county councils had abandoned their market-oriented models, there was an increasing interest in the quality of health care. Different models of quality improvement were introduced – for example, the Swedish model called QUL, an acronym for quality, development and management (Swedish Federation of County Councils, 2000). These models were derived from the producer model. At the same time, however, there was a growing awareness that all health care did not have conditions equal to manufacturing industry. Instead, it was pointed out that health care provision is based on a complex mixture of patient needs, which require contributions from many different departments and organisations. This means an interorganisational rather than intra-organisational context.

These considerations were important also for the development of 'chains of care' (Ahgren, 2003). This is a Swedish concept of integration and collaboration in health care, which includes all the services provided for a specific group of patients within a defined geographical area. Chains of care are interorganisational networks based on clinical guidelines – that is, agreements on the content and distribution of the clinical work between different health care providers and professionals. Most chains of care can be described as co-ordinated networks, where the financial and clinical responsibilities of the parties involved remain separated. Furthermore, binding contracts, regulating the activities performed, usually are not in place (Ahgren, 2007).

The main objective of the chains of care was to bring together health services operating at different, or the same, hierarchical levels. In this sense, chains of care seem to be similar to 'managed clinical networks' in Scotland, Wales and Northern Ireland, which predominantly aim to bridge organisational and professional barriers, and thereby achieve cohesive health care provision for specific patient groups. Despite the possible literal association with 'integrated clinical pathways', chains of care have not so much in common with this kind of protocol-based care (Ahgren, 2003).

The chain of care concept has a clear patient focus, sometimes also expressed as a 'customer orientation' (Lindberg and Trägårdh, 2001).

Because of this orientation, the concept was considered to be part of the New Public Management in the 1990s. Within the framework of the purchaser-provider split, there were also some experiments of commissioning a whole chain of care. The aim was to create incentives for providers to develop cost-effective care through the whole chain. In spite of these experiments, however, chains of care have remained a concept for improving the quality rather than the cost-effectiveness of health care (Ahgren, 2010a).

ON THE PATH TO THE NEW MILLENNIUM

The development of integrated health care in Sweden has continued in the new millennium. In the beginning of the 2000s, chains of care were well-established in many county councils. Some of them had quite an impressive record, with 25 or more chains of care, most of them focusing on chronic diseases (Ahgren, 2003). At the same time, however, a majority of county councils were dissatisfied with their development of integrated health care, because of difficulties in implementing sustainable solutions in a predominantly non-integrative context (Ahgren, 2010a) and negative reactions from health care professionals to top-down development approaches (Ahgren and Axelsson, 2007).

The development of integrated health care has not been limited to chains of care. During the 2000s, many Swedish county councils also restructured their health services and introduced a system of 'local health care', which can be described as an upgraded family- and community-oriented primary health care within a defined local area, supported by flexible hospital services. The ambition has been to create an integrated provision of health care that matches the needs of a local population. In practice, this means an orientation towards common diseases and needs of major population groups – for example, the elderly and patients with chronic diseases. Thus, the content and organisation of local health care often differ from one area to another (Ahgren, 2010b). According to the National Board of Health and Welfare, two out of three county councils, including the largest ones, have implemented local health care, which means that 80% of the Swedish population is covered by this form of integrated care (National Board of Health and Welfare, 2003).

Because of different local needs and circumstances, there is no single model of local health care to be applied everywhere (Ahgren, 2010b). In most county councils, however, the introduction of local health care has not involved any large-scale organisational changes. Rather, it has been a question of combining existing organisations, resources and competences to secure adequate responses to the most frequent needs of the local population. This means quite a loose integration, which has been achieved mainly by chains of care (National Board of Health and Welfare, 2003). Thus, there seems to be a mutual relationship between local health care and chains of care. Local health care needs chains of care as integrating mechanisms and the chains of care are strengthened by the integrative context of local health care (Ahgren, 2010a).

The implementation of local health care has been important also for the integration of health and social services. This is the case particularly in the care of the elderly and long-term psychiatric care, which were also the targets of national reform in the 1990s. Local health care has facilitated collaboration between health professionals and social workers – for example, in 'dementia teams' (Haraldsson and Wånell, 2009), 'multidisciplinary home care teams', different forms of 'case management' and 'rehabilitation teams' (National Board of Health and Welfare, 2005; 2007a; 2008a).

These forms of collaboration have not been restricted to local health care. Health professionals have collaborated with social workers also in other contexts – for example, in teams for 'assertive community treatment' of mental illness (Malm, 2002), in centres for treatment and prevention of addiction and dependency, and in support of vulnerable children and young people (National Board of Health and Welfare, 2007b; 2008b). Another area of multiprofessional collaboration has been in health care for refugees (Lindencrona *et al.*, 2009). There also have been experiments with a common organisation for health and social service in one municipality (Ovretveit *et al.*, 2010) and a consortium for mental health and social care in another (Hansson *et al.*, 2010).

Furthermore, extensive experiments in interorganisational integration have been carried out in the field of vocational rehabilitation, where health professionals have collaborated with social workers and officials from the social insurance administration and the national employment service (Wihlman *et al.*, 2010). The positive outcomes of these experiments and projects have resulted in legislation that makes it possible for county councils and municipalities to form 'local associations' for financial co-ordination together with the local offices of the social insurance administration and the national employment service (SFS, 2003). Today there are 82 associations of this kind (Finsam, 2011).

Financial co-ordination means that resources from the different organisations are pooled into a common budget for the local association. This budget may be used for different rehabilitation projects, which are managed by the association. These projects usually are aimed at individuals with multiple problems that require collaboration between professionals from the different organisations involved (Bihari Axelsson and Axelsson, 2009).

WHERE HAS THE SWEDISH PATH TAKEN INTEGRATED CARE?

When responsibility for the care of the elderly and long-term psychiatric care was transferred from the county councils to the municipalities, there was an incentive to allocate patients to the most cost-effective care possible. As a result, the number of hospital beds in Sweden was reduced by 45%, during the 1990s, while Ireland had a reduction of 11% during the same period, which is equivalent to most other European countries (McKee, 2004). Thus, the integration of health and social services may have improved cost-effectiveness, but it also created new problems related to a lack of physicians in municipal nursing homes and parallel organisations for home health care in the county councils and the municipalities (Rom, 2006).

The integration of health and social services in the 1990s was problematic also for other reasons. There were many 'territorial' conflicts between the different organisations and professions involved (Axelsson and Bihari Axelsson, 2006). However, with the introduction of local health care, the provision of integrated care for the elderly and the mentally ill has been improved. Gaps between the different services can be bridged, and the quality of care and rehabilitation surely benefit from multiprofessional collaboration within the framework of local health care (Andersson and Karlberg, 2000).

Concerning the chains of care, a national survey has shown that seven out of 10 county councils in Sweden were disappointed with their development work (Ahgren, 2003). As mentioned before, it seems that the chains of care had been implemented mainly through a top-down approach, which was not appropriate in an environment dominated by strong professional groups. In such an environment, developments initiated from the top of the organisation often are resisted. If the development of chains of care had been initiated from below by dedicated professionals, it would probably have been more successful (Ahgren and Axelsson, 2007).

There also have been other reasons for resistance to the development of integrated health care. For instance, general practitioners have not supported the decentralisation of responsibility for the care of the elderly to the municipalities, since it has threatened their position as managers of nursing homes (Andersson and Karlberg, 2000). The implementation of local health care has aroused similar reactions among general practitioners, who have thought there is a risk that primary health care will disappear or become more anonymous (Anell, 2005).

In vocational rehabilitation, financial co-ordination between the different organisations involved has eliminated many obstacles to integration and collaboration. One of the main obstacles has been the fear of costs being transferred between the organisations involved (Hultberg *et al.*, 2007). Moreover, it seems that the local associations' use of financial co-ordination has improved the management and continuity of vocational rehabilitation (Andersson *et al.*, 2011). On the other hand, many of the rehabilitation activities of the local associations are temporary and regarded as projects, which means that they are separated from the different organisations involved. The integration is limited to these projects and is not really influencing ordinary work (Löfström, 2010).

According to organisation theory, the level of integration in health care should be related to the degree of differentiation of services. A high degree of differentiation requires a high degree of integration (Lawrence and Lorsch, 1967). Therefore, the degree of integration varies between different organisations and services, depending on their need for integration, and also depends on the possibility of attaining 'collaborative advantage' (Huxham, 1999). Organisational researchers have pointed out that it is important for stakeholders to discover and recognise the possible advantages of collaboration. Unless there is potential for such advantages, collaboration should be avoided (Huxham and Vangen, 2005).

The development of integration may be destructive when collaborative advantages are concealed or lacking, since professionals as well as managers tend to defend their territories when these are believed to be threatened (Bihari Axelsson and Axelsson, 2009). Such a shift of focus, from joint activities to protection of boundaries, may have very negative effects. In Sweden, there have been many examples, such as resource battles between health care providers (Trägårdh and Lindberg, 2004), threats against the position of the physicians (Anell, 2005), and unwillingness to collaborate in general (Adamiak and Karlberg, 2003).

Although there have been many setbacks in the development of integrated health care, it seems that more favourable conditions have emerged during the past decade. As described before, there is a 'mutualistic' relationship between chains of care and local health care (Ahgren, 2010a). Chains of care have become the building blocks of local health care, and they have benefited also from being embedded in such an integrative context. This context has been favourable also for other forms of integration and collaboration between health and social services. In addition, integration in vocational rehabilitation has been facilitated by new legislation encouraging county councils, municipalities and state agencies to collaborate and to create local associations of financial co-ordination (SFS, 2003: 1210).

BARRIERS TO BYPASS

Despite the fact that integrated health care has been high on the political agenda during the last two decades, counteracting policies have been, and still are, promoted. The increasing privatisation and the period of purchaser-provider split have been mentioned before. Both of these developments were based on political, as well as economic, considerations. Lately, a new system of free choice for patients in primary health care has been proposed by a parliamentary committee and is expected to be introduced in all the county councils (SOU, 2008). According to the proposal, the free patient choice will generate a capitation payment to the chosen primary health care centre. This system is based mainly on political convictions. Policy-makers believe that, as a result of competition between health centres, strong providers will survive while unprofitable ones will be eliminated (Ahgren, 2010b).

In order to implement the new system, different models of patient choice have been developed. In some county councils, the patients can choose among comprehensive local health care arrangements whereas, in other county councils, they register for a specific general practitioner (Anell, 2008). There is a great challenge for the health authorities to simultaneously manage both competition and collaboration, although it is easier when patients choose among networks of integrated health care and not among individual general practitioners. Models of the latter kind tend to fragment the provision of health care services, a problem that also has been addressed in the Irish *Primary Care Strategy* of 2001 (McDaid *et al.*, 2009).

Although interorganisational integration has been promoted, developed and implemented during the last two decades, intra-organisational integration still has a strong foothold in Swedish health care. In recent years, there have been a number of mergers of hospitals and creation of hospital groups under joint management. These mergers are aiming at large-scale production and motivated by economies of scale. They have been strongly endorsed also by policy-makers. In spite of bad experiences, related to the size and complexity of the new hospital organisations, the mergers are spreading to more and more county councils (Ahgren, 2008). As a result, the number of hospitals has been halved since the beginning of the 1990s. Today, there are only 53 general hospitals in Sweden and many of them are multi-sited hospital groups. This equals the number of hospitals providing acute care in Ireland (McDaid *et al.*, 2009). The restructuring of Swedish hospitals is proceeding in spite of the fact that the multi-sited hospitals have not been systematically evaluated, neither in Sweden nor internationally (Posnett, 1999).

Regardless of this lack of evidence, the hospital mergers have been followed by proposals about a merger of the Swedish county councils. A parliamentary committee has proposed that the present 21 Swedish county councils should be merged into six to eight more equally-sized regional councils (SOU, 2007). The committee apparently mistrusts the willingness and ability of the county councils to integrate their services and collaborate with each other. Confidence in mergers and large-scale solutions appears be widespread among policy-makers (Ahgren, 2008).

CONCLUSION

To conclude, it is clear that Swedish policy-makers have been supporting the development of integrated health care during the last decade but, at the same time, they also have been promoting contrary strategies, implying a fragmentation of health services and mistrust in collaborative advantages. Even if consistency is not necessarily a political virtue, the contradictory policies possibly could be linked to the lack of evidence about the benefits of integrated health care (Nies, 2004). In any case, more efforts should be placed on the evaluation of integrated health care, as well as on the other developments described, in order to replace political convictions with evidence on the benefits of different forms of health care provision.

REFERENCES

Adamiak, G. and Karlberg, I. (2003). 'The Situation in Sweden', in van Raak, A., Mur-Veeman, I., Hardy, B., Steenbergen, M. and Paulus, A. (eds.), *Integrated Care in Europe: Description and Comparison of Integrated Care in Six EU Countries* (pp.41-72), Maarssen: Elsevier Gezondheidszorg.

Ahgren, B. and Axelsson, R. (2007). 'Determinants of Integrated Health Care Development: Chains of Care in Sweden', *International Journal of Health Planning and Management*, 2: 145-157.

Ahgren, B. (2003). 'Chain of Care Development in Sweden: Results of a National Study, *International Journal of Integrated Care* [serial online], 3, 7 October.

Ahgren, B. (2007). *Creating Integrated Health Care*, NHV-report 2007:2, Göteborg: Nordic School of Public Health.

Ahgren, B. (2008). 'Is It Better To Be Big? The Reconfiguration of 21st Century Hospitals: Responses to a Hospital Merger in Sweden', *Health Policy*, 87: 92-99.

Ahgren, B. (2010a). 'Mutualism and Antagonism within Organisations of Integrated Health Care', *Journal of Health Organization and Management*, 24(2): 396-411.

Ahgren, B. (2010b). 'Competition and Integration in Swedish Health Care', *Health Policy*, 96(2): 91-97.

Andersson, G. and Karlberg, I. (2000). 'Integrated Care for the Elderly: The Background and Effects of the Reform of Swedish Care of the Elderly', *International Journal of Integrated Care* [serial online], 1, 1 November.

Andersson, J., Ahgren, B., Bihari Axelsson, S., Eriksson, A. and Axelsson, R. (2011). 'Organizational Approaches to Collaboration in Vocational Rehabilitation: An International Literature Review', *International Journal of Integrated Care* [serial on line], 11, 18 November.

Andreasson, S., Brommels, M. and Sarv, H. (1995). *Det måste finnas ett annat sätt* [There Must Be Another Way], Stockholm: Swedish Federation of County Councils [in Swedish].

Anell, A. (2005). *Primärvård i förändring* [Primary Health Care in Change], Lund: Studentlitteratur [in Swedish].

Anell, A. (2008). *Vårdval i primärvården – modeller och utvecklingsbehov* [Choice of Care in Primary Care – Models and Needs for Development], Lund: KEFU [in Swedish].

Anthony, R.N., Dearden, J. and Bedford, N.M. (1989). *Management Control Systems*, 6th edition, Homewood, IL: Irwin.

Axelsson, R. and Bihari Axelsson, S. (2006). 'Integration and Collaboration in Public Health: A Conceptual Framework', *International Journal of Health Planning and Management*, 21(1): 75-88.

Axelsson, R. (2000). 'The Organizational Pendulum: Healthcare Management in Sweden 1865-1998', *Scandinavian Journal of Public Health*, 28: 47-53.

Baroni, E. and Axelsson, R. (2011). *Pensions, Health and Long-term Care, ASISP Annual National Report 2011: Sweden*, Brussels: European Commission.

Bihari Axelsson, S. and Axelsson, R. (2009). 'From Territoriality to Altruism in Interprofessional Collaboration and Leadership', *Journal of Interprofessional Care*, 23(4): 320-330.

Danermark, B. and Kullberg, C. (1999). *Samverkan – Välfärdsstatens nya arbetsform* [Collaboration – The New Working Method of the Welfare State], Lund: Studentlitteratur [in Swedish].

Deming, W. (1986). *Out of the Crisis*, Cambridge, MA: MIT Center for Advanced Engineering Study.

Finsam (2011). *Översikt över samordningsförbunden* [Overview of the Associations for Financial Co-ordination] 2011, available http://www.susam.se/finsam/oversikt_forbund, accessed 15.12.2011.

Hallin, B. and Siverbo, S. (2003). *Styrning och organisering inom hälso- och sjukvården* [Management and Organisation in Health Care], Lund: Studentlitteratur [in Swedish].

Hammer, M. and Champy, J. (1994). *Reengineering the Corporation: A Manifesto for a Business Revolution*, London: Nicholas Brealey.

Hansson, J., Ovretveit, J., Askerstam, M., Gustafsson, C. and Brommels, M. (2010). 'Co-ordination in Networks for Improved Mental Health Service', *International Journal of Integrated Care* [serial online], 10, 25 August.

Haraldsson, U. and Wånell, S.E. (2009). *Demensteam: en nationell överblick* [Dementia Team: A National Overview], Stockholm: Stockholm Gerontology Research Centre [in Swedish].

Harrington, H.J. (1991). *Business Process Improvement: The Breakthrough Strategy for Total Quality, Productivity and Competitiveness*, Columbus, OH: McGraw-Hill.

Hood, C. (1991). 'A Public Management for All Seasons?', *Public Administration*, 69: 3-19.

Hultberg, E., Lönnroth, K. and Allebeck, P. (2007). 'Effects of a Co-financed Interdisciplinary Collaboration Model in Primary Health Care on Service Utilisation among Patients with Musculoskeletal Disorders', *Work*, 28(3): 239-247.

Huxham, C. and Vangen, S. (2005). *Managing to Collaborate: The Theory and Practice of Collaborative Advantage*, London: Routledge.

Huxham, C. (ed.) (1999). *Creating Collaborative Advantage*, London: Sage.

Kodner, D. and Spreeuwenberg, C. (2002). 'Integrated Care: Meaning, Logic, Applications and Implications: A Discussion Paper', *International Journal of Integrated Care* [serial online], 2, 14 November.

Lawrence, P.R. and Lorsch, J.W. (1967). *Organization and Environment: Managing Differentiation and Integration*, Cambridge, MA: Harvard University Press.

Lindberg, K. and Trägårdh, B. (2001). 'Idén om vårdkedja möter lokal praxis' ['The Chain of Care Concept Faces Local Practice'], *Kommunal ekonomi och politik*, 5(2): 51-68 [in Swedish].

Lindencrona, F., Ekblad, S. and Axelsson, R. (2009). 'Modes of Interaction and Performance of Human Service Networks', *Public Management Review*, 11(2): 191.

Löfström, M. (2010). 'Interorganizational Collaboration Projects in the Public Sector: A Balance between Integration and Demarcation', *International Journal of Health Planning and Management*, 25(2): 136-155.

Malm, U. (2002). *Case Management: Evidensbaserad Integrerad Psykiatri* [Case Management: Evidence-based Integrated Psychiatry], Lund: Studentlitteratur [in Swedish].

McDaid, D., Wiley, M., Maresso, A. and Mossialos, E. (2009). *Ireland: Health System Review*, Copenhagen: European Observatory on Health Systems and Policies.

McKee, M. (2004). *Reducing Hospital Beds: What Are the Lessons To Be Learned?* Vol.6, Copenhagen: European Observatory on Health Systems and Policies.

National Board of Health and Welfare (2003). *Kartläggning av närsjukvård* [Survey of Local Health Care], Stockholm: National Board of Health and Welfare [in Swedish].

National Board of Health and Welfare (2005). *Personligt ombud på klientens uppdrag – förhandlare och gränsöverskridare* [Personal Representative by Order of the Client – Negotiator and Exceeder of Limits], Stockholm: National Board of Health and Welfare [in Swedish].

National Board of Health and Welfare (2007a). *Rehabilitering för hemmaboende äldre personer* [Rehabilitation of Elderly Persons Living at Home], Stockholm: National Board of Health and Welfare [in Swedish].

National Board of Health and Welfare (2007b). *Strategi för samverkan – kring barn och unga som far illa eller riskerar att fara illa* [Strategy for Collaboration – About Children and Youngsters in Trouble or Who are Risking Getting into Trouble], Stockholm: National Board of Health and Welfare [in Swedish].

National Board of Health and Welfare (2008a). *Hemsjukvård i förändring* [Home Care in Change], Stockholm: Socialstyrelsen [in Swedish].

National Board of Health and Welfare (2008b). *Missbruks - och beroendevårdens öppenvård (ÖKART): en nationell kartläggning* [Outpatient Care of Addiction and Dependency: A National Survey], Stockholm: National Board of Health and Welfare [in Swedish].

Nies, H. (2004). *A European Research Agenda on Integrated Care for Older People*, Dublin: European Health Management Association.

Ovretveit, J., Hansson, J. and Brommels, M. (2010). 'An Integrated Health and Social Care Organisation in Sweden: Creation and Structure of a Unique Public Health and Social System', *Health Policy*, 97: 113-121.

Pollitt, C. (1990). *Managerialism and the Public Services: The Anglo-American Experience*, Oxford: Blackwell.

Posnett, J. (1999). 'The Hospital of the Future: Is Bigger Better? Concentration in Provision of Secondary Care', *British Medical Journal*, 319: 1063-1065.

Rom, M. (2006). *Närvård i Sverige 2005* [Local Health Care in Sweden 2005], Stockholm: Swedish Association of Local Authorities and Regions [in Swedish].

Siverbo, S. (2004). 'The Purchaser-Provider Split in Principle and Practice: Experiences from Sweden', *Financial Accountability and Management*, 20(4): 401-420.

Statens offentliga utredninger (SOU) (2007). *Hållbar samhällsorganisation med utvecklingskraft* [Sustainable Organisation of Society with Development Power, 2007:10], Stockholm: Ministry of Finance [in Swedish].

Statens offentliga utredninger (SOU) (2008). *Vårdval i Sverige* [Choice of Care in Sweden, 2008:37], Stockholm: Ministry of Health and Social Affairs [in Swedish].

Svensk författningssamling (SFS) (2003). *Lag om finansiell samordning av rehabiliteringsinsatser* [The Act on Financial Co-ordination of Rehabilitation Measures between the Social Insurance Office, the County Labour Boards, Municipalities and County Councils, 2003:1210], Stockholm: Svensk författningssamling [in Swedish].

Swedish Federation of County Councils (2000). *Kriterier och anvisningar för Qvalitet Utveckling Ledarskap 2000/2001 – ett instrument för verksamhetsutveckling* [Criteria and Instructions of Quality Development and Management 2000/2001 – A Tool for Activity Development], Stockholm: Landstingsförbundet [in Swedish].

Trägårdh, B. and Lindberg, K. (2004). 'Curing a Meagre Health Care System by Lean Methods – Translating Chains of Care in the Swedish Health Care Sector', *International Journal of Health Planning and Management*, 19: 383-398.

Wihlman, U., Stålsby Lundborg, C., Holmström, I. and Axelsson, R. (2010). Organising Vocational Rehabilitation through Interorganisational Integration: A Case Study in Sweden', *International Journal of Health Planning and Management*; published online: 10 October.

SECTION II: THE BIOMEDICAL AND SOCIAL INTERFACE OF INTEGRATED CARE: THEORY, POLICY AND SERVICE USERS' NEEDS

6: INTEGRATED DIABETES CARE: "IT MEANS DIFFERENT THINGS TO DIFFERENT PEOPLE"

Sheena McHugh and Ivan Perry

INTRODUCTION

This chapter examines the concept of integrated care for chronic diseases, using the case of diabetes management to explore what integrated care means, what it looks like and whether it is implemented. We begin with an overview of the problem to which integrated care is proposed as the solution: fragmented and unco-ordinated care for chronic illnesses. This is followed by a qualitative analysis of what constitutes integrated care in an effort to distinguish the concept from other models of care. The chapter will chart the evolution from shared and structured diabetes care initiatives in Ireland to the emergence of a national model of integrated care. The current level of integration between settings will be examined, as well as the physical and attitudinal barriers to implementing a national model. Finally, we will consider the tension between the planned model of integrated care, in which primary care is a cornerstone, and the capacity at present to manage routine diabetes management in primary care.

A SEA OF CHALLENGES – CO-ORDINATION, CONTINUITY AND CHRONIC ILLNESS CARE

Today, most health care reforms, both nationally and internationally, propose to re-organise the way health care is delivered. Poor organisation and a lack of co-ordination within the health system are cited as primary causes of the quality chasm surrounding health care delivery (Institute of Medicine, 2001). The cracks in the delivery of health care are particularly precarious for those with complex chronic conditions who require planned, structured, multidisciplinary care that is integrated across professions and settings, including social and health care (Wagner *et al.*,

1996; Bodenheimer *et al.*, 2002). The challenges to seamless co-ordinated chronic illness care in Ireland are well-documented, including an under-developed primary care infrastructure, poor communication between primary and secondary care settings and a lack of access to specialist and allied health professionals. In a recent survey of chronic disease management in Ireland, almost one-third of general practitioners (GPs) felt the health system needed to be rebuilt entirely to manage chronic disease appropriately (Darker *et al.*, 2012).

Diabetes "exemplifies the complex nature of chronic disease" (McKee and Nolte, 2009: 409) and epitomises one of the major challenges facing health systems: how to effectively and efficiently integrate care across multiple health care professionals, in several settings, with different funding and governance arrangements. This prevalent and costly chronic disease highlights the need for health systems to re-organise health care from acute reactionary services to structured planned management that meets the changing needs of patients. As a result, diabetes has become the condition of choice for modelling health care reform (Kahn and Anderson, 2009). A number of care arrangements for the management of diabetes have emerged that combine system-level, organisational, professional and patient-level strategies in an effort to deliver integrated diabetes care. We will now examine what this integrated care looks like.

WHAT CONSTITUTES INTEGRATED DIABETES CARE?

While there is consensus on the need to reform and improve the delivery of services for people with diabetes, what is not as obvious or consistent is how best to achieve this aim. Integrated care is one of a plethora of terms used to describe the way diabetes care is organised across and within settings. Other terms commonly used include transmural care, shared care, integrated care pathways, 'managed care', chronic disease management programmes, and 'structured care' (Vrijhoef *et al.*, 2001a; Gröne and Garcia-Barbero, 2001; Kodner and Spreeuwenberg, 2002). The individual terms are often ill-defined, the components implemented as part of these care arrangements are not uniform, and over time the terms have developed multiple meanings and connotations. One of the reasons for the lack of consistent opinion on how best to integrate care is the diversity across health systems in terms of infrastructure, organisational processes, providers and professional cultures (Saltman *et al.*, 2006). The variability, even within our own country, has led to the emergence of several subtly different models of care.

Untangling Models of Care

Shared care was one of the first examples of efforts to co-ordinate the delivery of diabetes care. The Netherlands has been a pioneer of the shared care approach, with health care providers working together in regional networks under the term 'transmural care' (Maier *et al.*, 2008; Branger *et al.*, 1999). When shared care was introduced as a pilot project in the Maastricht region, Type 2 diabetes care shifted from the outpatient clinic delivered by endocrinologists, to the general practice setting delivered by nurse specialists. The endocrinologist continued to review patients annually. The GP was ultimately responsible for patient care and took on a greater role, co-ordinating care with patients and other care providers. The nurse specialist had an interfacing role, co-ordinating care between the two settings, which had a positive impact on HbA1c levels and was as good as the traditional model on other clinical outcomes (Vrijhoef *et al.*, 2001b). The establishment of shared care led the way for a more formal disease management model in the region. This disease management model was proposed as an integration of shared and traditional care models that had been operating, in the hope of providing structured, integrated care for all patients (Eijkelberg *et al.*, 2001). Thus concepts of shared and structured care were combined in an effort to provide more comprehensive disease management. The merging of structured and shared care is reflected also in a recent systematic review of shared care interventions that included organisational and professional components such as "pre-specified clinical protocols, referral guidelines, continuing education of participating clinicians, specifically designed information systems and ongoing audit and evaluation of services delivered" (Smith *et al.*, 2007: 2).

The experience in The Netherlands suggests the concept of shared care was regarded as a precursor to fully-developed chronic disease management programmes (Vrijhoef *et al.*, 2001a), designed to deliver structured, pro-active, integrated care. In the US, there is a distinction among chronic disease management programmes between those based on primary care and integrated within the health system and commercial plans developed by companies to which employers and health care plans contract out disease management (Casalino, 2005). The latter format of disease management is a for-profit service marketed to customers as a cost containment strategy. The focus is often on patient education and self-management, employing e-health technology and tele-medicine without having to engage the physician in behaviour change or re-organisation (Geyman, 2007).

Chronic disease management programmes often are based on the Chronic Care Model (CCM) (Casalino, 2005). The CCM is a framework that outlines the components necessary for high quality chronic disease management (Bodenheimer *et al.*, 2002). First, there are three overlapping spheres in which chronic illness care takes place: the practice is embedded in a health system, which is embedded within a wider community of resources and policies. There are six 'pillars' of effective chronic illness care: community resources and policies; health care organisation; self-management support; delivery system design; decision support; and clinical information systems (Wagner *et al.*, 1996). Community resources include policies and negotiated relationships or links with other care providers to enhance the continuity of care. Health system organisation relates to the structure, values and goals of a system, including the promotion and prioritisation of chronic care and payment structures to support service delivery. The remaining four components – self-management support; delivery system design; decision support; and clinical information systems – exist within the practice setting. The evidence-based framework is intended to be used as a guide for the design of chronic illness care (Wagner *et al.*, 2001).

While the term structured care is associated with chronic disease management programmes, the term often is used by itself to describe interventions. In the literature, structured care is defined largely by the strategies it incorporates to improve care delivery. Hence structured care can be considered as an approach to care delivery applicable in many care settings. For example, a systematic review by Griffin and Kinmonth (1998) differentiated between structured and unstructured care by the presence or absence of an organised system for recall and prompting for patients and doctors. In the more recent TRANSLATE trial, a structured care intervention involved the use of guidelines and prompts for GPs, continuing education, regular patient follow-up, individualised patient goal-setting and feedback for both patients and GPs. Hence the model of structured care was characterised by a series of "multifaceted disease management strategies" (Olivarius *et al.*, 2001: 8). Finally, a study examining the impact of a nurse facilitator-enhanced intervention on Type 2 diabetes included training for GPs and practice staff in the use of guidelines, encouraging structured care and providing performance feedback (van Bruggen *et al.*, 2008). This intervention was conducted in The Netherlands using locally adapted shared care guidelines.

In Ireland, 'structured care' has particular connotations with primary care diabetes management. There are a number of primary care initiatives in Ireland that have adopted this approach with positive results (Brennan *et al.*, 2008; McHugh *et al.*, 2011). Providing structured care in this context refers to a systematic approach to management, including maintaining patient registers, regular audit, continuing professional education, and the routine review and management of patients in general practice. Traditionally, the term has been used to distinguish GP-led initiatives from shared care schemes; however, this is not to imply that shared care or hospital-led care is unstructured in its delivery. In Ireland, shared care has been defined as the "joint participation between hospital consultants and general practitioners in the planned delivery of care for patients with a chronic condition, informed by an enhanced information exchange over and above routine discharge and referral notices" (Irish College of General Practitioners Task Group, 2000). Currently, this model is provided formally by the East Coast Area Diabetes Shared Care Programme (ECAD), which was established jointly by a GP and an endocrinologist. The underlying and somewhat diminishing distinction between shared and structured care in Ireland is becoming less of a fixation as emphasis is placed on the need for regular integrated care for people with diabetes in Ireland.

DELINEATING INTEGRATED CARE

Integrated care is sometimes considered an umbrella term covering shared care arrangements, teamwork, delegation, substitution and re-organisation. For example, a review of integrated care programmes for chronic diseases included interventions that involved patient-focused strategies (education), professional-focused strategies (education), organisational strategies (case management) and co-ordination strategies (multidisciplinary teams) (Ouwens *et al.*, 2005). An integrated care programme was defined as an organisational process of co-ordination with the aim of achieving continuous care.

The evolution of terminology and its interchangeable use muddies the waters for those seeking to understand and implement 'integrated care'. There is substantial overlap in terms of the studies included in reviews of integrated care, shared care and chronic disease management programmes. While all of the interventions seek to improve the delivery and co-ordination of services, the scope of the strategies varies (Gröne and Garcia-Barbero, 2001). Interventions and reforms in this area typically involve changes to enhance integration *within* the practice setting and/or changes to enhance integration *between* providers and settings.

This distinction has been conceptualised as vertical *versus* horizontal integration – for example, horizontal integration includes strategies to link services for people with chronic diseases on the same level (for example, an electronic patient registration system within a practice), while vertical integration might involve a shared protocol between primary and secondary care services and providers for the management of people with Type 2 diabetes. This is just one taxonomy of integration – the concept has been delineated along other dimensions, including the breadth and degree of integration (Nolte and McKee, 2008).

Given the quagmire of terms, aims, scope, components and applications, the World Health Organization (WHO) has proposed the following broad system-based definition:

> Integrated care is a concept bringing together inputs, delivery, management and organisation of services related to diagnosis, treatment, care, rehabilitation and health promotion. Integration is a means to improve the services in relation to access, quality, user satisfaction and efficiency (Gröne and Garcia-Barbero, 2001, p.7).

According to Kodner and Spreeuwenberg, definitions such as that put forward by the WHO are system-based and therefore focus on improving efficiency and cost-effectiveness. Their definition on the other hand reflects integration that is aimed at providing a high-quality *patient-sensitive* service:

> A coherent set of methods and models on the funding, administrative, organisational, service delivery and clinical levels designed to create connectivity, alignment and collaboration within and between cure and care settings (Kodner and Spreeuwenberg, 2002, p.3).

The definition is accompanied by a continuum of mechanisms or strategies to enhance integration at various levels of the health system cited above – for example, joint commissioning at the administrative level, case management at the service delivery level or shared clinical records at the clinical level. In Ireland, efforts to enhance integration tend to concentrate on the service delivery and clinical levels of the health system, the levels over which local stakeholders have more flexibility to make changes depending on local circumstances such as the closing of a local hospital, the availability of a consultant endocrinologist or the interest of a group of local GPs. These factors have acted as catalysts for a number of diabetes initiatives (**Figure 6.1**) that have emerged since the late 1990s, as captured by this quote from an urban GP:

> Some of our small inner city hospitals closed and moved out to the suburbs. So a group of GPs all formed a sort of partnership with the

then Health Board to share some services like podiatrists, like dieticians trained in diabetes ... Then we decided to enter negotiations with the hospital ... and we started off with educational sessions for ourselves and reasonably frequent meetings with the hospital team. So we educated ourselves, we wrote a set of guidelines ... In the beginning, we also shared a diabetes specialist nurse with the hospital.

Figure 6.1: Diabetes Initiatives in Ireland

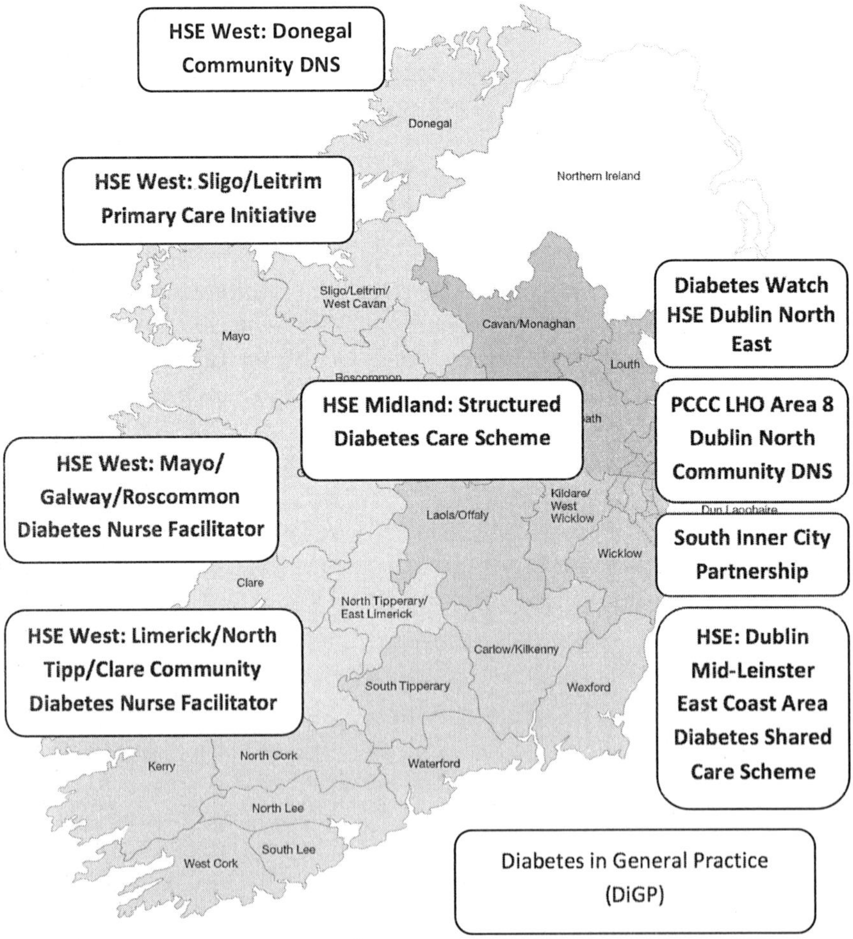

Reproduced with permission from the Health Service Executive.

THE EMERGENCE OF A NATIONAL MODEL OF INTEGRATED CARE

The structure and format of the initiatives in **Figure 6.1** is context-specific and, as such, there are differences in the organisation and co-ordination of care, the underlying model of funding and the availability of resources. However, it is envisaged that all of the initiatives would form part of a national model of integrated care for diabetes.

A model of integrated care was proposed by the Expert Advisory Group for Diabetes (EAGD) in 2008, a multidisciplinary group established by the Health Service Executive (HSE) (EAGD, 2008). The model of care also was endorsed in the national guidelines for the management of Type 2 diabetes (Harkins, 2008). Responsibility for implementation, due to start in late 2012, rests with the Clinical Care Programme for Diabetes, part of the Quality and Clinical Care Directorate in the HSE. In practice, the national model of diabetes care will see the majority of routine diabetes care for uncomplicated Type 2 diabetes taking place in primary care. The current proposal is for three four-monthly visits to primary care for uncomplicated cases of Type 2 diabetes and one visit in secondary care. Patients with complicated Type 2 diabetes, as defined by the national programme, will be managed by both primary and secondary care. All patients with Type 1 diabetes and those with gestational diabetes or genetic causes of diabetes will be managed in secondary care (Oireachtas, 2012; Ryan, 2012).

While this is the first time a model of care has been agreed at a national level, the concept of integrated care has been part of the policy lexicon for over decade and has been advocated time and again as a solution to fragmented and disjointed chronic disease care. In 2001, the national health strategy, *Quality and Fairness: A Health System for You* (Department of Health and Children (DoHC), 2001a), which prioritised 'high performance' as one of its four goals, proposed protocols and planning between health care providers as mechanisms for enhanced integration. The result would be planned regular interaction between the patient and health care provider, and primary care was deemed the appropriate setting for continuous co-ordinated chronic illness care. In the same year, the national primary care strategy, *Primary Care: A New Direction* (DoHC, 2001b), proposed the establishment of primary care teams across the country as a way of providing multidisciplinary integrated care. Teams would comprise GPs, nurses and other health care professionals within a wider network of professionals, such as dieticians and community pharmacists. A major selling point of this proposal was the expected improvement in integration between primary and secondary settings, particularly relevant for the management of diabetes. Integration would be facilitated by investment in communication and information technology, as well as the development of local referral protocols, discharge plans and shared care arrangements for chronic conditions such as diabetes.

In 2008, the Chronic Disease Management Framework (DoHC, 2008) identified the lack of integration between settings as one of the key challenges to effective chronic illness care in Ireland. The tools promoted within the framework were congruent with the elements of optimal chronic illness care outlined in the CCM (Bodenheimer *et al.*, 2002; Wagner and Groves, 2002): enhanced self-management support; information systems and patient registers to support monitoring and communication; a model of shared care to integrate settings; and the need for multidisciplinary care teams. This model of system changes has been used by many other countries to guide the re-organisation and improvement of chronic illness care (Epping-Jordan *et al.*, 2004; Rosemann *et al.*, 2008).

Looking at the organisation of diabetes care specifically, a number of multidisciplinary working groups and committees have advocated a formal model of diabetes care in Ireland. One of the earliest calls for integrated care came in response to the *St. Vincent Declaration* of 1989, a landmark set of standards and goals agreed internationally to improve diabetes care and outcomes (Diabetes Care and Research in Europe, 1990). The Irish St. Vincent Group highlighted the disorganised nature of diabetes care outside the major cities and the lack of service planning, citing integration between providers as an area in need of attention (Firth, 2000). This priority was to re-emerge in several reports over the course of the next decade.

In 2002, the Diabetes Service Development Group (DSDG) (Barragry *et al.*, 2002) re-iterated the need for structured shared care across settings. As part of the proposed model of care, the group recommended the establishment of local DSDGs to monitor and advise on services. This report was followed soon after by recommendations from the DoHC's working group (DoHC, 2006) which emphasised, among other priorities, the need for a diabetes register and an integrated model of care. Once more, local DSDGs were recommended to assess needs and plan services at local level. Yet again in 2008, the EAGD recommended the adoption of "a new integrated, planned, shared and structured model of care" for diabetes in Ireland (EAGD, 2008: 10).

Applying an Integrated Model of Care to the Existing Service Structure

The endorsement of integrated diabetes care in the national guidelines and the devolution of responsibility for improving diabetes care to the Clinical Care Programme and regional Diabetes Services Implementation Groups, goes some way towards a long-awaited national strategy for diabetes care in Ireland (Firth, 2000; International Diabetes Federation - Europe and Federation of European Nurses in Diabetes, 2005). However, the progress and success of integrated care for diabetes depends on the structure, organisation, resources and capabilities of those who will be expected to implement this model of care on the ground.

The traditional approach to diabetes care in Ireland was to refer patients to specialist hospital-based care upon a diagnosis of diabetes, where patients were managed indefinitely (Smith, 2007). While this tradition still exists for a number of patients, over the last decade there has been a shift towards greater primary care involvement in routine diabetes management. A survey of diabetes care in general practice in Ireland, conducted prior to the establishment of the HSE, found that up to 60% of Type 2 diabetes care was being provided by the GP as well as up to 24% of Type 1 diabetes care (O'Sullivan and Smith, 2006). However, the balance of care between general practice and the hospital setting is not always straightforward and, as mentioned previously, there are a variety of diabetes care arrangements in Ireland.

A survey of diabetes care in general practice in 2008 illustrated the lack of formal integration within and between settings (McHugh *et al.*, 2009). In terms of integrating care within the general practice setting, less than half the GPs surveyed maintained a diabetes register (46%, n=157) and 55% reported using guidelines (n=140). While 30% had a formal call/recall system for review (n=78), a further 20% indicated that an informal yet regular approach was in place (n=54). Almost one-quarter of GPs did not employ *any* of these organisational features within the practice (24%, n=62). There was a significant association between maintaining a diabetes register and other aspects of care delivery, such as engaging in formal recall, that suggests organisational processes, such as patient registration, are part of a wider integrated structured approach to diabetes management in the practice.

Looking at integration between settings, most GPs did not have a formal shared protocol with their local hospital-based specialist diabetes team (90%, n=232). Only 10% of GPs reported having *ever* had a joint meeting with the hospital-based team (n= 25), while only 3% had regular meetings with the hospital-based team (n=7). Of those who had regular meetings, the meetings usually were held every four to six months (n=5). Access to auxiliary services also was deficient, as 43% of GPs did not have direct access to chiropody services and 37% reported having no direct access to a dietician. These results contrast with findings from the UK, where 39% reported a formal protocol and 14% had regular joint meetings with the hospital-based specialist diabetes team (Williams *et al.*, 2002).

Integrated Diabetes Care = Our Own Primary Care Paradox

The current landscape of diabetes care delivery in Ireland, set against the ambitious policy proposals for universal integrated care by 2014 and routine management in the primary care setting, represents our very own version of the primary care paradox. This paradox has been described as the tension between "the relative weakness" of primary care *versus* the intention to assign critical strategic functions to it"(Boerma, 2006: 16), such as the co-ordination of routine diabetes management for patients with Type 2 diabetes in Ireland, for example. A number of the persistent barriers to optimal diabetes care delivery in the primary care setting originally were highlighted in the 2001 national primary care strategy (DoHC, 2001b). 'Inadequacies' in primary care included poor primary care infrastructure, fragmented services, lack of availability of certain professional groups, poor liaison between settings and the failure to fully realise the potential of primary care to ease the pressure on secondary care (DoHC, 2001b). These barriers hinder the provision of high quality care across all chronic conditions.

From our national survey, most GPs feel that training and education is the key priority for developing diabetes care (**Figure 6.2**) (McHugh *et al.*, 2009). Other priority areas include easier access to specialist advice (65%), better access to community services, such as dieticians and ophthalmology services, guidelines and protocols. Each of these elements is essential for the success of an integrated model of care that is built on routine management taking place in the primary care setting.

Figure 6.2: Principal Opportunities for Developing Diabetes Care in a Practice

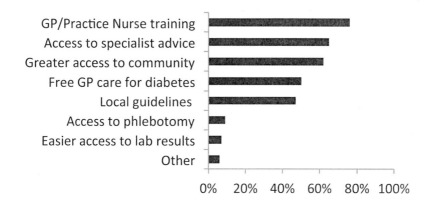

Source: McHugh, 2009.

CONCLUSION

A model of integrated care should encompass integration from the upper levels of policy, planning and funding, through administration and organisation of services, down to service delivery and the clinical management of people with diabetes. At present in Ireland, we have somewhat isolated islands of shared and structured care with different levels of funding, reimbursement and resources. These initiatives are surrounded by a sea of unknowns in terms of the quantity and quality of integration between health care professionals and settings. Some have questioned whether the models of disease management discussed in this chapter truly represent shared care or are simply shifting the burden from one setting to another (Overland *et al.*, 1999; Maher and Millar, 2003).

It is important to identify and anticipate physical and attitudinal barriers to integrated care. These hurdles highlight the need for flexibility within a national model of care, to allow for varying levels of interest, but also uneven capacity to manage the majority of people with diabetes. Flexibility, depending on local circumstances, does not negate the need for clarity surrounding the realms of responsibility and the standard of care to be delivered. Responsibility for co-ordinating care needs to be assigned to prevent wasteful duplication and gaps in care that could prove costly for the patient (Bodenheimer, 2008).

REFERENCES

Barragry, J., Forde, R., Shelley, E., McKenna, T. and Quirke, R. (eds.) (2002). *Diabetes Care: Securing the Future, Report of the Diabetes Service Development Group*, Dublin: Diabetes Service Development Group.

Bodenheimer, T. (2008). 'Co-ordinating Care: A Perilous Journey through the Health Care System', *New England Journal of Medicine*, 358: 1064-1071.

Bodenheimer, T., Wagner, E.H. and Grumbach, K. (2002). 'Improving Primary Care for Patients with Chronic Illness', *Journal of the American Medical Association*, 288: 1775-1779.

Boerma, W. (2006). 'Co-ordination and Integration in European Primary Care', in Saltman, A., Rico, A. and Boerma, W. (eds.), *Primary Care in the Driver's Seat? Organisational Reform in European Primary Care*, Maidenhead: Open University.

Branger, P.J., Vant Hooft, A., Van der Wouden, J.C., Moorman, P.W. and Van Bemmel, J.H. (1999). 'Shared Care for Diabetes: Supporting Communication between Primary and Secondary Care', *International Journal of Medical Informatics*, 53: 133-142.

Brennan, C., Harkins, V. and Perry, I. (2008). 'Management of Diabetes in Primary Care: A Structured Care Approach', *European Journal of General Practice*, 14: 117-122.

Casalino, L.P. (2005). 'Disease Management and the Organization of Physician Practice', *Journal of the American Medical Association*, 293: 485-488.

Darker, C., Martin, C., O'Dowd, T., O'Kelly, F., O'Kelly, M. and O'Shea, B. (2012). 'Chronic Disease Management in General Practice: Results from a National Study', *Irish Medical Journal*, 105: 102-105.

Department of Health and Children (DoHC) (2001a). *Quality and Fairness: A Health System for You*, Dublin: Stationery Office.

Department of Health and Children (DoHC) (2001b). *Primary Care: A New Direction*, Dublin: Stationery Office.

Department of Health and Children (DoHC) (2006). *Diabetes: Prevention and Model for Patient Care*, Dublin: Stationery Office.

Department of Health and Children (DoHC) (2008). *Tackling Chronic Disease: A Policy Framework for the Management of Chronic Disease*, Dublin: Stationery Office.

Diabetes Care and Research in Europe (1990). 'The St. Vincent Declaration', *Diabetic Medicine*, 7: 360.

Eijkelberg, I., Spreeuwenberg, C., Mur-Veeman, I. and Wolffenbuttel, B. (2001). 'From Shared Care to Disease Management: Key Influencing Factors', *International Journal of Integrated Care*, 1.

Epping-Jordan, J.E., Pruitt, S.D., Bengoa, R. and Wagner, E.H. (2004). 'Improving the Quality of Health Care for Chronic Conditions', *Quality and Safety in Health Care*, 13: 299-305.

Expert Advisory Group for Diabetes (EAGD) (2008). *Diabetes Expert Advisory Group First Report: April 2008*, Dublin: Health Service Executive.

Firth, R. (2000). 'Existing Facilities for Diabetes Care in the Republic of Ireland and Developments Required', *Irish Journal of Medical Science*, 169: 2-7.

Geyman, J.P. (2007). 'Disease Management: Panacea, Another False Hope, or Something In Between?', *Annals of Family Medicine*, 5: 257.

Griffin, S. and Kinmonth, A.L. (1998). 'Systems for Routine Surveillance for People with Diabetes Mellitus', *Cochrane Database of Systematic Reviews*, 1.

Gröne, O. and Garcia-Barbero, M. (2001). 'Integrated Care: A Position Paper of the WHO European Office for Integrated Health Care Services', *International Journal of Integrated Care*, 1.

Harkins, V. (2008). *A Practical Guide to Integrated Type 2 Diabetes Care*, Dublin: Health Service Executive, in association with Irish College of General Practitioners, Department of Health and Children and Irish Endocrine Society.

Institute of Medicine (2001). *Crossing the Quality Chasm: A New Health System for the Twenty-first Century*, Washington: Washington Academic Press, available http://www.iom.edu/Reports/2001/Crossing-the-Quality-Chasm-A-New-Health-System-for-the-21st-Century.aspx.

International Diabetes Federation in Europe and Federation of European Nurses in Diabetes (2005). *Diabetes - The Policy Puzzle: Towards Benchmarking in the EU 25*, Brussels: International Diabetes Federation-Europe and Federation of European Nurses in Diabetes.

Irish College of General Practitioners Task Group (2000). *Guidelines for Diabetes Care in the Community*, Dublin: Irish College of General Practitioners.

Kahn, R. and Anderson, J.E. (2009). 'Improving Diabetes Care: The Model for Health Care Reform', *Diabetes Care*, 32: 1115-1118.

Kodner, D. and Spreeuwenberg, C. (2002). 'Integrated Care: Meaning, Logic, Applications, and Implications: A Discussion Paper', *International Journal of Integrated Care*, 2.

Maher, E. and Millar, D. (2003). 'Shared Care: Step Down or Step Up?', *Quality and Safety in Health Care*, 12: 242-242.

Maier, M., Knopp, A., Pusarnig, S., Rurik, I., Orozco-Beltran, D., Yaman, H. and Van Eygen, L. (2008). 'Diabetes in Europe: Role and Contribution of Primary Care, Position Paper of the European Forum for Primary Care', *Quality in Primary Care*, 16: 197-207.

McHugh, S., Marsden, P., Brennan, C., Murphy, K., Croarkin, C., Moran, J., Harkins, V. and Perry, I.J. (2011). 'Counting on Commitment: The Quality of Primary Care-led Diabetes Management in a System with Minimal Incentives', *BMC Health Service Research*, 11.

McHugh, S., O'Keeffe, J., Fitzpatrick, A., De Siún, A., O'Mullane, M., Perry, I. and Bradley, C. (2009). 'Diabetes Care in Ireland: A Survey of General Practitioners', *Primary Care Diabetes*, 3: 225-231.

McKee, M. and Nolte, E. (2009). 'Chronic Care', in Smith, P., Mossialos, E., Papanicolas, I. and Leatherman, S. (eds.), *Performance Measurement for Health System Improvement*, New York: Cambridge University Press.

Nolte, E. and McKee, M. (2008). 'Integration and Chronic Care: A Review', in Nolte, E. and McKee, M., *Caring for People with Chronic Conditions: A Health System Perspective*, European Observatory on Health Systems and Policies, Brussels: World Health Organization.

Oireachtas (2012). *Parliamentary Question No 721-722*, Dublin: Stationery Office.

O'Sullivan, T. and Smith, S. (2006). 'National Survey of Diabetes Care in General Practice', *Irish Medical Journal*, 99: 104-106.

Olivarius, N., Beck-Nielsen, H., Andreasen, A., Horder, M. and Pedersen, P. (2001). 'Randomised Controlled Trial of Structured Personal Care of Type 2 Diabetes Mellitus', *British Medical Journal*, 323: 970-975.

Ouwens, M., Wollersheim, H., Hermens, R., Hulscher, M. and Grol, R. (2005). 'Integrated Care Programmes for Chronically Ill Patients: A Review of Systematic Reviews', *International Journal for Quality in Health Care*, 17: 141-146.

Overland, J., Mira, M. and Yue, D.K. (1999). 'Diabetes Management: Shared Care or Shared Neglect', *Diabetes Research and Clinical Practice*, 44: 123-128.

Rosemann, T., Laux, G., Szecsenyi, J. and Grol, R. (2008). 'The Chronic Care Model: Congruency and Predictors among Primary Care Patients with Osteoarthritis', *Quality and Safety in Health Care*, 17: 442-446.

Ryan, V. (2012). 'Total Coverage for Diabetes by 2014', *Irish Medical Times*, 27.04.12.

Saltman, A., Rico, A. and Boerma, W. (2006). *Primary Health Care in the Driver's Seat?: Organisational Reform in European PHC*, European Observatory on Health Systems and Policies, Maidenhead: WHO and Open University Press.

Smith, S.M. (2007). 'Primary Care Diabetes in the Republic of Ireland', *Primary Care Diabetes*, 1: 207-208.

Smith, S.M., Allwright, S. and O'Dowd, T. (2007). 'Effectiveness of Shared Care across the Interface between Primary and Specialty Care in Chronic Disease Management', *Cochrane Database Systematic Reviews*, 3, CD004910.

van Bruggen, R., Gorter, K.J., Stolk, R.P., Verhoeven, R.P. and Ruttien, G.E.H.M. (2008). 'Implementation of Locally-adapted Guidelines on Type 2 Diabetes', *Family Practice*, 25: 430-437.

Vrijhoef, H., Diederiks, J., Spreeuwenberg, C. and Wolffenbuttel, B. (2001a). 'Adoption of Disease Management Model for Diabetes in Region of Maastricht', *British Medical Journal*, 323: 983-985.

Vrijhoef, H., Diederiks, J., Spreeuwenberg, C. and Wolffenbuttel, B. (2001b). 'Substitution Model with Central Role for Nurse Specialist is Justified in the Care for Stable Type 2 Diabetic Outpatients', *Journal of Advanced Nursing*, 36: 546-555.

Wagner, E.H., Austin, B.T., Davis, C., Hindmarsh, M., Schaeffer, J. and Bonomi, A. (2001). 'Improving Chronic Illness Care: Translating Evidence into Action', *Health Affairs*, 20: 64.

Wagner, E.H., Austin, B.T. and Michael Von, K. (1996). 'Organizing Care for Patients with Chronic Illness', *Milbank Quarterly*, 74: 511-544.

Wagner, E.H. and Groves, T. (2002). 'Care for Chronic Diseases', *British Medical Journal*, 325: 913-914.

Williams, D.R., Baxter, H.S., Airey, C.M., Ali, S. and Turner, B. (2002). 'Diabetes UK Funded Surveys of the Structural Provision of Primary Care Diabetes Services in the UK', *Diabetic Medicine*, 19(Suppl.4): 21-26.

7: AN EXAMINATION OF THE NDRIC FRAMEWORK OF INTEGRATED CARE FOR DRUG USERS

Laura Desmond and Tom O'Connor

INTRODUCTION

This chapter is focused on the rehabilitation of addicted persons and, in this context, it examines a model that may offer hope: the National Drug Rehabilitation Implementation Committee (NDRIC) Framework Model (Doyle and Ivanovic, 2010). The chapter includes a discussion of recent research conducted on the implementation of the NDRIC model in the Cork area, which compares the views of those who are charged with its operation, alongside the views of service providers and practitioners.

The chapter is structured into five parts: first, a description of the scale of the problem of drug use in Ireland is provided; the second section reviews Irish government policy to tackle drug addiction; section three details the new integrated care approach to delivering addiction services within the NDRIC framework document (Doyle and Ivanovic, 2010); the fourth section gives an account of the methodology employed to examine the early stages of roll-out of this framework within the South of the country; the fifth section discusses the results of this research in terms of evaluating the participants' views on the workability of the NDRIC framework. Finally, conclusions and recommendations are provided.

The focus here is essentially on an evaluation of the still relatively new NDRIC framework for delivering addiction services; the research results are used in that context. The objectives do not include an attempt at praxis with any other established evidence, other than the NDRIC document itself. As such, for example, this chapter does not tease out NDRIC by way of comparison on theoretical and substantive best practice grounds with the growing literature in the area, given that the objective of this study is only to evaluate the current NDRIC framework against the views of practitioners and policy-implementers.

DRUG USE IN IRELAND

Drug use is a worldwide phenomenon, occurring in almost every country in the world. According to the United Nations Office on Crime and Drugs (UNOCD):

> Globally, UNOCD estimates that in 2009 between 149 and 272 million people, or 3.3% to 6.1% of the population aged 15 to 64, used illicit substances at least once in the previous year (UNOCD, 2011: 13).

Cannabis, opiates and cocaine are the most commonly-used drugs worldwide. Cannabis was consumed by approximately 125 to 203 million people globally in 2009 (UNOCD, 2011).

One of the reasons why drug use has increased globally is that the production of opium has been shifting. Afghanistan now produces 79% of all opium production and is the predominant supplier worldwide by means of trafficking across Asia and through other continents. Afghanistan and many other countries across the world engaged in the supply of drugs have developed supply to match demand, particularly in the economically-developed world. The problem of addiction and related social, economic and health problems has resulted. However, the focus of this chapter is not to outline solutions to the demand for drugs.

Any model that attempts to provide a framework for drug rehabilitation must operate in the context of national drug use patterns. This includes not alone the ready supply of illegal drugs, but also the widespread availability of very cheap alcohol products nationwide. Ireland has felt the effects of the continuous supply of drugs, for which there has been ready demand. The National Advisory Committee on Drugs (NACD) carried out a survey in 2010/2011, the aim of which was to provide accurate and current data on the prevalence and patterns of illicit and licit drug use among the general population in terms of age, gender and region (NACD, 2012). The survey sampled a number of people aged between 15 and 64. Some of the findings in this survey were:

- 27% of Irish people reported using illegal drugs in their lifetime, including:
  - Cannabis, at 25%, the most common drug used amongst the adult population;
  - After cannabis came cocaine, ecstasy, and magic mushrooms, at 7%;
  - LSD at 5%;

o   Less than 1% reported ever having used crack (0.6%), heroin (0.8%) and methadone (0.5%) (NACD, 2012: 1).

Illegal drug consumption was highest (at 42%) amongst people aged 25 to 34, while the report showed that women reported higher levels of use of sedatives and anti-depressants than men (NACD, 2012: 2).

One of the most striking findings is that:

Half of all new cases entering into treatment services had started to use drugs at the age of 15 in the period between 2005 and 2010 (NACD, 2012).

These statistics give a brief description of drug use amongst the general population in Ireland. There are also issues of alcohol use and treatment for alcohol misuse has become more prevalent in recent years. According to a report by the Health Research Board (HRB):

In the period of 2005 to 2010 a total of 42,333 cases presented to a drug and alcohol service with alcohol being their main problem substance, accounting for more than half (52.7%) of all cases treated for problem substance use during that period. (HRB, 2011).

Among 35 European countries, Ireland is ranked as having the highest number of adolescents who regularly binge-drink; also Ireland is the second highest for general drunkenness (European Monitoring Centre for Drugs and Drug Addiction, 2007).

Media reports also have shown the extent of the drug problem in Ireland. Take, for example, an article by Carl O'Brien in *The Irish Times*, entitled, *Ireland among worst for drug deaths*, which states:

Ireland has one of the highest drug deaths in Europe according to the United Nations. The report shows that Ukraine, Iceland and Ireland experienced some of the highest death rates in Europe with over 100 drug-related deaths per million inhabitants aged between 15 and 64 (O'Brien, 2011).

The article also reports that heroin is on the increase in Ireland and Sweden, although it is stabilising in most European countries (O'Brien, 2011).

In another article, HRB senior researcher Dr. Suzi Lyons states:

The figures on drug deaths accurately reflect the problem in Ireland. One of the reasons why the Irish rate is so high is because our monitoring systems were not as comprehensive (HRB, 2011).

GOVERNMENT POLICY TO TACKLE DRUG ADDICTION

So what has the government done to tackle the problem of drug addiction in Ireland? The Department of Community, Rural and Gaeltacht Affairs (DoCRGA) developed the *National Drugs Strategy 2009-2016* (2009). The four pillars in this strategy are:

- **Supply reduction:** Strategies to reduce the supply of illegal substances in Ireland – for example, looking into ways to improve measures to stop drug trafficking;
- **Prevention:** Ways in which services can prevent a service user from falling into addiction;
- **Treatment and rehabilitation:** Ways to improve services around treatment and rehabilitation;
- **Research/information:** Ways of dealing with drug abuse (DoCRGA, 2009).

These four pillars deal with all aspects of the drug problem in Ireland. They are administered *via* statutory drug and alcohol services and also community and voluntary drug and alcohol services.

What progress has been made in rolling these out? According to the *National Drugs Strategy Progress Report* (Department of Health and Children (DoHC), 2012), 52 actions in the National Drugs Strategy have been implemented to date or progress has been made on them. The following four are particularly pertinent:

- **Action 2:** Establish a local police forum – guidelines for this have been sent out to the relevant drug task forces for implementation;
- **Action 22:** Promote the establishment of substance misuse policies – this is being considered and yet to be finalised;
- **Action 32:** NDRIC has developed a framework for integrated care and training has begun;
- **Action 52:** A unique reporting system is currently being drafted (DoHC, 2012: 1-24).

The government also funds a number of projects around the country to tackle the drug problem. In Cork alone, there are 33 people employed within the Local Drugs Task Force and there are 22 in the Southern Regional Drugs Task Force Project.

A four-tier system/model (Doyle and Ivanovic, 2010) is used within addiction service for service users. This maps out services, based on the severity of the drug addiction problem of the service user. This model is being piloted as a perceived gold standard for addiction services. Based on an adaptation of the UK model, the four tiers are:

• Education and health service;

• Drug and alcohol service;

• Specialist practitioners;

• Dedicated stabilisation and detoxification services (Doyle and Ivanovic, 2010).

So, for example, a service user may enter a tier 1 service: seeing their local GP, or mentioning his/her drug use to a teacher in school. The service user then would be referred to a tier 2 service, normally a community-based drugs project. An assessment would be conducted here; if the drug use is particularly problematic, then he/she would be referred to a tier 3 specialised drug and alcohol service. Having been assessed at that level, if it was found that the drug and alcohol problem was beyond the scope of tier 3, then he/she would be referred to a tier 4 service, which is likely to be a residential setting. The NDRIC (Doyle and Ivanovic, 2010) framework is based on integrated care pathways within addiction services across all four tiers.

THE NDRIC MODEL AND INTEGRATED CARE: A 'GOLD STANDARD'?

The NDRIC framework on integrated care is perceived among policy-makers as an excellent model. Why? Currently, within the field of addiction, there is little integration with other services and most of it is done on an informal basis. The current framework has designed ways to standardise the integration of services to benefit the service user and the service provider. This has been achieved by:

• Key working, case management and care planning;

• Developing protocols and service level agreements; and

• Organisational standards for alcohol and drug treatment services and care planning (known as 'QuADS' – for 'quality in alcohol and drugs services') (Doyle and Ivanovic, 2010).

These aspects have been put in place to benefit the service user/provider, but they are also there to protect both the service user and provider.

NDRIC has introduced what are called 'common assessment forms'. Each agency attached to the service user will have two types of common assessment forms:

- **Initial assessment form**: This is used when the service user makes his/her first point of contact with a service and the initial assessment is carried out. From this assessment, it is decided what tier service would suit the service user best;
- **Comprehensive assessment form**: This is normally completed by the case manager, who will give further information on what the service user requires in terms of all elements of his/her life, not just the drug and alcohol issue. This again blocks out more similar assessments (NDRIC, 2011).

From the initial assessment, the services that the service user requires are established. It is within these services then that key workers are assigned. This basically means that the social worker attached to the service user is a key worker equivalent to the addiction counsellor. From this group of key workers, a case manager is decided. The case manager then will decide on what action needs to be taken and by whom. He/she will follow up to make sure that what needs to be done is being done.

NDRIC has developed five protocols to support collaborative working between services:

- Initial assessment and matching the service user to the most appropriate service;
- Comprehensive assessment and developing an interagency care plan;
- Referral between agencies;
- Interagency care plan meetings;
- Gaps and blocks (NDRIC, 2011: 7-13).

Overall, NDRIC is committed to:

- Overseeing and monitoring the implementation of the recommendations from the rehabilitation report;
- Developing agreed protocols and service level agreements;
- Developing a quality standard framework which builds upon existing standards;
- Overseeing case management and care planning processes; and
- Identifying core competencies and training needs and ensuring that such needs are met (Doyle and Ivanovic, 2010).

The Model as Integrated Care

This model fits into integrated care in terms of getting all services attached to the service user communicating and integrating, in order to create a 'shared care plan' or a collaborative care plan for the service user. This is done by each service provider acting as a key worker to the service user; one of these key workers then takes on the role of the case manager, who ensures that each key worker is following up on their part of the shared care plan. This is mentioned in protocol 2: "Comprehensive assessment and developing an interagency care plan" (NDRIC, 2011: 8). Integrated care is the outcome of getting all agencies to discuss together what the service user needs and to come up with a collaborative care plan.

In a seminal journal article on integrated care in Ireland (Doocey and Reddy, 2010), the authors point to a significant debate worldwide on the need for integrated care amongst health care services to achieve a better service delivery through integrated pathways and final outcomes for patients. The NDRIC model attempts to move service provision forward in this direction. The framework evidences integrated care within the care system and is capable, if implemented correctly, of removing unnecessary blockages and bureaucratic procedures within different strands of the service. This makes the patient's journey seamless. It is clear that the overall drive for integrated care is for a better delivery of service to benefit the service user and to reach Doocey and Reddy's 'touchstone':

> Ensuring that patients are able to move easily through entire care systems requires a service to be well organised ... integration between primary and secondary care with the development of care pathways and protocols, guidelines and shared care arrangements (Doocey and Reddy, 2010: 27).

Integrated care for the full spectrum of patients and clients has been policy for the Health Service Executive (HSE) for at least six years. The HSE has introduced the Integrated Services Programme (ISP), *Integrating Hospital and Community Services* (2010), which shows some vital reasons to change from an individualised reflective practice to a more structured and democratic one, by integrating hospital and community services:

- To drive and support safe, quality care for clients;
- To organise to meet increasingly complex client needs;
- To remove barriers to integrated care (HSE, 2010: 1).

The need for change came about due to the increasing prevalence of conditions such as diabetes, obesity, heart disease, asthma, etc, which have put pressure on hospitals to deliver services. Consequently, by integrating within primary care and community services in particular, service provision can happen at the most appropriate level for the client or patient, halving case-loads and reducing the risk of burn-out for many health and social care professionals (HSE, 2010).

Given that integrated care is a general population health commitment within Ireland at present (HSE, 2010) and that the NDRIC (Doyle and Ivanovic, 2010) models seem to represent a useful addition to the treatment of addiction, the remainder of this chapter outlines research conducted in Cork in 2012.

The question of whether the enthusiasm of policy-makers and administrators for the NDRIC model would be matched by those working in the field of drug addiction services in Cork was of foremost concern for the research. Thus, a comparison was made between the views of 'policy-makers' and of 'policy-implementers' within the interviews conducted for this research.

RESEARCH METHODOLOGY

Design

This research was based on a qualitative approach. The researcher took an interpretive approach and interviewed 'key stakeholders' within the framework, as the researcher wanted to get some idea as to what the service providers involved in this framework thought of it. The stakeholders were broken into two groups: 'policy-makers' and 'policy-implementers'. The research design was cross-sectional, due to the fact that the framework was based on integration of services within the area of addiction. Having a cross-section design meant that people from a range of services could be interviewed to show whether integration was possible/successful/unsuccessful. The structure of this research was based on interviews and observing a focus group.

Because the framework is relatively new, workers from all sectors are still being trained on three aspects of the framework:

- Key working;
- Care planning;
- Case management.

After a discussion with the Drugs and Alcohol Services Co-ordinator of the HSE South, it was decided that an examination of training also would be beneficial to the research on the NDRIC integrated model as it is currently rolled out in Cork.

Participants

There were five interviews, with three policy-makers and two policy-implementers. For the purpose of this research, acronyms will be used as shown here:

- Policy-makers:
  - o Drugs and Alcohol Co-ordinator of the HSE South: D&AC;
  - o Cork Local Drugs Task Force Co-ordinator: CLDTFC;
  - o Rehabilitation Co-ordinator: RC;
- Policy-implementers:
  - o Link Worker Cork and Kerry: LW;
  - o Senior Addiction Counsellor: SAC;

A non-participant observation study was conducted also in order to get an in-depth interagency perspective on this framework. This was done through observation of training sessions conducted for practitioners within the field of addiction. The agencies involved, and the sectors they represented, included:

- Drug and alcohol services: HSE;
- Social workers: HSE;
- Probation officers: HSE;
- Housing: Community and voluntary;
- Link workers: HSE;
- Youth workers: Community and voluntary;
- Education and training officers: Community and voluntary;
- Rehabilitation Co-ordinator: HSE.

The interviews asked questions covering the following broad areas and the observed training was consistent also with these four areas:

- Co-ordination;
- Key working, care planning and case management;
- Four-tier system/model;
- Protocols/service level agreements/QuADS.

RESEARCH RESULTS

Observation Study

The following results were obtained from the interactive training sessions observed, covering the practitioners' views on the new NDRIC protocols for the Key Worker, Case Manager and Shared Care Plan.

Table 7.1: Observation Study Results

Occupation	Protocols		
	Key Worker	Case Manager	Shared Care Plan
Addiction counsellor	√	√	√
Social worker	√	√	X
Probation officer	√	√	*
Educational officer	*	√	*
Housing officer	√	√	*
Youth worker	√	√	√
Voluntary workers	√	√	*
Drugs project workers	√	√	√

Symbols: Agreed √ , disagreed X , unsure * .

From the table, it is clear that most organisations were in agreement on all three protocols. For those who were unsure, this was only due to basic confusion as to how this role would work. Everyone agreed with the case manager role, as they felt it would take pressure away from them, although what they did not seem to realise was that one of them could be acting as case manager depending on the case.

For those who were unsure on the care plan, their reasons revolved around the need for resources and the timing of the interventions, in that it seemed impossible to them to find a convenient time and place to discuss with all key workers and develop a shared care plan for the service user. The probation officer (with a social work background) did not agree with the shared care plan. This was mainly due to her assertion that she would not be happy to change her style of practice, in terms of moving from an individualised practice to a more structured practice.

There were three main issues arising amongst all agencies:

- Confidentiality;
- Confusion of role;
- Increased workload if they bought into this model.

Interviews

The fieldwork for the interviews was ethnographic and was conducted in the workplace, a 'naturalistic' setting. The subjects were encouraged to be reflective, with a particular emphasis on the practical applicability of the policy at the macro level and how it would impact at the micro level of practice in working with drug abusers. As such, this reflects the in-built methodological commitment to the use of a 'critical' approach to social research. This overall type of research methodology is consistent with the best practice recommendations for critical ethnographic research, sometimes referred to as critical ethno-methodology (Harvey and McDonald, 1993). Further, a thematic analysis was brought to bear on the interview results, which is presented across the five themes below.

Theme 1: Co-ordination

The researcher interpreted co-ordination in terms of the NDRIC model of integrated care as being the integration of services into a plan and coming up with service level agreements in order to deliver a cohesive, integrated care plan for the service user. All interviewees had slightly different interpretations of co-ordination in relation to the framework: D&AC gave a great explanation as to what he viewed co-ordination within the framework to be:

> I would interpret the co-ordination as an orchestra playing music. Within an orchestra, you have a whole range of different instruments. You'd have violins, percussion, wind, etc. How this is related is that many of the key workers would act as those musicians – for example, somebody in an addiction service would be helping a service user with counselling or medical treatment, etc or likewise in the educational sector, you have the likes of FÁS which would look at developing vocational skills with service users. They have that specific remit, like a violinist will have within the orchestra: a job to do in terms of playing the violin, likewise the pianist will have that job to play that instrument within the orchestra. So they all have their little job to do, so the framework is a little like the orchestra in terms of co-ordination, which is about the conductor of that orchestra bringing it all together to make incredible music. The way I see it is that the key workers are the musicians and the conductor is the case manager who co-ordinates all the little jobs that need to be done in an interagency care plan for a greater outcome for the client.

Other interviewees gave differing interpretations:

CLDTFC: Co-ordination is about the client at the end of the day ... it's about services being able to have a continuum of services for a service user who hits any of the four tiers, and making it as seamless as possible through means of protocols, QuADS, key working, case management and shared care planning.

RC: There are six parts to co-ordination in relation to this framework. They are: case management/key working; QuADS process, all drug and alcohol services in the Cork region are becoming QuADS-compliant; they are also piloting an integrated database system and an electronic patient system (EPS); protocols; and common assessment forms.

LW: Co-ordination within this model is vitally important in terms of creating a more integrated cohesive delivery of service for the service user.

SAC: Co-ordination in relation to this model in my opinion is a best practice idea but the practicality of it may differ slightly historically ...

The interviewees were asked: 'Can anybody act as the case manager?'. The answer to this question was twofold: the interviewees said, on a technical basis, yes, anybody can act as the case manager but then they explained that what will happen is that the case manager usually will be somebody who knows the case really well and who may have established a relationship with the service user. The case manager must have the correct skills and competencies in order to carry out this role. LW said:

In my opinion, the case manager would be the person who may have the most engagement with the client and has built up a relationship with the client. Also the case manager's role is to ensure all the key workers are fulfilling their part of the shared care plan, which means the case manager will need to have the skills and competencies to ensure that all of this is happening and including the service user in the process at all times.

Theme 2: Functions of Key Worker, Case Manager and Shared Care Plan

A list of the functions of the key worker and case manager were shown according to the NDRIC model, as per **Tables 7.2** and **7.3**. The tick marks then indicate what each interviewee mentioned or failed to mention as key functions.

Table 7.2: Functions of the Key Worker

Functions	D&AC	CLDTFC	RC	LW	SAC
Engaging with the service user	✔	✔	✔	✔	✔
Ensuring consent	✔	✔	✔	✔	
Completing assessments & developing care plans within the service	✔	✔	✔	✔	
Advocating on behalf of the service user	✔	✔	✔	✔	
Engaging and sharing information with other agencies as required	✔	✔	✔	✔	✔
Keeping relevant case notes/records			✔	✔	✔
Working to fulfil care plan actions relating to their direct service provision	✔	✔	✔	✔	✔

Table 7.3: Functions of the Case Manager

Functions	D&AC	CLDTFC	RC	LW	SAC
Ensuring a care plan is in place and SMART objectives are set	✔	✔	✔	✔	✔
Arranging regular reviews to monitor and assess the progression of the care plan	✔	✔	✔	✔	✔
Reviewing the care plan with the service user, all key workers/agencies involved, and where appropriate with the service users' families	✔	✔	✔	✔	✔
Have the skills and competencies to act as a case manager	✔	✔	✔	✔	✔
Be familiar with the case/established a relationship with the client	✔	✔	✔	✔	✔

There was a clear mixture of views in regard to the stated positions. SAC made a valid point about the case manager's role, pointing out that the NDRIC framework failed in some respects:

> The first issue I would have is the practicality of these roles in terms of the sums. There are massive amounts of case-loads and limited number of staff so that would make it difficult in carrying out these roles effectively/efficiently… also I would like to add that I don't see in the framework anything about team management, in terms of who is auditing the case manager's role in ensuring that he/she is carrying out the role effectively and efficiently?

On the question on the shared care plan: What should be happening from this model?, interviewees said:

> D&AC: The great thing about the shared care plan is that bringing all key workers together to create the care plan will highlight all issues in relation to the service user that can then be worked on in the delivery of service required.

> CLDTFC: A shared care plan is essential to any service user for their care; otherwise services are just stumbling around in the dark.

> RC: Shared care plans are a relatively new addition to drug and alcohol services ... this hasn't happened before, due to agencies having a fear of other agencies feeding into their service ... a shared care plan is the way to go forward ... it is the best possible solution for the service user.

> LW: My opinion is that a shared care plan is designed from all the key worker's own individual care plans; from a shared care meeting, it is then decided what goes into the shared care plan in order of priority.

Theme 3: Four-tier Model

The four-tier model is essential within addiction services in relation to matching a service to the needs of the service user. The general view amongst all interviewees was that the four-tier model was in place as a mapping for the service user; for example, somebody with experimental drug use would be best suited at a tier 1 service and somebody with chaotic use would be best in a tier 3 or tier 4 service, depending on their needs:

> D&AC: The four-tier model is not just about the treatment of the service user; it's about the severity of the case i.e. dual diagnosis: mental health issues as well as addiction issues ... Tier 3 and 4 are still not fully resourced ... A tier 4 service is not just about residential treatment; it's about the specialised services that are required which are not there to date, such as specialised consultants ... tier 1 and 2 are much broader scale ... tier 1 and 2 are the usual first point of contact and need the correct assessment tools.

> CLDTFC: I think that the four-tier system is an excellent model in terms of correctly assessing clients ... if I am a nurse or a guard in a tier 1 service through NDRIC, I will have been trained in the relevant assessing tools so I will know what tier this particular client needs to be at and then can refer correctly ... the four-tier system is great for

systematically working with clients through each necessary tier to ensure the best treatment and outcome possible.

RC: It's good in that it maps services and service providers can place themselves on the continuum of care .... The problem is that it can cause argumentative points in that service providers aspire to be a certain tier and may not have the skills, resources or services to do so.

LW: I try to work as much as possible from the four-tier model ... I think it can be misunderstood ... I think if we all understand the model then it'll be a lot easier to know our limitations and to make the correct referrals.

SAC: I sort of understand the model in terms that treatment happens in all tiers yet the culture here in Cork is that you're only in treatment if you're in a residential setting and a residential setting is a tier 4 service which actually isn't the case.

Of particular note was the following question: In your professional opinion, do you think there will be any gaps or barriers when integrating the NDRIC model into the four-tier model? All interviewees said "Yes". The view was that each agency might be a bit hesitant in communicating with other agencies for a number of reasons. One being that it has been done on an informal basis all along and now NDRIC has brought in standard policies and procedures around doing so, so agencies may feel confusion around their current role. Also all interviewees mentioned trial and error in saying that, when an evaluation is done on the integration into the four-tier system, agencies will know in more detail about gaps and barriers and work on those. RC mentioned:

In my opinion, an immediate gap/barrier is that some services just aren't available for integration ... also some services in some regions don't have all four tiers locally so that would be a barrier in integrating the NDRIC model.

Theme 4: Protocols/service level agreements/QuADS

Protocols
The general view about protocols was very positive. All interviewees explained that protocols created processes that staff can follow to ensure a better quality in service and also as a structured way in carrying out tasks that previously may have had no protocols attached:

D&AC: Protocols are critically important ... the clearer the protocol, the better the service delivery will be.

RC: Protocols are essential in ensuring that workers and the service users are safe and also ensure that information-sharing is done correctly ... not everybody needs to know everything.

CLDTFC: Protocols create accountability and take away personalities. By that, I mean a service user can't access a service because of the 'type' of client he is; there will be a protocol in place that will lay out a clear process in which this service can be accessed for that service user.

LW: In my line of work, I always practice confidentiality. I believe that protocols are a great thing to be brought into services as they ensure safe sharing of information. I strongly believe that every service attached to the client does not need to know everything. Protocols will ensure that information is shared on a need-to-know basis.

SAC: Protocols will progress standards in the service ...

Service Level Agreements
The view on service level agreements (SLAs) was again quite positive. However, all interviewees mentioned that the theory of these SLAs was great but putting them into practice might create some difficulty:

D&AC: Service level agreements have been in the addiction services of the HSE for a couple of years and what I found is that they were very legalistic, which leads to people not fully understanding what they were ... NDRIC needs to avoid this and create clarity and understanding around SLAs.

RC: QuADS and SLAs link and they both need to be transparent ... SLAs need to be evidence-based i.e. working off a QuADS policy and creating value for money ... SLAs haven't come into effect through NDRIC in Cork as of yet but will be enforced in the very near future.

CLDTFC: SLAs are wonderful ... Some services have very clear SLAs, others not so clear ... They are really all about keeping our house in order to benefit the client!

LW: SLAs are critical in the sense that it's the way how each service works with each other and they need to be clear and understood in order to ensure better results for the client.

SAC: Theory is good but practice is yet to be proved ... my opinion is that they require a huge amount of management and monitoring ... not enough resources within the HSE to ensure that this happens ...

QuADS

That putting these standards and procedures in place would improve drug and alcohol services was the general view from all interviewees:

> D&AC: Within addiction services, we have a strong history of having clear policies and procedures in place ... QuADS are a great thing that has been introduced to addiction services as they pick up on policies that may not have been in place already and create a good quality standard in the delivery of practice ... they protect the service provider and the service user.

> CLDTFC: We are currently going through the QuADS process ... QuADS create good practice and quality in service and in my professional opinion are the best thing ever to come into Cork.

> SAC: QuADS are a slow-burning reality and will take a long time to put into place a record of protocols, policies and procedures ... We have to have these in place to protect us (the service provider) and the service user.

> LW: No experience of QuADS within my organisation, but I do hope they come into effect sooner rather than later.

CONCLUSION

The NDRIC framework is a ground-breaking model to provide a fully integrated service for dealing with drug and alcohol rehabilitation. It is sufficiently robust to deal with health treatments – for example, from detox to counselling to recreation to education to housing, all of which have a strong social care/social educational/social pedagogy focus. It also has SLAs for these areas and areas such as training for the client and advocacy. These should be in place in all drug and alcohol services.

Integrated care pathways are the way forward. This can only happen if people are educated in the success of integrated care so the NDRIC model could be very useful as a tool to foster integrated health and social care education for social care educators.

There is a clear and urgent need to implement this model in full as soon as possible. It has been shown from this research that other areas in the health care systems have gradually become integrated under government policy. The government should make it mandatory that all addiction services buy into the NDRIC model where possible.

The NDRIC model is a clear example of an integrated services model and the learning from its implementation can be diffused to other plans for integration at the micro level to benefit patients and clients across the whole continuum, including mental health patients, disabled service users, older people and many others.

REFERENCES

Department of Community, Rural and Gaeltacht Affairs (DoCRGA) (2009). *National Drugs Strategy 2009-2016*, Dublin: Stationery Office.

Department of Health and Children (DoHC) (2012). *National Drugs Strategy 2009-16: Implementation of Actions Progress Report End 2011*, Dublin: Health Service Executive.

Doocey, A. and Reddy, W. (2010). 'Integrated Care Pathways: The Touchstone of an Integrated Service Delivery Model for Ireland', *National Transformation Programme 1*, Dublin: Health Service Executive.

Doyle, J and Ivanovic, J. (2010). *National Drugs Rehabilitation Framework Document*, National Drugs Rehabilitation Implementation Committee, Dublin: Health Service Executive.

European Monitoring Centre for Drugs and Drug Addiction (2007). *Annual Report 2007: The State of the Drugs Problem in Europe*, Lisbon: European Monitoring Centre for Drugs and Drug Addiction.

Harvey, L. and McDonald, M. (1993). *Doing Sociology*, London: Macmillan.

Health Research Board (HRB) (2011). *Trends in Treated Problem Drug Use in Ireland 2005-2010*, Dublin: Health Research Board.

Health Service Executive (HSE) (2010). *Integrated Services Programme: Integrating Hospital and Community Services*, Overview to Irish Pharmaceutical Healthcare Association, September.

National Advisory Committee on Drugs (NACD) (2012). *General Population Survey on Drug Use in Ireland*, survey by Ipsos MORI, Dublin: NACD.

National Drugs Rehabilitation Implementation Committee (NDRIC) (2011). National Protocols and Common Assessment Guidelines, Dublin: Health Service Executive.

O'Brien, C. (2011). 'Ireland amongst worst for drug deaths', *The Irish Times*, 23 June.

O'Connor, T. and Murphy, M. (2006). *Social Care in Ireland: Theory, Policy and Practice*, Cork: CIT Press.

United Nations Office on Crime and Drugs (UNOCD) (2011). *World Drug Report 2010*, New York: United Nations Publications.

8: THE FUTURE OF INTEGRATED CARE IN IRELAND

Vanessa Hetherington, Faisal Shaikh and Sean Tierney

INTRODUCTION

This book explores many of the aspects of integrated care, including an analysis of a wide range of initiatives in Ireland. However, it is clear that, despite some isolated examples and pilots, the system of health care delivery in Ireland is both highly fragmented and poorly co-ordinated. A partial mix of public and private procurement and delivery has not resulted in the spontaneous evolution of anything approaching an integrated health care system. The *Programme for Government: Towards Recovery, Programme for a National Government 2011-2016* (Fine Gael/ Labour, 2011) sets out a range of measures for reform of the Irish health system based on the Dutch model. In the *Programme for Government*, it is proposed to manage (and increase) competition between public and private health insurers and public and private health care providers. The stated aim of the reform is to develop:

> … a universal, single-tier health service, which guarantees access to medical care based on need, not income. By reforming our model of delivering health care, so that more care is delivered in the community, and by reforming how we pay for health care through Universal Health Insurance, we can reduce the cost of achieving the best health outcomes for our citizens, and end the unfair, unequal and inefficient two-tier health system (Fine Gael/Labour, 2011).

In this chapter, we will examine the challenges that will need to be overcome in transforming Ireland's health care delivery system into a fully-integrated model. In particular, we will explore the challenges in using a market-based model to drive integration.

GOVERNMENT PROPOSALS 2011-2016

Under Universal Health Insurance (UHI), based on the Dutch model of competing private insurers, the Health Service Executive (HSE) will cease to exist. The functions of the HSE as a service commissioner would be taken over by insurance companies. Public health functions, presumably, would return to the Minister for Health and the Department of Health (DoH). Service provision would be taken over by service providers, funded either directly by the insurers under a service level agreement or on a 'fee per item' system of reimbursement. In the case of primary care, exchequer funding would be transferred initially to a primary care fund but then phased out as mandatory insurance is phased in. While insurance will be compulsory, payment will be related to ability to pay and the State will subsidise in whole or in part insurance premiums for people on low incomes.

Primary care will be made universally available, funded by insurance, but there may well be some co-payments at the point of use. However, general practitioners (GPs) would be paid primarily by capitation for the care of their patients. Public hospitals would be amalgamated into independent, not-for-profit trusts, and funded on the basis of activity ('money follows the patient'). These trusts would compete for contracts with other (for profit) providers.

There is some tension between the stated goals of creating an integrated system of primary and hospital care and the use of the market model of care with competing insurers and competing providers to achieve this. Integration, as we have seen in this book, is usually managed centrally whether by a public body or a private insurer. While the *Programme for Government* (Fine Gael/Labour, 2011) does provide for an Integrated Care Agency to oversee the flow of centrally (tax) funded resources between the different arms of the system, the intent appears to rely primarily on competitive market forces. Previous experience in Ireland of rebalancing funding between insurers (risk-equalisation) and service users (community rating) have been largely ineffective in the private insured health care sector (Irish Medical Organisation (IMO), 2012).

The theme of providing integrated care runs through the implementation plan for the *Programme for Government* in the Department of Health *Statement of Strategy 2011-2014* (DoH, 2012), which includes a number of measures intended to enable integration of care, including:

- The development of electronic health information systems to deliver more integrated and more cost-effective patient care with legislation to enable the use of unique patient identifiers;

- The re-organisation of hospital services, including through the development of the Smaller Hospitals Framework, so that patients receive high quality care in the most appropriate setting, resulting in the best possible outcomes for their health;

- The development of the National Clinical Programmes system, promoting service integration between the acute hospital sector and primary care primarily in a disease- or speciality-based approach;

- The introduction of programme-based budgeting and a 'money follows the patient' financing mechanism for hospital services;

- The development of primary care services and the building of primary care centres;

- The development of clinical care pathways and chronic disease management programmes throughout the primary care sector, to be facilitated by new contractual arrangements with GPs.

SPECIFIC CHALLENGES AND CONSIDERATIONS

Clearly, there is a wide range of issues to be considered and addressed if the government is to deliver on its stated policy of providing integrated care to the population. Among those issues, we consider the most critical to be:

- Effective use of information;

- Appropriate standardisation of care through the use of protocols;

- Effective management of resource allocation (particularly for primary care); and

- Appropriate incentivising of care providers.

Many of the other issues have been considered in specific contexts elsewhere in the book. In this chapter, we will consider these key issues in detail.

Information and Communications Technology

Information and communications technology (ICT) is widely considered a key tool for supporting/assisting integrated health care systems and the 'seamless' transfer of patients between clinical settings. Electronic patient records can be stored centrally or in the 'cloud', retrieved at the point of care (wherever this may be) and updated much more effectively, leading to administrative and clinical efficiencies. The use of ICT in health care (e-health) allows for the more efficient transfer of patient information between health care settings, enhancing patient safety and quality of care, by reducing repetition and errors in diagnostics and treatments. Collection of individual patient data supports the effective application of disease management protocols. In addition, aggregate data can be used for medical research, and health service planning.

While the benefits of e-health are considerable, these cannot be realised unless issues of interoperability, patient safety and patient confidentiality are addressed.

A report prepared for the European Commission DG Information Society and Media (Kenny *et al.*, 2010) on the development and progress of e-health solutions in Ireland, found:

> Overall, in order to resolve remaining obstacles for the development and deployment of interconnected system for patient data transfer, a governance structure is needed, which provides the framework for:
> - Legitimate uses of an individual's medical data;
> - Access rights of the main actors;
> - Security policies and standards that will need to be applied;
> - Patient consent policy;
> - Standards that must be applied to all data extracts/clinical findings and other observations;
> - Legal framework that will govern the new EHR service (Kenny *et al.*, 2010).

While many health care organisations are reaping the advantages of e-health, the development of ICT systems in Irish health care is taking place in an *ad hoc* fashion. In the absence of a single national system of electronic health records, the interoperability of ICT systems used in different health care settings is essential if the wider benefits of e-health are to be realised in Ireland. The interoperability of ICT systems requires:

- The data structure and minimum data set within the systems to be standardised;
- Convergence of taxonomy and terminology; and
- Messaging standards for the exchange of data between systems to be adopted.

Without the early adoption of interoperability standards, considerable wastage may occur as current ICT projects require upgrading or replacement.

The responsibility to define and mandate standards falls to the Health Information and Quality Authority (HIQA) and while there has been some progress made in addressing these issues, such as the HIQA *General Practice Messaging Standard* (HIQA, 2011a) and the establishment of the e-Health Standards Advisory Committee within HIQA to develop National e-Health Interoperability Standards for Ireland (HIQA, 2011b), the issues have yet to be addressed comprehensively.

In addition to interoperability standards and secure communication, the use of e-health to support integrated care raises obvious issues of patient safety and confidentiality. As patient data is transferred between settings, it is important that individuals accessing the data are securely identified. In addition, they should be able to access only appropriate parts of the health care record. Confidentiality is central to the doctor-patient relationship and disclosure of patient information to others is only allowed under strict conditions (Medical Council, 2009). Unique identifiers for patients and practitioners would help resolve issues of patient and practitioner identity. However, there is an urgent need for legislation to clarify issues of confidentiality, access and security in relation to electronic health records and secondary use of data. Much of this must be addressed in the *Health Information Act*.

Standardised Care Delivery through Shared Protocols

Shared protocols, such as those developed by the HSE's clinical care programmes and care pathways, contribute to integrated care by standardising care across services and sites. These protocols also promote continuity of care by defining roles and responsibilities for all team members/providers involved in the care process (Suter *et al.*, 2009). Strong leadership and clinician engagement (across providers) in the process are essential in the successful development and deployment of clinical protocols. Performance measurement (of processes and outcomes) and management (linking outcomes to reimbursement) are important aids in ensuring these protocols are applied effectively (Suter *et al.*, 2009). However, protocols also may have unintended consequences in discouraging individualised care and promoting 'gaming', such as manipulation of waiting lists, etc.

Currently, under the Hospital Transformation Programme, the HSE is developing a range of clinical programmes and the National Clinical Effectiveness Committee within the DoH is aggregating a National Suite of Clinical Guidelines.

While the goal of clinical protocols is to improve quality of care and cost-effectiveness, there is a danger, due to resource constraints or the time lag involved in the gathering of evidence and incorporating it into formal quality-assured clinical guidelines, that protocols may not be up to date nor result in the optimal clinical outcome. The burden of ensuring that the guidelines and protocols are regularly revised in the light of outcome and best practice data may be considerable.

Clinical protocols also usually are disease-focused and thus designed to be applied to population groups with similar morbidity. However, they may not factor in co-morbidity or the impact of individual patient characteristics that may make the protocolised care inappropriate. Furthermore, patient-centred care is about patients being involved and making informed decisions about their own care, based on their own values rather than population norms (Mulsow *et al.*, 2012). The development of clinical programmes and performance measurement systems place an emphasis on standard processes and outcomes and do not consider the needs and wishes of individual patients. In a recent review of 16 pilot integrated care projects in the UK (Rand Europe, Ernst and Young LLP (REEY), 2012), staff reported process-related improvements in care but patients did not appear to share the same sense of improvement.

In that study (REEY, 2012), the review team found strong leadership and staff engagement were key facilitators of success of integrated care pilots. Health care providers reported that teamworking, communication and work patterns had improved. Many had taken on extra responsibilities and felt that their job was more interesting, though there was a need for extra training. Patients did report receiving care plans more frequently and that their care was better co-ordinated on discharge from hospital. However, patients found it significantly more difficult to see a nurse of their choice, felt they were listened to less frequently and less involved in decisions about their care. The reviewers concluded that:

> The focus on the needs and preferences of end users can easily be lost in the challenging task of building the organisational platform for integration and in organising new methods of delivering professional care (REEY, 2012).

Adequate Resourcing of Integrated Primary Care

The development of an integrated, team-based, user-friendly primary care system for Ireland was adopted as government policy in the 2001 strategy *Primary Care: A New Direction* (Department of Health and Children, 2001). The key objective of this strategy was to provide patients with 'one-stop-shop' access to a range of health care providers, including GPs, psychologists, physiotherapists, public health nurses, social workers, practice nurses, midwives, community mental health nurses, dieticians, dentists, community welfare officers, occupational therapists, home helps, health care assistants, speech and language therapists, chiropodists, community pharmacists, and others. Primary care teams (PCTs) were to have direct access to diagnostic services and shared care arrangements were to be put in place for patients with chronic disease.

There have been a number of problems with the delivery of these PCTs from which important lessons should be learned. At the end of 2008, less than 100 PCTs were in place (HSE, 2009). While the HSE reported having increased the number of teams to 425 by 2011 (HSE, 2011), these vary considerably in the level of implementation and some merely hold a multi-disciplinary meeting. In contrast, a study by the Irish College of General Practitioners (ICGP) in 2011 found that only 58% of GPs are part of a PCT and the majority (64.6%) felt the team functioned poorly (ICGP, 2011). Just 8% of PCTs are fully co-located and there is wide variation in access to ancillary services both within and outside PCTs. Even successful teams are starting to feel the pressure of reduced funding and an embargo on recruitment leading to community waiting lists.

At the same time, public expenditure on health has been cut by over 11% from €15.073bn in 2009 to €13.317bn in 2012. Hospital services, particularly non-urgent services, also are being curtailed as staff numbers are cut. A complex mix of funding means that many patients, who are entitled to free hospital care (which may not, in fact, have been adequately funded), have to pay out-of-pocket for certain services when they are provided in the community, even if they have private health insurance. In some cases, community services are provided only to those with medical cards, meaning some patients cannot access those services at all.

There is a perception that many of these services will be developed in primary care as resources are transferred from the hospital sector. However, many of these services have never been adequately funded in the hospital sector. Nor is it certain that the transfer of allied health professionals to community clinics will be cost-neutral, due to the loss of some of the economies of scale and the greater resilience of larger services to cope with absences, staff turnover, and training.

While it is expected that integrated care systems can lead to both administrative and clinical cost savings, integration processes may require additional initial investment before any savings become apparent (Suter *et al.*, 2009). Integrated care will not resolve inadequate resourcing of services (World Health Organization (WHO), 2008) and new activities cannot be integrated successfully without an increase in resources (WHO, 2008). Seeking to raise these resources directly from patients, in the form of co-payments, (particularly where the amounts are large) may deter patients from seeking appropriate medical care and lead them to rely on more complex (and expensive) care later.

A key element of effective integration is seamless programmes of chronic disease management based in primary care rather than specialist units. Chronic disease management programmes have been operational in the US for over a decade, particularly in managed care systems. More recently, they have spread to health systems in Western Europe and their introduction have been proposed in Ireland. Exemplar programmes have shown improvements in service utilisation, reduction in cost and improvements in quality of care. The main benefits are reduction in unplanned hospital admissions, length of hospital stay, urgent care visits and significant reductions in medication utilisation. Moreover, patient and family satisfaction has been shown to be increased (HSE, 2012).

Such programmes require substantial resources in primary care. Ireland has approximately 58 GPs per 100,000 population (FÁS, 2009), which is below the EU average and well below those systems operating effective integrated care systems. In addition, those GPs that we do have are unevenly distributed geographically, a situation that may be exacerbated by recent deregulation of general practice under the terms of the EU/IMF bailout.

Incentivising Providers

Traditional payment models tend either to promote 'activity' (fee per item) or to penalise it (fixed budgets), neither of which may be matched to patient needs. In the context of integrated care, an alternative model of bundled payments has emerged, particularly in The Netherlands and among Accountable Care organisations in the US (Struijs and Baan, 2011).

Bundled payment systems provide a single fee to a health care provider for all services related to a specific treatment or condition. The contracting entity either provides all the services or manages the subcontracting of some services to other providers. Bundled payments systems are intended to drive cost reduction, as they provide an incentive to eliminate unnecessary services. Effective care may reduce long-term costs as complications are avoided or at least delayed. However, the exact content of the care bundle must be carefully defined as there is an incentive for both payers and providers to stint on care in order to contain costs.

In 2007, bundled payments were introduced in The Netherlands on an experimental basis for diabetes care and expanded in 2010 to COPD and CVD risk management. Insurers pay a single fee to a 'care group' to cover a full range of integrated chronic disease care services. A care group usually consists of a number of care providers (often exclusively GPs), who assume clinical and financial responsibility for all assigned patients, delivering care themselves or subcontracting with other care providers. The price of the bundle is freely negotiated between insurers and care groups and between care groups and subcontracted providers (Struijs and Baan, 2011).

A one-year review of bundled payments to diabetes care groups found that rates charged under bundled payment contracts varied widely from €258 to €474 per patient per year and were explained in part by differences in care provided (Struijs *et al.*, 2010). All bundle payments conformed to standards of care as established by the Dutch Diabetes Federation in terms of recommended number of check-ups, laboratory examinations and annual eye and foot examinations, while differences lay in additional GP consultations, guidance on smoking cessation or foot care. Inexperience of both insurers and providers in setting prices is thought also to have contributed to the price variation. However, variations persisted in 2008, 2009 and 2010, perhaps due to differing interpretation of the standards by insurers seeking to avoid costs. The appropriate cost of these diabetes care bundles is not known.

In addition:

- All providers reported that the care delivery process had improved, as care groups were fully responsible for organisational arrangements defining who is responsible for what care at what price and for the co-ordination of care;
- Subcontractors complained that the negotiating power of care groups distorted the market and that, by working with preferred providers, patient choice was limited;
- No considerable changes in outcomes were found after one year. Performance on most quality indicators was already good at baseline;
- Transparency of care improved due to record-keeping obligations.

While the bundling model is based on process with an assumption that this will result in better outcomes, there is an alternative strategy of payments based on 'performance' (P4P). In reality, outcomes are difficult to measure effectively or are too remote to be useful in determining reimbursement. Many systems of P4P rely, in fact, on measuring process. Mullen *et al.* have shown that, rather than encouraging providers to shift resources toward quality improvement, P4P is likely to encourage providers to focus on narrow (incentivised) areas (Mullen *et al.*, 2010). The authors concluded that they failed "to find evidence that a large P4P initiative either resulted in major improvement in quality or notable disruption in care".

In contrast, a large study in the UK of the introduction of the Quality Outcomes Framework in over 8,000 GP practices found that there was a high rate of compliance with targets (83%). The study used over 100 indicators across 10 chronic diseases and GPs were well incentivised, as practice earnings increased by an average of over 30% (Doran *et al.*, 2006). Such incentives are not likely to be sustained, as indicators and targets are continuously revised but it is likely that some measures of performance will form part of the basis for payment in integrated care systems in future.

CONCLUSION

In general, Ireland's health care system currently is fragmented and poorly co-ordinated. While government policy has consistently defined an integrated care model as being desirable, the challenges of aligning ICT systems, shared care protocols, resources and payment incentives without losing focus on patient-centred care should not be underestimated. The deployment of UHI in and of itself will not ensure that care delivery becomes more integrated. Indeed, funding systems based on market forces, competing insurers and competing providers may militate against the effective integration of care, especially in a small market. Tight regulation may ameliorate this problem but it is difficult to be sure how effective or affordable this approach will be. Centrally-managed systems (like Kaiser Permanente in the US or the NHS in the UK) that are not-for-profit arguably are more effective at controlling costs while maintaining quality.

REFERENCES

Department of Health and Children (2001). *Primary Care: A New Direction*, Dublin: Stationery Office, available http://www.dohc.ie/publications/primary_care_a_new_direction.html.

Department of Health (DoH) (2012). *Department of Health Statement of Strategy 2011-2014*, Dublin, available http://www.dohc.ie/publications/pdf/Statement_of_Strategy_2011-2014.pdf.

Doran, T., Fullwood, C., Gravelle, H., Reeves, D., Kontopantelis, E., Hiroeh, U. and Roland, M. (2006). 'Pay-for-Performance Programs in Family Practices in the United Kingdom', *New England Journal of Medicine*, 355: 375-384.

FÁS (2009). *A Quantitative Tool for Workforce Planning in Health Care: Example Simulations*, Dublin: FÁS Skills and Labour Market Research Unit, available http://www.fas.ie/ NR/rdonlyres/9ABC5EE1-CF20-4AA5-ACA4-

C5B81DD9FE5E/792/SLMRU_FAS_EGFSN_Final_Version_Report_AQuantit
ative.pdf.

Fine Gael/Labour (2011). *Programme for Government: Towards Recovery, Programme for a National Government 2011-2016*, Dublin: Fine Gael/Labour.

Health Information and Quality Authority (HIQA) (2011a). *General Practice Messaging Standard Version 2.0*, Cork: HIQA, available http://www.hiqa.ie/publications/general-practice-messaging-standard-version-20.

Health Information and Quality Authority (HIQA) (2011b). *Developing National eHealth Interoperability Standards for Ireland: A Consultation Document*, Cork: HIQA, available http://www.hiqa.ie/publications/ developing-national-ehealth-interoperability-standards-ireland-consultation-document.

Health Service Executive (HSE) (2009). 'Opening Statement to the Joint Committee on Health and Children on Primary Care Team Developments' by Ms Laverne McGuinness, National Director, PCCC HSE, available http://www.hse.ie/eng/ News/National_Tab/Opening_Statement_to_the_Joint_Committee_on_Health_and_Children_on_Primary_Care_Team_Developments_by_Ms_Laverne_McGuinness,_National_Director,_PCCC_HSE.shortcut.html, accessed June 2009.

Health Service Executive (HSE) (2011). *Performance Report on National Service Plan, December 2011*, available http://www.hse.ie/eng/services/Publications/corporate/ performancereports/2011prs.html.

Health Service Executive (HSE) (2012). *HSE Model of Care*, available http://www.hse.ie/ eng/staff/Resources/FactFile/Health_Status_Reports/Population_Health/HSE_Model_of_Care/.

Irish College of General Practitioners (ICGP) (2011). *Primary Care Teams – A GP Perspective*, Dublin: ICGP, available http://www.icgp.ie/go/about/news/CF613CF0-19B9-E185-83176841131F682B.html.

Irish Medical Organisation (IMO) (2012). *IMO Position Paper on The Market Model of Health – Caveat Emptor*, Dublin: IMO, available http://www.imo.ie/policy-international-affair/research-policy/imo-position-papers/.

Mulsow, J.J.W., Feeley, M.T. and Tierney, S. (2012). 'Beyond Consent – Improving Understanding in Surgical Patients', *American Journal of Surgery*, 203(1): 112-120.

Kenny, T., Giest, S., Dumortier, J. and Artmann, J.E. (2010). *Health Strategies: Country Brief: Ireland*, Bonn/Brussels: European Commission, DG Information Society and Media, ICT for Health Unit, available http://ehealth-strategies.eu/database/documents/ Ireland_CountryBrief_eHStrategies.pdf.

Medical Council (2009). *Guide to Professional Conduct and Ethics for Registered Medical Practitioners*, 7th edition, Dublin: Medical Council, available http://www.medicalcouncil.ie/Information-for-Doctors/Professional-Conduct-Ethics/.

Mullen, K.J., Frank, R.G. and Rosenthal M.B. (2010). 'Can You Get What You Pay For? Pay-for-performance and the Quality of Health Care Providers', *RAND Journal of Economics*, 41: 64-91.

Rand Europe, Ernst and Young LLP (REEY) (2012). *National Evaluation of the Department of Health's Integrated Care Pilots Prepared for the Department of Health*, Cambridge: RAND Europe, available http://www.dh.gov.uk/en/

Publicationsandstatistics/Publications/PublicationsPolicyAndGuidance/DH
_133124.

Struijs, J.N. and Baan, C.A. (2011). 'Integrating Care through Bundled Payments –
Lessons from The Netherlands', *New England Journal of Medicine*, 364: 990-991.

Struijs, J.N., van Til, J.T. and Baan, C.A. (2010). *Experimenting with a Bundled
Payment System for Diabetes Care in The Netherlands - The First Tangible Effects*,
Bilthoven: National Institute for Public Health and the Environment, available
http://www.rivm.nl/Bibliotheek/Wetenschappelijk/Rapporten/2010/
oktober/Experimenting_with_a_bundled_payment_system_for_diabetes_car
e_in_the_Netherlands_The_first_tangible_effects.

Suter, E., Oelke, N.D., Adair, C.E. and Armitage, G.D. (2009). 'Ten Key Principles
for Successful Health Systems Integration', *Health Care Quarterly*, 13(Special):
16-23.

World Health Organization (WHO) (2008). *Integrated Health Services – What and
Why? – Technical Brief No.1*, Geneva: WHO, available http://www.who.int/
healthsystems/technical_brief_final.pdf.

SECTION III: INTERPROFESSIONAL CHALLENGES: POLICY TRANSLATION AND PRACTICAL DELIVERY

9: CHALLENGES FOR PRIMARY CARE ON THE ROAD TO INTEGRATED CARE

Diarmuid Quinlan and Joe Moran

INTRODUCTION

General practice is crucial in the delivery of high quality, cost-effective health care in Ireland. The challenge facing government, physicians and patients is to satisfy increasing demand for high quality health care, at a time of spiralling costs and diminishing financial resources. General practitioners (GPs) provide care across the spectrum of patients and pathology, from antenatal care right through to terminal illness. We never discharge our patients. General practice is the first point of contact for patients with acute, undifferentiated illness. GPs play a crucial role as both gatekeepers and navigators of the health care system. We are key agents in health promotion, and carry an increasing role in management of chronic disease. For general practice to prosper, we need sufficient GPs, spending sufficient time with patients, with the appropriate training to equip GPs with the necessary competencies to deliver high quality care in the 21st century. General practice is increasingly centre stage and mission critical to drive and implement service quality improvement.

Consequently, this chapter examines some key challenges that need to be addressed within the new era of higher expectations for primary care set out in the Department of Health and Children's (DoHC) *Primary Care Strategy* (2001). The chapter starts by outlining the history and structure of GP services in Ireland alongside the unique role and functions of the GP.

It then discusses the status of the GP within the field of medicine and the organisational structure of health delivery across the different levels of care. It proceeds with a discussion of the role of the GP in family and community life and the GP's role as a patient advocate.

Following on, the chapter comments on the importance of new technology for GP practice in recent years, most notably the mobile phone. The pivotal importance of the out-of-hours (OOH) service and the Continuous Medical Education (CME) network for GPs is also highlighted.

The focus then moves on to highlight the rationale for the increased emphasis on GP care, alongside inconsistent public policy challenges that continue to impact on primary care. In the context of a population health approach, this starts with the model of GP remuneration. Case studies of three significant diseases posing particular challenges to public health are then examined: asthma, diabetes and haemochromatosis. This discussion will highlight the poor record of progress within public health policy to date in incentivising and enhancing the role of GPs in the treatment of these conditions, which pose consistently high demands on GP practice. Finally, consideration is given to the feminisation of GP practice and the appropriate model for a GP OOH service.

The approach in this chapter is to use our experience as GPs over a considerable number of years to highlight issues 'at the coal face' and to point to published evidence where significant improvements can be made in Ireland that could positively impact on patients and would help in the process of delivering the proposed new era for primary care in Ireland as suggested in numerous policy documents in recent years by the Health Service Executive (HSE) and the Department of Health (DoH).

THE HISTORICAL BACKGROUND TO GENERAL PRACTITIONER SERVICES IN IRELAND

In Ireland, the Choice of Doctor/General Medical Services (GMS) scheme introduced in 1972 replaced the old Dispensary Doctor scheme. GPs now operated on a fee per item basis and patients had a choice of GP, for the first time. This removed the differences between public and private patients. All patients were free to attend the doctor's surgery. Prior to this, public patients were seen in the local dispensary and private patients usually attended the local doctor's private house or surgery. This barrier was now removed. This contract was amended in 1989. GP units were set up by the Health Boards and GP unit doctors were retained to help advise the DoH on matters relevant to general practice. The importance and role of these units seems to have lessened in recent years and they do not appear to have any function in policy-making. They seem to function primarily as a local 'problem-solving' resource for local HSE issues.

However, the introduction of 'drug budgeting' was the first widespread effort to provide funding for the development of general practice. This was introduced in the mid-1990s. Subsequently, the *Primary Care Strategy* was introduced (DoHC, 2001) and all DoHC/DoH plans since then for GP or primary care development have been referenced to this in the areas of: sole practice/group practice; practice nursing; and special interest – for example, family planning/surgery/diabetes.

THE CURRENT MODEL OF GENERAL PRACTICE

In the current hierarchical structure of Irish medicine, general practice has the lowest 'status' among the rest of the medical profession, HSE management and the public. This has resulted in underfunding of general practice education, training, research and, most importantly, service delivery. One of the basic problems facing general practice at present is the serious gap between primary care and secondary and tertiary care services. Primary, secondary and tertiary care all have their own, seemingly autonomous worlds and associated agendas. These worlds do not embrace each other and do not seem to have a shared mission or value system. There are many gaps between the three organisational layers of service delivery. Many of these gaps have their origins in attitudinal or cultural issues and will not necessarily be solved by 'throwing money at the problem'. This situation compromises the quality of patient care in many ways – for example, unnecessarily long waiting lists; limited GP access to diagnostic services; and poor quality communication when patients are being admitted and discharged from the hospital system, to name a few. We believe that a 'cultural shift' needs to occur throughout the current health care system in order for these problems to be resolved. Paradoxically, the current economic crises may provide the catalyst for these changes. This shift needs to occur also among other health care professionals, the DoH, the HSE management and politicians. Otherwise, the current high level of confusion is unlikely to facilitate high quality clinical care.

A GP is primarily a skilled front-line clinician able to respond in an appropriate, patient-centred manner to whatever problem the patient presents with. The GP aims to work with patients and their families to obtain the optimum result for the patient. The GP is community-based and is skilled in working with other health care providers, where appropriate, for their patients' benefit. The GP is a generalist and recognises the strengths and weaknesses of generalist knowledge. GPs are a resource to the wider community and make themselves available to their communities – for example, presenting at health information sessions or giving classes in their local schools. Finally, the GP is an expert on the 'doctor-patient' relationship and uses this expertise to improve the care to their patients. The care provided by GPs to an individual frequently extends over many years and even generations. This 'continuity of care' is generally valued by patients and GPs. It usually, but not always, facilitates the provision of high quality care. As a result of this long-term relationship, the GP is frequently in a position to act as an advocate for his/her patients.

GENERAL PRACTICE: SOME INNOVATIONS

The local GP is enmeshed in family and community life. Prior to the introduction of the mobile phone in the 1990s, the GP's extended family, particularly in rural areas, were involved in providing services to the patient. They 'manned' the home phone and made themselves available to the public 24/7. Their contribution to the provision of front-line health services has not been recognised and should be. The introduction of the mobile phone liberated these people from this thankless task. At this time, again particularly in small towns and rural areas, patients would frequently call to the doctor's house, especially after hours. Indeed the concept of 'after-hours' did not exist at this time. It fell to the members of the doctor's family to meet and initially 'triage' these patients, often without any medical training or background. The recent professionalisation of OOH care, combined with the spread of mobile phone technology, has moved patient contact away from the local GP's house to local call centres. This has been a major change for many patients and not without its difficulties.

A further tangible benefit to GP practice has been the introduction of the CME network to facilitate ongoing GP education. CME network development has had the effect of reducing the professional isolation of single-handed GPs. It also had the effect of uniting GPs and reducing some of the competition between them. Ironically, the current Competition Authority wants to foster competition between GPs. However, the authors feel that this reveals a lack of understanding of the role and functions of general practice and that this increased competition will result in lowered standards of patient care, not increased standards as they envision. Clinical Societies around the country have also been a source of CME and social contact for many GPs over the past 25 years.

PUBLIC POLICY CHALLENGES FOR GENERAL PRACTITIONER SERVICES

Rationale and Remuneration

In this context of the current model of GP practice as outlined, there is increasing emphasis on delivering health care in the community, partly to improve access for patients and partly to curtail healthcare costs. Unfortunately this shift in workload often is not accompanied by a simultaneous migration of resources. Further, the current model of remuneration for GPs, where they are mainly self-employed small businesspeople, in competition with each other, needs to be critically examined within Irish public health policy. In our view, this model can create conflicts of interest for the doctor. Of great significance is the fact that no other health care professional is remunerated in this manner. There is an urgent need for a public policy debate around this anomalous situation, which is unfavourable to patients and practitioners alike.

Asthma

Within the population health approach, the GP has a key role to play. The GP is the first point of contact for most users of the health services and deals with diseases that are often particularly acute and affect significant proportions of the population. In order to underline the critical importance of the GP in this context, asthma is the first of three illnesses examined.

Ireland has the fourth highest prevalence of asthma in the world, at 14% (Masoli *et al.*, 2004). Ireland had 62 reported asthma deaths in 2011 (Central Statistics Office, 2011). This is more than one person dying of asthma every week! Ireland is reported as having the highest rate of paediatric admissions and prevalence of an asthma attack in the previous 12 months (European Federation of Allergy and Airways Diseases Patients Association, 2004). In the years 2005-2009, Ireland had an average of 4,753 hospital admissions *per annum*, with an average length of stay of 3.1 days (Economic and Social Research Institute (ESRI) and HSE, 2005-2009). Attendances at emergency departments are estimated at 19,000 *per annum* for the same period (ESRI and HSE, 2005-2009). The primary care reimbursement service 2005-2009 reports an average of 50,559 emergency nebuliser treatments provided yearly for acute asthma attacks, costing in excess of €2 million (HSE, 2009). This is a staggering number of emergency asthma treatments in a small country.

Asthma treatment in Ireland can learn from the UK, where the National Health Service (NHS) introduced the Quality and Outcomes

Framework (QOF) in 2004 (NHS Employers, 2011). Diseases chosen were those that are common and/or important, where chronic management rests primarily with the GP and which were both evidence-based/ guideline-driven to deliver improved management results. The QOF explicitly rewards practices for objective provision of high quality care. It standardises the delivery of medical care, helping reduce regional variations in quality of care – what is sometimes called 'post code medicine'. The indicators of quality are patient-focused and evidence-based, whereby data collection is minimised and never duplicated (NHS Employers, 2011). An important feature of the QOF is establishing and maintaining disease registers (NHS Employers, 2011).

The quality indicators for asthma, which generate payment in practices, are:

• Establishment of an asthma register;

• Objective measurement of airway function;

• Documentation of smoking status;

• Asthma review undertaken and documented in the preceding 15 months.

These quality markers are derived from both the British Thoracic Society and the Scottish Intercollegiate Guidelines Network (SIGN) guidelines. The guidance explicitly states:

> It is important that resources in primary care are targeted to patients with greatest need – in this instance, patients who will benefit from asthma review rather than insistence that all patients with a diagnostic label of asthma are reviewed on a regular basis (NHS Employers, 2011).

The success in the UK lies in sharp contrast to the documented outcomes in Ireland, as outlined above: almost 20,000 A&E attendances and nearly 5,000 hospital admissions, and 62 asthma deaths in 2011 (ESRI and HSE, 2005-2009). The UK system rewards clinical excellence; the Irish system does not. The sole payment for asthma management under the GMS is a fee for nebulisation of a patient with asthma. This is a perverse disincentive to high quality structured care.

One of the authors currently is participating in a joint Irish Asthma Society/Irish College of General Practitioners (ICGP) asthma initiative. This initiative is modelled on the Finnish Asthma programme. Finland has a population size similar to Ireland. The Finns initiated high quality, research-based, and primary care-delivered asthma management commencing in 1994 (Haahtela et al., 2006). Over the following decade, the Finns reduced asthma deaths by over 50% and reduced hospitalisation by 69%, while halting the previously inexorable rise in asthma medication costs (Haahtela *et al.*, 2006):

> The essence of long term success is to keep alive the network of contact persons, GPs, nurses, and pharmacists ... the shift in care from specialist to primary health providers has taken place over the whole country (Finland) (Haahtela *et al.*, 2006).

Is it unreasonable to ask that, almost two decades later, we could tentatively imitate such a successful and cost-effective model of asthma care?

Diabetes and Structured Care

The NHS QOF makes the following observations:

> Diabetes mellitus is one of the common endocrine diseases affecting all age groups in the UK. Effective control and monitoring can reduce mortality and morbidity. Much of the management and monitoring of diabetic patients, particularly patients with Type 2 diabetes is undertaken by the GP. The quality indicators for diabetes are based on widely recognised approaches to the care of diabetes (NHS Employers, 2011).

In acknowledging the complexity of management, 15 quality indicators are described, each attracting a different payment. No such incentives are available across Ireland.

In Ireland, McHugh *et al.* made a comparison between the performance of three primary care-led diabetes schemes in Ireland with the relative results available from England and Scotland (McHugh *et al.*, 2011). The findings clearly demonstrated that a similar proportion of patients achieved relevant clinical targets in both Ireland and the UK, in that:

> The quality of primary care-led diabetes management in the three initiatives studied appears broadly consistent with results from the UK (McHugh *et al.*, 2011).

Nonetheless, the need within Irish primary care for continuing professional education, the establishment and maintenance of diabetes registers, together with the enhanced use of guidelines and audit is highlighted. Allied to this is the availability of other professional supports, endocrinologists, dieticians, podiatry, diabetic nurse specialists, in a timely and focused fashion. The lack of incentives to participate in high-quality structured care in Ireland is a barrier, which in other countries has been addressed.

The alternative model of care is to refer these patients with diabetes into the secondary care system. Within the hospital system, the HSE then will fund care at much greater cost. The ease of access provided by a local GP is highly valued by our patients. They can choose a date and time to receive their diabetes review, rather than the date and time determined by a hospital outpatient clinic. The continued delivery of such care and expansion to other patients is critically dependent on state funding, as happens in the NHS. Primary care delivers on quality, access and cost. Primary care is mission critical in diabetes management.

Haemochromatosis and Structured Care

"Too much iron nearly killed me". (*Irish Independent*, February 2008)

Hereditary haemochromatosis (HHC) is a hereditary condition in which excessive amounts of iron are absorbed from the diet and stored in a variety of organs, including the liver, heart, pancreas and joints. HHC is more common in Ireland than anywhere else in the world and has been dubbed 'the Celtic mutation'. Approximately 1% of Irish people have HHC; most are unaware of this ticking time bomb (House, 2009). Based on prevalence of 1 in 100, and with a population of 4 million, some 40,000 individuals in Ireland are estimated to have HHC (DoHC, 2006).

A DoHC working group on HHC was established in March 2006, and reported just three months later (DoHC, 2006). The chairman, Dr. Manning, reported:

> HHC is a potentially life-threatening illness, which affects a sizeable number of Irish people. It is also an illness which can be easily and inexpensively detected. If caught on time HHC responds to relatively easy and inexpensive treatment. This is an illness which exists largely below the radar; its existence is unknown to many people, including some people in the medical profession, policy-makers and opinion-formers (DoHC, 2006).

The report attempts to establish the extent of HHC in Ireland and the steps needed to accurately identify, quantify and manage the condition, especially since current figures almost certainly underestimate the extent of the problem. The report examines such issues as the need for screening and awareness programmes, support for existing sufferers of HHC, the role of the Irish Haemochromatosis Association, the use of blood donated by HHC patients, discrimination by insurance companies and other related issues. This report represents a serious opportunity to focus public attention on HHC and to put in place, at relatively low cost, a series of measures that will have positive consequences at a far greater level than the costs incurred. It is clear that, in most cases, once detected, the disease can be effectively treated. Identification of the predisposition early in the course of the disease permits effective prevention. This report is a wake-up call, proposing a series of easily implementable recommendations which need to be implemented with urgency (DoHC, 2006). A deafening silence followed the publication of the report.

In the absence of treatment, liver disease is the commonest cause of death in patients with HHC. Hepatocellular carcinoma accounts for 30% of all deaths in HHC, while other complications of cirrhosis account for an additional 20% (DoHC, 2006). The morbidity and mortality of HHC can be reduced by early diagnosis and treatment to remove excess iron (venesection). Early diagnosis is therefore important, as life expectancy in treated non-cirrhotic patients is normal. Lack of early detection is a concern, as treatment does not reverse damage such as cirrhosis or diabetes.

The report makes 20 recommendations. The following are amongst the most important of the report's recommendations (and numbered accordingly):

2. The Health Service Executive should aim to ensure early diagnosis of HHC in order to prevent the onset of a range of serious medical conditions.

4. Funding must be prioritised to develop a HHC screening programme.

17. Venesection services should be established by the Irish Blood Transfusion Service at the earliest date and not later than during 2007.

19. The cost of up to €600 for venesection treatment in public hospitals is a dissuasive element. The Department of Health and Children should consider introducing a standard fee (or removing this fee altogether) in order to attract more people to attend for regular venesection.

20. Venesection is currently not covered by the GMS if undertaken by a GP. Arrangements should be made by the HSE to reimburse GPs for providing venesection in their surgeries. This would help to reduce the number of persons attending hospital unnecessarily. (DoHC, 2006: 8, 10, 22)

To date, none of the recommendations above have been fully implemented. The absence of a national programme six years later is indefensible. The HSE provides venesection free of charge to holders of medical cards in hospital only. However, in using hospitals to provide venesection, access is inconvenient and the financial cost to the HSE substantial. The role of general practice is ignored. This goes against the published reports by DoH and HSE which put primary care and integrated care as a central public health priority.

The Increasing Feminisation of General Practice

The growing importance of primary care, integrated care and population health means that a continuous supply of well-qualified GPs going forward is vital. For this reason, apart from the obvious need to ensure gender equity, the increased participation of women in family practice is very welcome. Family practice can only benefit from this increased participation, with both Ireland and the UK moving firmly in this direction. Dr. Clare Gerada is a London GP and chair of the Royal College of General Practitioners (RCGP). She is the first female to hold this post since 1961. The RCGP chair changes every three years, so Dr. Gerada represents a relatively recent departure within the hierarchy of general practice. The chairing of the RCGP by a woman in the UK for the first time in 50 years is clearly consistent with recent evidence for Ireland whereby almost three-quarters of the ICGP graduates in 2010 and 2011 were female. In 2009, 65% were female. This coincides with an internationally recognised increasing feminisation of general practice (Howe, 2007).

The career obstacles facing all female doctors are well-documented, reducing the contribution of women in many medical disciplines, but especially in the upper echelons of medicine, as one UK study has pointed out in particular (RCGP, 2007). Documented obstacles include rigid career structures, domestic responsibilities and discrimination (RCGP, 2007). In the UK, female consultants outnumber males in certain specialities (GP, psychiatry, paediatrics, dermatology, and genitourinary medicine). However, if we examine the UK experience, women are outnumbered at consultant level in cardiology, gastroenterology and renal medicine. Just 10% of surgical consultants under 45 years of age are women, and only 12% of clinical professors are women (RCGP, 2007). This segregation of women, both horizontal (women over-/under-represented in certain fields) and vertical (women underrepresented at senior level) is slowly reversing to achieve a more equitable balance. The desire of women for flexible working conditions, compatible with family life and earlier retirement, seems eminently sensible. General practice offers women excellent opportunities both to work part-time and to become a principal in practice (McKinstry *et al.*, 2006). Despite this, the RCGP noted that, in 2005, most GP partners were men, while most women GPs were either salaried or sessional workers.

In Scotland, there is an increasing proportion of women GPs who work fewer hours in all age groups than their male colleagues. Male doctors spend almost 20% more time in clinics and almost 50% more time on teaching, research and administrative duties than female GPs (McKinstry *et al.*, 2006). This raises the spectre of insufficient clinicians available for patients, coupled with a deficit in research and practice development. Irish research suggests that these concerns are overstated, that feminisation will not significantly impact on service provision, yet it voices similar concerns pertaining to females in leadership roles (Teljeur and O'Dowd, 2009). The feminisation of general practice, and medicine, continues apace. Nonetheless, we need more female GPs, with enhanced vertical integration.

GENERAL PRACTICE AND OUT-OF-HOURS CARE: AN EVOLVING MODEL OF CARER

If the current Irish health policy expectations that reduced secondary care admissions are to be achieved, to a large extent by enhancing primary care services, then of necessity, OOH GP services need to be majorly improved.

When one of the authors started his GP training in Kent in 1992, the GPs in the practice did the OOH care. When he left England in 1996, over 50% of all practices had moved to a different model of OOH care. This generally involved large groups of GPs combining resources to deliver OOH care to a defined patient cohort.

In Ireland, Southdoc is an OOH service covering Cork and Kerry in the south of the country. It is a GP co-op established in 2001, now comprising almost 500 GPs, and providing care to more than 600,000 patients widely dispersed across Cork and Kerry (Southdoc, *n.d.*). Southdoc undertakes approximately 200,000 patient consultations *per annum*. It has 26 treatment centres, with cars to facilitate domiciliary visits where necessary. This high rate of use, as the 200,000 consultations demonstrate, needs to be examined by the DoH and the HSE and in consultation with the general public. Is the service being used as an emergency OOH service or as a convenience service? (The 'McDonaldisation of general practice' as it has been called). The use of the ambulance service also requires examination and consultation. Further, the effect of alcohol abuse on the A&E services is frequently discussed in the media but its impact on GP OOH services is seldom examined – for example, GP attendance at brawls and in Garda stations.

In the context of the need for an enhanced OOH service, Southdoc clearly provides a strong working model for accessibility and quality GP care out-of-hours. As an OOH service, the methodology it employs is extremely robust:

- The call is answered by a trained receptionist who takes essential demographic details;
- A nurse with specialised telephone triage skills subsequently gathers relevant medical details;
- This determines subsequent management, most often a timed appointment to see a GP at a treatment centre;
- This service ensures that the patient is seen by a qualified GP in an appropriate facility;
- The service is available evenings and overnight, every night, 365 days a year.

This is in clear contrast to another provider of OOH care: VHI Swiftcare, which has just three treatment centres in the Republic of Ireland, charges €125 and closes at 10 pm (VHI, *n.d.*). Swiftcare will not assess children under the age of one. Nor will Swiftcare assess adult patients with chest pain, severe breathing difficulty, acute stomach pain, severe burns, pregnancy-related conditions or those requiring a domiciliary visit. It will assess "minor injuries or illness that requires urgent treatment" (VHI Swiftcare, *n.d.*). However, minor illness by definition does not require urgent treatment!

Most of Ireland is now covered by OOH GP co-operatives. This is an effective use of a skilled workforce, much in demand during the ordinary working day. It ensures the patient sees an appropriately qualified GP when unwell. It further ensures that GPs can achieve a reasonable work-life balance, essential to recruitment and retention of GPs, especially in more remote areas. A substantial investment in IT allows timely email of all information from the call centre to the treating GP. A copy of the entire encounter is sent by email to the patient's own GP. Next morning, the GP knows in detail about those patients who became unwell in the OOH period.

In little over a decade, this new model of OOH care has become established and accepted. It is reliant on a highly trained workforce, from those who first answer the phone, nurse and GP, to the administrator who finally emails the outcome to the patient's own GP, and dependent on modern IT systems.

CONCLUSION

Primary care is centre stage and mission critical for current and future health care delivery. The enhancement of primary care is a *sine qua non* for the provision of integrated care in the community. This chapter has stressed the role of the GP as a medic, advocate and source of social support within the community. Yet, it also has outlined significant challenges that need to be resolved with regard to the GP model of funding and the need for financial incentivisation towards clinical excellence across three areas of chronic illness that would improve patient health outcomes. It has pointed to the welcome participation of women in GP practices but has warned also against the hierarchical statuses in different areas of medicine. The chapter has stressed also the difficulties that gaps and blockages create between primary and secondary care, all of which work against an integrated care system. It has highlighted the continued underfunding and poor diagnostic services available at primary care, together with a culture within medicine generally that leads to sub-optimal levels of communication between primary and secondary care systems. It has urged for an urgent need to review and consult with the public on the administration of OOH services. All these factors create further impediments to integrated care. We face a period of unprecedented financial challenges against a backdrop of increasing demand for high-quality health care for all. General practice is well placed to deliver, now and into the future.

REFERENCES

Central Statistics Office (2011). *Vital Statistics, Fourth Quarter and Yearly Summary 2011*, Cork: Central Statistics Office.

Department of Health and Children (DoHC) (2001). *Primary Care Strategy*, Dublin: Stationery Office.

Department of Health and Children (DoHC) (2006). *Report of Working Group Set Up by the Tánaiste in March, 2006 to Examine the Nature and Extent of Haemochromatosis in Ireland and to Advise Her on the Action Necessary to Address the Problems Caused by Haemochromatosis*, Dublin: Stationery Office.

Economic and Social Research Institute (ESRI) and Health Service Executive (HSE) (2005-2009). *Hospital Inpatient Enquiry (HIPE), 2005-2009*, Dublin: ESRI and HSE.

European Federation of Allergy and Airways Diseases Patients Associations (EFA) (2004). *Fighting for Breath: A European Patient Perspective on Severe Asthma*, available at http://www.efanet.org/wp-content/uploads/2012/07/Fighting_For_Breath1.pdf.

Haahtela, T., Tuomisto, L.E., Pietinalho, A., Klaukka, T., Erhola, M., Kaila, M., Nieminen, M.M., Kontula, E. and Laitnen, L.A. (2006). 'A Ten Year Asthma Programme in Finland: Major Change for the Better', *Thorax*, 61: 663-670.

Health Service Executive (HSE) (2009). *PCRS Financial and Statistical Analyses*, available http://www.hse.ie/eng/staff/PCRS/PCRS_Publications/.

House, J. (2009). 'Women in Medicine: A Future Assured, *The Lancet*, 13 June, 373: 1997.

Howe, A. (2007). 'Why Family Medicine Benefits from More Women Doctors', *British Journal of General Practice*, 57(535): 91–92.

Masoli, M., Fabian, D., Holt, S., Beasley, R. and Global Initiative for Asthma (GINA) Program (2004).'Global Initiative for Asthma (GINA) Program: The Global Burden of Asthma: Executive Summary of the GINA Dissemination Committee Report', *Allergy*, 59: 469-478.

McHugh, S., Marsden, P., Brennan, C., Murphy, K., Croarkin, C., Moran, J., Harkins, V. and Perry I.J. (2011). 'Counting on Commitment: The Quality of Primary Care-led Diabetes Management in a System with Minimal Incentives', *BMC Health Services Research*, 11: 348.

McKinstry, B., Colthart, I., Eliott, K. and Hunter, C. (2006). 'The Feminisation of the Medical Work Force: Implications for Scottish Primary Care: A Survey of Scottish General Practitioners', *BMC Health Services Research*, 6: 56.

NHS Employers (2011). *Quality and Outcomes Framework Guidance for GMS Contract 2011/12: Delivering Investment in General Practice*, available at http://www.nhsemployers.org/Aboutus/Publications/Documents/QOF_g uidance_GMS_contract_2011_12.pdf.

Royal College of General Practitioners (RCGP) (2007). *The Future Direction of General Practice: A Roadmap*, London: RCGP.

Southdoc (*n.d.*). http://www.southdoc.ie/, accessed 4 September 2012.

Teljeur, C. and O'Dowd, T. (2009). 'The Feminisation of General Practice: Crisis or Business as Usual?', *The Lancet*, 374 (9696): 1147.

VHI Swiftcare (*n.d.*). https://www.vhi.ie/swiftcare/index.jsp, accessed 4 September 2012.

10: INTERPROFESSIONAL EDUCATION: APPLYING AN INTENSIVE PROGRAMME IN AN IRISH CONTEXT

Ona McGrath

"Coming together is a beginning. Keeping together is progress. Working together is success." **Henry Ford**

INTRODUCTION

In this chapter, an educational programme on health and social care professionals is considered. First, the author will consider some relevant background information relating to interprofessional education (IPE) – for example:

- What is meant by IPE?
- Does teamwork and collaboration have the best outcome for the patient/service user?
- Can cohesive teamwork improve the work environment for the carer/professional?
- How effective is IPE?

An overview of a current international educational model, involving undergraduate students from various health and social care disciplines and from different countries, will be elucidated upon. Finally, a brief consideration of how this programme may be applicable to an Irish context will be offered.

THE BACKGROUND TO INTERPROFESSIONAL EDUCATION

Currently, IPE appears to be the preferred terminology to describe health and social care professionals working together within an educational framework. However, the terms 'multiprofessional education', 'interdisciplinary studies' or 'multidisciplinary education' are used frequently and are widely referred to in many situations, particularly in practice.

The following definition provides a useful and broadly-recognised description that captures the essence of IPE:

> Interprofessional education occurs when two or more professions learn with, from and about each other to improve collaboration and the quality of care (Centre for the Advancement of Inter Professional Education (CAIPE), 2002).

The notion of learning 'with', 'from' and 'about' each other will be developed further throughout the chapter. IPE supports interactive learning and engagement between different professions as opposed to a uniprofessional education model where professions learn separately from one another.

CAIPE uses the term 'interprofessional education' to include all such learning in academic and work-based settings before and after qualification, adopting an inclusive view of 'professional' (CAIPE, 2002).

The concept of structured IPE was first mooted over four decades ago in North America and Europe but in an *ad hoc* occasional approach (Barr, 2003). In 1988, the World Health Organization (WHO) published a report, *Learning Together to Work Together for Health*, which laid the foundation for the current international impetus of IPE and endorsed interprofessional education and collaboration among health and social care professions:

> It is the policy of the WHO to foster a type of educational programme for health personnel … During certain periods of their education students of different health professions learn together the skills necessary for solving the priority health problems of individuals and communities that are known to be particularly amenable to teamwork. The emphasis is on learning how to interact with one another" (WHO, 1988: 5).

The benefits and advantages of IPE are put forward in the following summary of the report:

- It develops the ability of students to share knowledge and skills collaboratively and thereby provides individuals and the community with health care more efficiently;

- It enables students to become competent in the teamwork needed for the solution of priority health problems;
- It helps to develop mutual respect and understanding between health team members;
- It helps to 'decompartmentalise' curricula;
- It permits the integration of new skills and areas of knowledge that have a role to play in health care;
- It helps teachers, learners and service staff of different disciplines to communicate more easily among themselves;
- It generates, establishes and promotes new roles, competencies, responsibilities and areas of interest;
- It promotes multiprofessional research;
- It requires and promotes interdepartmental and interdisciplinary understanding and co-operation within institutions responsible for training and research;
- It permits collective consideration of the allocation, use and assessment of educational and service resources according to ascertained needs;
- It helps to ensure consistency and to avoid contradiction or conflict in curriculum design (WHO, 1988: 16-17).

At the time, WHO used the term 'multiprofessional' but since has adopted the term 'interprofessional education'.

More recently, WHO reiterated its confidence and belief in IPE and collaborative practice with the publication of *Framework for Action on Interprofessional Education and Collaborative Practice* (2010). Amongst its key messages are:

> The World Health Organization (WHO) and its partners recognise interprofessional collaboration in education and practice as an innovative strategy that will play an important role in mitigating the global health workforce crisis.
>
> Interprofessional education is a necessary step in preparing a 'collaborative practice-ready' health workforce that is better prepared to respond to local health needs. Integrated health and education policies can promote effective interprofessional education and collaborative practice (WHO, 2010: 7).

It appears that international policy and thinking favours the notion that patient/service user care will improve if collaboration and teamwork among health professionals is strengthened. The literature suggests that, when healthcare professionals collaborate, a positive and rewarding practice environment is fostered (Barr, 2003; Freeth and Reeves, 2004; McNair *et al.*, 2005, cited in MacDonald *et al.*, 2010).

How Effective is IPE?

A number of studies have been carried out in an attempt to measure and evaluate the effectiveness of IPE. Zwarenstein *et al.* (1999) carried out a Cochrane systematic review of IPE evaluation studies using strict inclusion criteria of randomised controlled trials, controlled before and after and interrupted time series designs. However, they found no studies at the time that met the aforementioned inclusion criteria. An update of this review was carried out which searched data from 1999 to 2006 (Reeves *et al.*, 2010) using the same inclusion criteria. The updated review identified six IPE studies, concluding that:

> Four out of the six studies reported a range of positive outcomes (which) provides further incentive to continue to understand, in more comprehensive terms, the effects of IPE (Reeves *et al.*, 2010: 240).

It is important to emphasise that there is a wealth of evaluation-type studies that do not meet the strict inclusion criteria of the Cochrane process. The more methodologically-inclusive reviews provide insight and knowledge on the effectiveness of IPE. These insights "include changes in learners' attitudes towards one another's professions, improvements in knowledge of interprofessional collaboration, enhancement of collaborative behaviour and gains in the delivery of patient care" (Cooper *et al.*, 2001; Barr *et al.*, 2005; Freeth *et al.*, 2005; Hammick *et al.*, 2007; Reeves, 2001, cited in Reeves *et al.*, 2010: 231).

There appears to be a consensus that studies need to reflect both a qualitative and quantitative approach to give an overall greater understanding of IPE. A review carried out in the UK (*Evaluations of Interprofessional Education*) appraised 19 selected evaluations and drew the following implications:

> ... we see the need to widen the range of methodologies employed and to strike a balance between evaluation of process and outcome. The former is essentially qualitative, the latter often quantitative. Where findings refer to outcomes, it is vital to explain the learning process in sufficient detail to permit the reader to make sense of them (Barr *et al.*, 2000: 28).

Reeves *et al.* (2010: 240) in their conclusion also refer to the "need to continue to strengthen the quality of studies employing both quantitative and qualitative methods to ensure they can provide comprehensive insights into the effects of IPE".

INTERPROFESSIONAL EDUCATION IN AN INTERNATIONAL SETTING

A current collaborative intensive programme (IP) between a number of different countries and different health and social care professionals will now be considered. An IP is an educational programme of short duration that brings together students and staff from higher education institutes (HEIs) of at least three participating countries. In this instance, the IP was a three-year (2010-2012) project hosted by Lahti University of Applied Sciences, Finland and funded by EU Erasmus grants. The other HEIs and participating countries were Frankfurt am Main University of Applied Science, Germany, Saxion University of Applied Sciences, Enschede, The Netherlands and Cork Institute of Technology (CIT), Ireland. The programme was designed to cater for junior students (first and second year Bachelor degree level) studying a health and social care discipline. The participating students came from nursing, social work, social care, physiotherapy and recreation/leisure undergraduate degree courses. The focus of the programme was on 'constructors of wellbeing' (COW) within an interprofessional and intercultural framework. The next section will focus on the 2010 and 2011 COW IP experience.

A preliminary meeting was held in Frankfurt University in early November 2010 with representative staff from each participating country. Feedback (student and staff) from the previous IP in 2010 was discussed and reviewed. Based on feedback and experiences of staff, the detailed planning and organisation for the 2011 programme was arranged. Having completed a worthwhile meeting, staff returned to their home HEI and recruited 10 students from the relevant health and social care degree programmes. Students then began their preparatory work in early spring of 2011 in their home country. This involved students carrying out research into the structure of health and social care delivery in their country: topics such as funding of health and social care services, population and life expectancy, health of the population, hospital care, primary care and community services were researched. Students also prepared an introductory presentation on the cultural aspects of their country. Staff too prepared lectures and workshops based on their allocated theme.

The programme took place in Lahti University in the faculty of Social and Health Care over a two-week period in April/May 2011. In all, 40 students participated.

Goals and Learning Outcomes

The main goals and learning outcomes for the students identified by the IP came under the headings of Knowledge, Skills and Attitudes.

Knowledge
The student:

- Is familiar with the social and health care structures, professions and their missions in different European countries as a constructor of human wellbeing;
- Understands the contribution of his own and different social and health care professions to the wellbeing structure nationally and Europe-wide;
- Understands the possibilities of entrepreneurial potential in producing wellbeing;
- Understands the concept of wellbeing in different contexts (physical, mental, psychological, social, cultural).

Skills
The student:

- Develops the competencies to study and work in an interprofessional and multicultural working group;
- Gains language skills and broadens vocabulary when discussing professional issues;
- Gains tools to argue and defend their own opinions;
- Improves linguistic and rhetoric competencies;
- Strengthens e-learning skills in an international context;

Attitudes
The student:

- Learns to respect other cultures and opinions: mutual acceptance;
- Is encouraged to study and work in the EU;
- Respects the work and ideas of different professions in the social and health care areas;
- Gains positive attitudes towards new and entrepreneurial approaches in the social and health care area and also towards new, innovative teaching methods.

In addition, participating students gained five European Credit Transfer and Accumulation System (ECTS) credits, recognised towards their degree in their home HEI.

Organisation and Learning Methods of the Programme

Bringing together 40 students and 10 teachers from different European HEIs and different professions in an intense learning environment presents quite a challenge. Clear structure and innovative pedagogical approaches are required for the programme to have any chance of success. On day one of the programme, a lecture on the concept of wellbeing was presented. Then the students participated in a number of introductory creative activities that were referred to as 'mix and mingle'. The focus of these activities was on teamwork, collaboration and getting to know each other in an interactive way. For the next 10 days, students and teachers worked together in a variety of learning environments. Keynote lectures were presented by a staff member from each of the four HEIs, focusing on their assigned theme (structure of health and social care services; ethics; entrepreneurial potential; and different health and social care professionals). Staff and students participated in workshops that were carefully designed to maximise interprofessional and intercultural teamwork. The staff endeavoured to be facilitators:

> The effective facilitator is committed to collaborative learning and to the learners as the most important resource, calls upon the experience of other professions, and respects and welcomes differences in all people and professions. No longer is the teacher the font of all wisdom (Barr, 2009: 190).

To ensure interprofessional and intercultural fusion, the four workshop groups consisted of different professions and a mix of students from different countries. The workshops explored the four main themes of the programme through discussion, case studies, role play, presentations, problem-solving and lively dialogue. Cultural influences played a large role throughout the programme – students reflected on their own values and beliefs. They appreciated differences between countries and also recognised the importance of service users'/patients' sets of values and beliefs. Particularly, in the ethics workshops, students realised the importance of respecting differences, showing empathy and keeping an open mind towards each other and, indeed, to the people in their care. During the ethics workshops, the 'dilemma' method was used to discuss and provide clarity around case studies in health and social care. This method involved a logical approach to the case, which assisted students in clarifying objective elements and subjective feelings. The methodological approach of the workshops was very much orientated towards problem-based learning, which "is perhaps the most widely-used interprofessional learning method" (Barr, 1996, cited in Barr, 2003: 271). Scenarios and case studies drawn from real health and social care situations were discussed, ideas stimulated and plans made.

Students visited a number of health and social care centres in Helsinki and Lahti during the programme. A school for children with disabilities that used an interprofessional approach in the classroom environment proved very interesting for the students. Also the director of a large centre for community mental health gave an insight into mental health provision and issues in Finland. An innovative centre for early school leavers, a day centre for older adults and a centre for people with physical disabilities also were visited within the context of observing good practice and professionals working together.

A number of people, both professionals and service users from the health and social care sector, visited the university and spoke to the students about their personal experiences within the area.

A secure e-learning environment was created for the IP for students and staff, using Moodle. This enabled exchange of ideas, student reports from workshops, interactive questions, queries, presentation of lectures, profiles of participants, social events and much more.

Thus a wide variety of learning methods were used in the programme, with both students and staff gaining a wealth of experience. Barr identifies the following frequently-used learning methods in IPE:

- Exchange-based learning – debates and case studies;
- Action-based learning – problem-based learning, collaborative enquiry and continuous quality improvement;
- Observation-based learning – joint visits to a patient by students from different professions, shadowing another profession;
- Simulation-based learning – role play, games, skills labs, and experiential groups;
- Practice-based – co-location across professions for placements, out-posting to another profession and interprofessional training wards;
- E-learning – reusable learning objects relating to the above;
- Blended learning – combining e-learning with face-to-face learning;
- Received or didactic learning – lectures (Barr, 2009: 189).

Barr emphasises the importance of interactive and co-operative exchanges and warns against overuse of didactic methods such as lectures.

The whole notion of active engagement and learning is very much promoted in the interprofessional context:

> An IPE intervention occurs when members of more than one health and/or social care profession learn interactively together, for the explicit purpose of improving interprofessional collaboration and/or the health/wellbeing of patients/clients. Interactive learning requires active learner participation, and active exchange between learners from different professions (Reeves *et al.*, 2008: 3).

The concept of learning 'with', 'from' and 'about' each other, referred to at the beginning of this chapter, is central for effective collaboration.

Curricular Themes of the Programme

As referred to earlier, the core themes framing the IP and encompassing the concept of wellbeing were: structure of health and social care services; ethics; entrepreneurial potential; and different health and social care professionals. The last theme – health and social care professionals – was the Cork (CIT) contribution and this will be developed here.

As previously mentioned, it is widely accepted that the practice care environment is most beneficial when professionals work together successfully and collaboratively (McNair *et al.*, 2005; Freeth and Reeves, 2004, cited in McDonald *et al.*, 2010). However, international evidence suggests that professionals do not collaborate well together in the complex activity of patient care (Reeves *et al.*, 2008). During discussions and feedback from the students, the various issues and problems arising between professionals in the care of individuals were identified. Areas such as professional role definition, hierarchy of roles, knowledge of each other's profession, interpretation of 'what is best for the patient', lack of respect for each other and lack of communication were suggested as potential areas of conflict. These issues were addressed through group problem-solving, case studies, role play situations, personal experiences and feedback to the group (McGrath, 2011).

In the lecture on different health and social care professions, six established key competencies of interprofessional collaborative practice for patient-centred care were cited:

• Communication;
• Strength in one's professional role;
• Knowledge of the professional role of others;

- Leadership;
- Team function;
- Negotiation for conflict resolution (McDonald *et al.*, 2010: 238).

These six competencies were identified from a Canadian study that used a grounded theory approach (Glaser, 1978). Participants in the study took part in interviews of 30 to 90 minutes in length and were drawn from:

> Students from a variety of health science programs who had completed an interprofessional clinical practical in their senior years were included. Interviews were conducted with seven undergraduate students, two graduate students, four faculty members from four different professions, and 11 practitioners, for a total of 24 participants (McDonald *et al.*, 2010: 239).

From the findings of the study, six key competencies (as mentioned previously) and a number of behavioural indicators for each competency were identified. The key competencies identified in this study are similar to those identified in the literature (Interprofessional Education Collaborative Expert Panel (IPECEP), 2011; Hammick *et al.*, 2009).

Each of these competencies were debated and discussed. Students were encouraged to draw on their personal experience and their academic reading to give examples of situations involving the aforementioned competencies. Clearly, knowledge of one's own profession and that of others became evident as important. In the European context, it emerged that each country had different structures for training and even different titles of professions. This linked to the notion of respect for other cultures and systems in a mutual acceptance. Communication is a central aspect of interprofessionalism – students easily identified with this competency. They were able to see within the programme how their own communication skills improved – language skills, debating skills and listening skills to name but a few.

Leadership and team function are two vital competencies that enable a positive working environment when functioning effectively. Within the workshops and, indeed, in some of the social programme activities, these competencies were illuminated in practice for the participants. Finally, the 'negotiation for conflict resolution' competency emerged throughout discussions, debates, cultural differences, arguments for and against various scenarios. The issues arising then were addressed and formulated in a best practice professional manner between the facilitator and participants (McGrath, 2011).

Subsequently, a report by an expert panel[4] identified four core interprofessional competency domains:

- Values/ethics for interprofessional practice;
- Roles/responsibilities;
- Interprofessional communication;
- Teams and teamwork (IPECEP, 2011: 16).

In this context, the following definition of interprofessional competency domain was given: "A generally-identified cluster of more specific interprofessional competencies that are conceptually linked, and serve as theoretical constructs" (ten Cate and Scheele, 2007).

In this report, a comprehensive review of existing literature pertaining to interprofessional competency domains was undertaken both nationally and internationally with the following outcome:

> Although the number of competency domains and their categorization vary, we found convergence in interprofessional competency content between the national literature and global literature, among health profession organizations in the United States, and across American educational institutions. Interprofessional competency domains we identified are consistent with this content (IPECEP, 2011: 15).

Evaluation and Conclusion of the Programme

An evaluation of any programme is vital to ascertain its effectiveness, as evaluations can support improvement and development within a programme. Students participated in a questionnaire designed to establish their opinion on various aspects of the programme. When asked if they felt that the programme would help them in their future studies/careers, 35% said 'very much', 35% said 'quite much' and 30% said 'somewhat'. On the question relating to overall evaluation of the programme, 46% rated it as excellent and 54% as good. An open-ended question relating to 'what should be done differently' gleaned some of the following student responses:

- Some days were a little too packed;
- I think it is good the way it is now;
- Less lectures, more workshops and excursions.

---

[4]   The IPECEP comprised representatives from the American Association of Colleges of Nursing, American Association of Colleges of Osteopathic Medicine, American Association of Colleges of Pharmacy, American Dental Education Association, Association of American Medical Colleges, and Association of Schools of Public Health.

When asked 'what did you enjoy most', the responses were:

- Meeting all new people from other countries;
- Interactive work during the workshops;
- Clients' perspective lecture.

Teaching staff contributed articles relating to their experience of the 2010 programme in a publication series of Lahti University:

> The intensive programme was intended to be a booster for interprofessional and multicultural learning experiences. This intention proved to be true to a large extent. It was a great experience with enormous value for lifelong learning; not only for the students, but also for participating teachers (Dielis, 2011: 56).

An external evaluation also was carried out.

THE IRISH CONTEXT

It appears that Irish policy is in line with international policies, referred to at the beginning of this chapter. Irish government policy supports the concept of interprofessional teamwork in its delivery of health and social care as expressed in the *Primary Care Strategy* (Department of Health and Children (DoHC), 2001) and in *Vision for Change* (Mental Health Commission (MHC), 2006a). In 2010, Damian McCallion (Integrated Services Programme director, HSE) emphasised the importance of effective interprofessional teamwork when referring to the HSE *National Service Plan* (HSE, 2010) for that year:

> … strong focus on effective working relationships across various services designed to ensure patients and clients receive the care they need supported by teams of health care professionals (McCallion, 2010: 55).

So the policy and intended practice appears to be in place … but is there a gap between rhetoric and reality? Let me take one example to highlight apparent gaps. The example is that of primary care teams in Ireland. In March 2011, the HSE "identified 519 Primary Care Teams and 134 Health and Social Care Networks to be developed by 2011" (DoHC, 2011). It is now 2013 and we are still waiting.

In order for interprofessionalism to advance, the process needs to start at the training and educational level. Again, the research recommends incorporating IPE into undergraduate and postgraduate programmes:

> In order to encourage this 'competency' across the various groups who will comprise a multidisciplinary team, some consideration needs to be given to ensuring this facet (multidisciplinary) of training is

included across all professional courses, at undergraduate and postgraduate level (MHC, 2006b: 18).

This notion is reiterated in the excerpt below from *Vision for Change*, the government's policy on mental health provision:

> Consideration should also be given to the option of providing joint training modules across the various disciplines to facilitate collective training in fundamental values and principles, to promote understanding of the unique role that each professional specialty plays in mental health, and to encourage recognition of the value of multidisciplinary teamwork (MHC, 2006a: 186).

The number of Irish Institutes of Technology and universities offering structured modules on IPE appears to be very limited. In order for IPE to occur, students from different disciplines need to engage actively with each other, to learn 'with', 'from' and 'about' each other's profession. It is fair to say that IPE is at an embryonic stage in the Ireland of 2012.

It is hoped that this snapshot chapter has given an insight into IPE, with particular reference to a working IP and a brief glimpse of the Irish context. It does seem incongruous that IPE can successfully take place between four countries, but appears to be problematic within an Institute of Technology or university catering for a number of health and social care professions. Of course, this is not only an Irish problem; indeed, when discussing same with some Dutch colleagues, they recounted how their physiotherapy and social work departments did not have any IPE, despite their close geographical proximity.

It is important for academics and programme leaders to endeavour to incorporate IPE in their courses, particularly in light of national and international policy:

> It is no longer enough for health workers to be professional. In the current global climate, health workers also need to be interprofessional (WHO, 2010: 36).

REFERENCES

Barr, H. (2003). 'Unpacking Interprofessional Education', in Leathard, A. (ed.), *Interprofessional Collaboration – from Policy to Practice in Health and Social Care*, London: Routledge, 265-279.

Barr, H. (2009). 'Interprofessional Education', in Dent, J. and Harden, R. (eds.), *A Practical Guide for Medical Teachers*, London: Churchill Livingstone, 187-192.

Barr, H., Freeth, D., Hammick, M., Koppel, I. and Reeves, S. (2000). *Evaluations of Interprofessional Education – A United Review for Health and Social Care*, Fareham,

Hamps.: Centre for the Advancement of Interprofessional Education with The British Educational Research Association.

Centre for the Advancement of Inter Professional Education (CAIPE) (2002). *Defining IPE*, available http://www.caipe.org.uk/resources/, accessed 01.02.2012.

Davies, C., Finlay, L. and Bullman, A. (2000). *Changing Practice in Health and Social Care*, London: Sage.

Department of Health and Children (DoHC) (2001). *Primary Care Strategy: A New Direction*, Dublin: Stationery Office.

Department of Health and Children (DoHC) (2011). *Primary Care Teams Fact Sheet*, available http://www.dohc.ie/fact_sheets/pcts_201103.pdf?direct=1, accessed 25.03.2012.

Dielis, W. (2011). 'Intensive Programme Constructors of Wellbeing' in Hatakka, H. (ed.), *Interprofessional and International Learning Experiences in Social and Health Care Higher Education in Lahti University of Applied Sciences*, Lahti, Finland: Lahti University of Applied Sciences, 54-56.

Glaser, B. (1978). *Theoretical Sensitivity*, Thousand Oaks, CA: Sage, cited in McDonald, M.B., Bally, J.M., Ferguson, L.B., Murray, B.L. and Fowler-Kerry, S.E. (2010). 'Knowledge of the Professional Role of Others: A Key Interprofessional Competency', *Nurse Education in Practice*, 10(4): 238-242, doi:10.1016/j.nepr.2009.11.012.

Hammick, M., Freeth, D., Copperman, J. and Goodsman, D. (2009). *Being Interprofessional*, Cambridge: Polity Press.

Health Service Executive (HSE) (2010). *National Service Plan 2010*, Dublin: HSE.

Interprofessional Education Collaborative Expert Panel (IPECEP) (2011). *Core Competencies for Interprofessional Collaborative Practice: Report of an Expert Panel*, Washington, DC: Interprofessional Education Collaborative.

McCallion, D. (2010). 'HSE: Moving to New Service Delivery Model', *Health Matters* (national staff magazine of the HSE), 6(1): 55-57.

McDonald, M.B., Bally, J.M., Ferguson, L.B., Murray, B.L. and Fowler-Kerry, S.E. (2010). 'Knowledge of the Professional Role of Others: A Key Interprofessional Competency', *Nurse Education in Practice*, 10(4): 238-242, doi:10.1016/j.nepr.2009.11.012.

McGrath, O. (2011). 'Constructors of Wellbeing Erasmus Intensive Programme: Interprofessional Education in Social and Health Care' in Hatakka, H. (ed.), *Interprofessional and International Learning Experiences in Social and Healthcare Higher Education in Lahti University of Applied Sciences*, Lahti, Finland: Lahti University of Applied Sciences, 65-67.

Mental Health Commission (MHC) (2006a). *A Vision for Change: Report of the Expert Group on Mental Health Policy*, Dublin: Stationery Office.

Mental Health Commission (MHC) (2006b). *Multidisciplinary Team Working: From Theory to Practice*, available http://www.mhcirl.ie/documents/publications/Discussion%20Paper%20Multidisciplinary%20Team%20Working%20%20From%20Theory%20to%20Practice%202006.pdf, accessed 25.03.2012.

Reeves, S., Zwarenstein, M., Goldman, J., Barr, H., Freeth, D., Hammick, M., Koppel, I. (2008). 'Interprofessional Education: Effects on Professional Practice and Health Care Outcomes, *Cochrane Database of Systematic Reviews*, 1, Art. No.: CD002213, doi: 10.1002/14651858.CD002213.pub2.

Reeves, S., Zwarenstein, M., Goldman, J., Barr, H., Freeth, D., Koppel, I. and Hammick, M. (2010). 'The Effectiveness of Interprofessional Education: Key Findings from a New Systematic Review', *Journal of Interprofessional Care*, 24(3): 230-241.

ten Cate, O. and Scheele, F. (2007). 'Competency-based Postgraduate Training: Can We Bridge the Gap between Theory and Practice?', *Academic Medicine*, 82: 542-547, cited in Interprofessional Education Collaborative Expert Panel (2011), *Core Competencies for Interprofessional Collaborative Practice: Report of an Expert Panel*, Washington, DC: Interprofessional Education Collaborative, 2.

World Health Organization (WHO) (1988). *Learning Together to Work Together for Health: Report of a WHO Study Group on Multiprofessional Education of Health Personnel: The Team Approach*,
http://whqlibdoc.who.int/trs/WHO_TRS_769.pdf, accessed 06.02.2012.

World Health Organization (WHO) (2010). *Framework for Action on Interprofessional Education and Collaborative Practice*, available http://whqlibdoc.who.int/hq/2010/ WHO_HRH_HPN_10.3_eng.pdf, accessed 06.02.2012.

Zwarenstein, M., Atkins, J., Hammick, M., Barr, H., Koppel, I. and Reeves, S. (1999). 'Interprofessional Education and Systematic Review: A New Initiative in Evaluation', *Journal of Interprofessional Care*, 13: 417-424.

11: PRIMARY CARE, SOCIAL WORK AND INTEGRATED CARE: A NEW WAY OF DELIVERING SERVICES?

Deirdre Jacob

INTRODUCTION

In the past 11 years, Irish health services have been subject to significant attempts to change the way health and social services are delivered. Fundamental to this change are the policies that direct the way health services are delivered. This chapter begins by giving an overview of specific policy documents that highlight the change needed to achieve the fundamental objective: integrated care.

Essential to this change is the acceptance of primary care as the fundamental basis for the provision of services that are locally accessible, that are population health-focussed but which are central to the process of health care management for all of those in need of services. As a core concept, the primary health care model is one that has been embraced by a number of societies across Central Europe and North America. Ireland, in its establishment of primary care teams (PCTs), also has demonstrated its intention to adhere to this model – however, often in developing services, the core concepts of such a model can become overlooked. This chapter will give an overview of the model of primary health care as it is seen through the social determinants of health lens with the fundamental aim of re-embracing a model of care that has significant potential as a guiding principle for helping to improve the health of communities.

In accepting a social determinants approach and indeed a primary health care approach, the policy documents recognised the inclusion of primary care social workers as core team members of PCTs. The potential for social workers, as a generically-trained profession with a broad skill mix, to improve the experience of patients is explored in international literature. The specific skills of social workers as 'systems specialists' is noted, with reference to their potential in integrated care. The development of primary care social work services has not been without its difficulties. The complexities of developing a generic community-based social work service for care groups other than children and families is acknowledged in this chapter, with reference to the specific experience of psychiatric social work services in the 1970s.

Giving specific regard to the potential for social workers to become instrumental in care integration between primary and secondary care services, this chapter explores some internationally-accepted guiding principles that should be in place to facilitate an integrated care approach. The chapter concludes by alluding to the report of the Comptroller and Auditor General (CAG) (2010), which outlines the number of posts in social work in primary care, which stand at only 22% of the original target.

The chapter then will conclude by discussing the implications of primary care developments for the future of integrated care in Irish health services.

IRISH HEALTH POLICY AND THE COMMITMENT TO PRIMARY CARE

In 2001, the Department of Health and Children (DoHC) published a document that outlined a 'new direction' in health service provision in Ireland. *Primary Care: A New Direction* recognised the need to change the way health services were delivered, in keeping with the primary health care rhetoric that echoed across North America and other developed nations (DoHC, 2001).

The strategy emphasised the contextual basis for primary care services as the 'appropriate setting' to meet 90% to 95% of the health and social services needs of the general population. Further, the strategy clearly stated that primary care services and resources had the potential to prevent the developments of conditions that might later require hospital admission. The strategy also outlined the potential capacity of primary care to 'facilitate earlier hospital discharge' under circumstances where primary care is the 'central focus' of the health system and, finally, it throws down the gauntlet by stating that:

> The development of a properly integrated primary care service can lead to better outcomes, better health status and better cost-effectiveness (DoHC, 2001).

The idealism of the *Primary Care Strategy* offered open access to 'all people regardless of who they are or where they live or what social problems they had'. It also acknowledged that, in situations of more 'complex and special needs' that could not be met within the primary care context, secondary care then would be required.

Much time and attention was paid in this document to the potential of primary care providers to 'achieve growth and development' in service provision but it also recognised the lack of accessibility of certain professional groups, the lack of teamwork in this context and the lack of adequate liaison between primary and secondary services. However, the strategy pointed to international literature that illustrated the success of 'team-based approaches with an appropriate skill mix' to primary care provision evident in other countries.

THE PRIMARY HEALTH CARE MODEL

The 'new direction' of the health strategy, in keeping with evidence from international literature, proposed the introduction of 'interdisciplinary teams' that would include general practitioners (GPs), nurses/midwives, health care assistants, home helps, physiotherapists, occupational therapists, social workers and administrative personnel, who then would be supported by a wider network of other services from other primary care professionals including speech and language therapists, community pharmacists, dieticians, community welfare officers, dentists, chiropodists and psychologists (Irish College of General Practitioners (ICGP), 2011).

It was further envisaged that these professionals in turn would provide services to 'an enrolled population' that could be determined by 'encouraging GPs to join their existing lists of enrolled patients within certain geographic considerations'. According to the strategy, this approach would 'strengthen the capacity of the primary care team to adopt a population health approach to service provision' (DoHC, 2001).

It was envisaged also that teams would be co-located 'where possible', giving ease of access not just on an interdisciplinary basis but also to those in need of services. The vision emphasised out-of-hours and extended hours service provision.

'Prevention and rehabilitation' would become the emphasis, in conjunction with the traditional approach of 'diagnosis and treatment'. There would be better 'liaison between primary and secondary care' and the team would have 'better access to hospital services' to improve discharge planning with the 'development of individual care plans along with the identification of key workers where appropriate'. Integration between primary care services and specialist services in the community thus would be strengthened, bringing natural positive consequences for those in need of services (DoHC, 2001).

Finally, the strategy highlighted that, in order to implement plans to develop adequate primary care services, major investment in human resources, physical infrastructure and new ways of working for providers who deliver the range of primary care services available in the community would be needed (DoHC, 2001).

The primary care strategy can be considered to be important from a number of perspectives that are pertinent to this chapter:

- Within the context of better health service provision by an interdisciplinary team with a mix of skills who are deemed appropriate to address 90% to 95% of the population's health needs, social workers are identified as core team members;
- In order to improve and integrate service provision, a number of conditions are needed – for example, proposed joining of GP lists to accommodate the enrolling of identified populations within specific geographical locations, co-location of services, major investment in human resources and physical infrastructure and new ways of working within the community;
- Population health approaches to service provision, emphasising prevention and rehabilitation.

In terms of integrated services, the *Primary Care Strategy* (DoHC, 2001) firmly commits to changing the emphasis of care management from secondary to primary services, with better integration between services already located within the community but with greater emphasis on 'teamwork' between professionals. It also emphasises that the change could facilitate earlier discharge from hospital and better integration between primary and secondary services.

In the intervening years and in recognition of the need for a change of culture within community-based services, the Health Service Executive (HSE) published the *Transformation Programme 2007-2010* (HSE, 2007). This, also against the back-drop of ageing populations, increasing demands for health services and declining resources, stated that:

> … change was not an option – it was a necessity (HSE, 2007).

The document pulls no punches in imparting to HSE professionals that continuing to do things in the same way that they have been done in the past will:

> … lead to health and social care systems that are unable to cope, financially unsound and unable to provide quality care (HSE, 2007).

In particular, the document asserts the 'need to develop integrated care across all stages of the care journey', outlines the ability of patients to move with ease through the care system and commits to a seamless service where integration is at the heart of service provision:

> Patients and clients will be able to move easily through the entire care system because we will have services that are well organised and connected seamlessly across the organisation. Integrated care will be at the heart of the way we work (HSE, 2007).

In general, the document indicates the need for change in the management of chronic health conditions, making the point that 'two out of every three patients' admitted through A&E departments are admitted as a result of issues relating to an existing chronic health condition. There is a clear commitment here to developing patient journey processes, along with the implementation of a 'national model for integrated care delivery' with 'shared care' between primary care and hospital services.

Giving specific regard to the need to 'reconfigure community resources' to provide a significant range of services within the local community in the context of a multidisciplinary team, the *Transformation Programme* touches on various aspects of change necessary to realise the 'new way' of delivering services within communities.

A number of HSE policy documents avow the need for integrated services in the years since the publication of the *Primary Care Strategy* (DoHC, 2001). Although it is not pertinent to discuss all of them here, the most recent document published by the HSE that provides a clear commitment to integrated care is the *2012 National Service Plan* (HSE, 2012).

The Plan outlines the following vision:

1. The health of the population will be managed, as far as possible, within a primary care setting, with the population very rarely requiring admission to a hospital.
2. Those with additional or complex needs will have plans of care developed with the local PCT, who will co-ordinate all care required with specialist services in the community and, for hospital attendance, through integrated care pathways.
3. The PCT will act as the central point and will actively engage on the medical and social needs of its defined population with a wider Health and Social Care Network (HSCN). The HSCN covers a number of PCTs and provides specialist and care group services such as dietetics, ophthalmology, audiology, podiatry, etc.

In keeping with the core components of the *Primary Care Strategy*, the plan clearly places the responsibility of care and health management of specific populations in the domain of primary care community-based professionals. The programme further suggests that care and health management would be conducted in a 'programmatic and systematic way, thus improving outcomes for patients' on three fronts:

- Patient care;
- Health status; and
- Reduced waiting lists.

A point that will be discussed later in this chapter is the Government's commitment in this plan to strengthen primary care services with the availability of an additional €20m funding to fill vacancies provided by allied health professionals (HSE, 2012). In general, what we see is a clear plan and financial commitment to further develop PCTs and the HSCNs that support them as a means of 'responding to the episodic care needs of the population' (HSE, 2012).

As previously stated, the Irish Government, under much of the same financial pressure as other developing countries, decided to take the 'primary care' or indeed the 'primary health care' approach to health service provision as a means of responding to the health and social care needs of populations but also, it seems, as a means of managing the spiralling costs of providing that health care to a diverse and changing demographic.

However, despite the rhetoric, little appears to be known about the approach that now underpins health service provision and care management. More specifically, what are the fundamentals of this approach as a model for responding to health needs of populations? Can this approach meet the expectations and complex care needs of service users and become the linchpin of an integrated system? Here, we will touch on some of these questions with reference to international literature.

Keleher (2004) provides the following definitions for primary care and primary health care:

> Primary care is clinically focused, and can be considered a sub-component of the broader primary health care system. Primary care is considered health care provided by a medical professional which is a client's first point of entry into the health system. Primary care is practised widely in nursing and allied health, but predominately in general practice …

> Primary health care (PHC) incorporates personal care with health promotion, the prevention of illness and community development. The philosophy of PHC includes the interconnecting principles of equity, access, empowerment, community self-determination and

intersectoral collaboration. It encompasses an understanding of the social, economic, cultural and political determinants of health.

Indeed, Loudon (1983) highlights the historical role of the GP as the principal provider of primary care. The GP, who was viewed as 'having the ability to adapt to scientific medical developments and related changing community needs', increasingly is being complemented in the community by nurses and other allied health professionals who are playing 'an increasingly expanded role in primary care provision' (Martin and Sturmberg, 2005).

Dimitrov and Fahey (2010) point to an analysis by Kuzel (2006), who examined the organisational structure of 28 models of primary health care delivery in a number of industrialised nations. The analysis identified four distinct models:

- **Professional contact / traditional model:** Care is provided by the GP as the sole primary care provider with little or no interaction with other allied health professionals;
- **Professional co-ordination model:** Care is provided by GPs and nurses; IT integrates with other sources of health care service; nurse liaison helps to integrate health care services;
- **Integrated community care model:** Population care is provided by health centres linked by IT to other health care providers serving the same population; continuity of care is assured by a team;
- **Non-integrated community care model:** Health care centre focus with a full range of services; no IT or other mechanisms to integrate services with other providers; no formal mechanism to ensure continuity.

Trotter (2008) also classifies primary care models in two categories:

- The traditional models (GPs);
- Newer models (PCTs).

According to Dimitrov and Fahey (2010), a good vision of primary care is one that:

- Focuses on the health of populations;
- Integrates services and practitioners;
- Promotes continuity of care;
- Focuses on health promotion and prevention;
- Encourages patients as advocates and navigators of their own care needs; and

- Where 'case management and discharge planning assist in keeping people healthy helping them manage their own care'.

It is suggested that a primary care approach that works towards this vision will yield savings in the longer term.

In an extended form, according to the World Health Organization (WHO), primary health care is defined as:

> ... essential health care based on practical, scientifically sound and socially acceptable methods and technology made universally accessible to individuals and families in the community through their full participation and at a cost that the community and country can afford to maintain at every stage of their development in the spirit of self-reliance and self-determination. It forms an integral part both of the country's health system, of which it is the central function and main focus, and of the overall social and economic development of the community. It is the first level of contact of individuals, the family and community with the national health system bringing health care as close as possible to where people live and work, and constitutes the first element of a continuing health care process (WHO, 1978).

The question that most often arises when looking at the international literature is which model is most appropriate within the context of the Irish health system? The policy documents published show a clear drive to what the international literature defines as the 'primary health care model' which, according to Trotter (2008), has five main functions:

- Provision of care at first contact within the health care system;
- Continuity of care;
- Co-ordination of care;
- Comprehensiveness of care (including prevention and health promotion);
- Gate-keeping role to the upper levels of the health care system.

However, within the context of the WHO (1978) definition described above, this model of health care shifts its focus from care provision seen in the 'professional contact model' of primary care provision to a new model of primary care that recognises health in a broader definition:

> Health is a state of complete physical, mental, and social wellbeing and not merely the absence of disease or infirmity (WHO, 1946).

This provides the basis for the next subject of discussion in this chapter.

SOCIAL DETERMINANTS OF HEALTH AS A BASIS FOR PRIMARY HEALTH CARE PROVISION

This ideal model of health care was adopted in the declaration of the International Conference on Primary Health Care held in Alma Ata in 1978 (known as the *Alma Ata Declaration*) (WHO, 1978), which became a core concept of the WHO's goal of 'health for all'.

The objective of 'health for all' was to ensure that health is brought within reach of everyone in a given country, where health is meant a personal state of wellbeing, not just the availability of health services – a state of health that enables a person to lead a socially- and economically-productive life. 'Health for all' aims to ensure the removal of the obstacles to good health, including the elimination of malnutrition, ignorance, contaminated drinking water and unhygienic housing, as much as it implies the solution to good health rests in addressing issues in health care provision where there exists a lack of doctors, hospital beds, drugs or vaccines (Halfden, 1981).

The Alma Ata conference mobilised a 'primary health care movement' of professionals and institutions, governments and civil society organisations, researchers and grassroots organisations that undertook to tackle the politically, socially and economically unacceptable health inequalities in all countries identified following systematic global research. Intrinsic in this movement is a paradigm shift that recognises that health for all involves a set of 'mutually interdependent concepts' including:

- Primary health care;
- Health promotion;
- Teamwork;
- Equity;
- Collaboration between sectors;
- Community development; and
- Research and technology (Thomas and Graver, 1997).

There is much literature relating to the personal, social, economic and environmental determinants of health and their impact on health inequality. Marmot and Wilkinson (2003) highlight the evidence that 'people's lifestyles and the conditions in which they live and work strongly influence their health'. They outline the following conditions that are known to impact on the broader aspects of individual health and wellbeing:

- **Social and economic circumstances:** These affect health throughout the lifespan; life expectancy is shorter and most diseases are more common the further down the social ladder;

- **Stress:** Lack of control over work and home can have powerful effects on health;

- **Early life:** Important foundations of adult health are laid in early childhood;

- **Social exclusion:** Life is short where the quality is poor ... people living on the streets suffer the highest rates of premature death;

- **Work:** Stress in the workplace increases the risk of disease ... people who have better control over their work have better health;

- **Unemployment:** Job security increases health, wellbeing and job satisfaction; higher rates of unemployment cause more illness and premature death;

- **Social support:** Friendship, good social relations and strong supportive networks improve health at home, at work and in the community;

- **Addiction:** Individuals who turn to alcohol, drugs and tobacco suffer from their use, but use is influenced by the wider social setting ... addiction and its consequences are closely associated with social and economic disadvantage;

- **Food:** Global market forces control the food supply and so healthy food and access to it is a political issue ... a good diet and adequate food are central to promoting health and wellbeing;

- **Transport:** Healthy transport means less driving and more walking and cycling, backed up by better public transport (Marmot and Wilkinson, 2003).

The value in recognising that health 'is not merely the absence of disease or infirmity' is the acceptance that health service provision not only must take account of the broader determinants of health but, if we are to find ways of alleviating and preventing some of the socio-economic and environmental conditions of ill-health, we must find new ways of engaging with, and providing services to, the populations who are in need of health services.

The recognition in the *Primary Care Strategy* (DoHC, 2001) of social workers as core team members could be described as one of the Irish Government's most intuitive responses, not simply to a changing demographic with complex health and social care needs but also as a direct acknowledgement of the wider determinants of health and their impact on health service demand.

PRIMARY CARE SOCIAL WORK

The social determinants of health have given health service providers the impetus to begin to understand that simply responding to the medical needs of patients through traditional treatment methods is not sustainable.

We have touched on the policy documents within the Irish context which have clearly stated that we need to begin to find new ways of delivering services to people in a way that fosters prevention and health promotion, with the end result being better outcomes and improved population health. We have noted also that the policy documents agree that, as with the general theoretical position of primary health care provision, community health needs must be served by a team of allied health professionals 'with an appropriate skill mix' that, according to the *Primary Care Strategy* (DoHC, 2001) now includes social workers.

As a profession in Ireland, social work has quite a recent history, with foundations in the philanthropic endeavours of religious orders. Some developments mirrored in many ways the developments in Britain albeit under different political circumstances and much harsher poor laws (Kearney and Skehill, 2005). Social workers have been, and continue to be, employed in a number of medical and social service settings. Historically, social work as a profession has been confronted with societal changes – in particular, demographic changes, which have demanded flexible and adaptable professional responses to more complex human problems (Kearney and Skehill, 2005). It could be said that yet another demand is currently being imposed on the profession within the developing context of primary health care as it plays out in the complex Irish health system.

Primary care social work under the model of primary health care provision now demands that we find new ways of providing for the 'medical and social needs of defined populations'. It is my contention here that primary health care social workers, in an attempt to adapt to the 'new way' of delivering services, have the opportunity to shape a role that is respectful of our roots as 'welfare workers or case workers' but is cognisant also of the fact that 'bread and butter' social work may not meet the demands of a primary health care model that places such importance upon prevention, health promotion, collaboration and community development.

Just as there is international recognition of the social determinants of health and their impact on the health of societies, so too is there much in the literature about the role of social work in the context of primary health care:

Social work brings the perspective of understanding the whole person and the environment in which they live as a crucial component of managing care. Traditional health care providers are not generally prepared to fully incorporate this concept into practice (Rock and Cooper, 2000; Lesser, 2000; Claiborne and Vandenburgh, 2001; Siefert and Henk, 2001).

However, Schmidt *et al.* (2001) noted a growing trend for nurses and occupational therapists to assume case management responsibilities and to receive increasing amounts of training in the area of the psychosocial aspects of health. This heightens the need for social work to be more pro-active and organised in promoting the skills and abilities of the profession.

There is a general consensus that social work has six primary roles, or types of services, that it can provide in the primary health care setting (Lesser, 2000; Salvatore, 1988; Wharf, 1992) to individuals, families, groups and communities. These roles are:

- Assessment of the biopsychosocial aspects of health and wellbeing;
- Concrete service provision;
- Counselling and therapeutic services;
- Consultation with other health care providers about the biopsychosocial factors and their implications for health and wellbeing;
- Education and training in biopsychosocial aspects of illness and intervention strategies;
- Community development and capacity-building (Canadian Association of Social Workers, 2003).

As stated in the research, this comprehensive, though not exhaustive, range of roles demonstrates the rich potential that a move towards primary health care reform has for social work as a profession.

As a chairperson of the Irish Association of Social Workers (IASW) Special Interest Group for Primary Care Social Workers and in the absence of any Irish research on the role of primary care social workers, members working in primary care have claimed anecdotally to me that their current management arrangements seemed to favour the more 'traditional roles' of social work practice (assessment and case management) in the context of primary health care at the expense of more diverse roles (community development and capacity-building). This is in contrast to the literature, which suggests that there is considerable evidence to support the position that the primary care social worker within the context of a primary health care system is required to draw upon a broader set of skills associated with 'generalist practice', while at the same time developing specialised expertise (Levin and Herbert, 2001; Siefert and Henk, 2001).

Further, the authors describe the dichotomous position adopted by the profession when defining practice orientation. While our professional roots are grounded in advocating for structural change and community development, our profession emphasises clinical practice such as therapy and counselling. Described as one of the unfortunate by-products of the 'professionalisation of social work', this has been a strategic movement away from what are often considered low status activities such as the provision of concrete services (Seifert and Henk, 2001).

The focus of primary care social work as a 'community-based' social work service has had implications also for the development of the service. This, coupled with the absence of an established primary care social work management structure, has meant that primary care social workers have struggled, and continue to struggle, to prioritise the role in line with the expectations of a primary health care model and the multidisciplinary team approach.

Butler (2005) noted that, following the introduction of the *Health Act, 1970*, which located social work within community care programmes, a vision of the delivery of personal social services that were to be delivered to the public by generically-trained social workers became over-shadowed by an apparent 'pre-occupation' with child protection and welfare, 'almost to the total exclusion of the needs of other vulnerable groups'.

Indeed, Butler (2005) highlights the position of the Committee on Social Work which stated that:

> … ideally, community-based social work should provide a broad range of service, encompassing the elderly, the disabled and the young (DoHC, 1985).

The Committee also noted that:

> … in most areas, community social work was confined to families of children at risk (DoHC, 1985).

Primary health care social work represents an attempt to adhere to an approach to community-based social work that is generalist in nature, and provides services to all of those groups in need of social work services, including the elderly, people with disabilities and those whose mental health is managed within the context of primary care. Indeed, primary care social workers can provide services to individuals and families living in the community whose health and wellbeing is impacted by social factors. Anecdotally, however, it appears that the 'pre-occupation with child protection and welfare' noted by Butler (2005) continues to impact on the development of primary care social work services for other care groups outside of the hospital and secondary health care systems.

Indeed, members of the IASW who work in primary care have noted that some understaffed statutory social work services have been unable to resist the opportunity to 'redirect' primary care social workers to the child protection and welfare system. In such instances, the needs of primary care services become secondary to the demands of service provision in statutory services, limiting the opportunity to develop primary care services and multidisciplinary team working.

The result for these social workers may be a case-load that is more reflective of working in a child welfare system but, even more disadvantageous, it demonstrates a general inability to commit to a move towards integrated care for vulnerable adults needing social work services in the community, in the face of pressurised statutory social work services for children and families.

It may be reasonable at this juncture to conclude that managing primary care social workers within the children and families structure, while initially seeming a reasonable solution to a very obvious lack of management opportunities within primary care, may be counter-productive in terms of primary care and integrated care development, in particular for the vulnerable adult population.

Systemic constraints aside, primary care social work continues to try to 'carve out a niche' (Butler, 2005) for itself in a health system that is committed to a multidisciplinary approach to care provision, but which has yet to accept clearly a definition of social work that departs from traditional notions of the profession based in the community. Primary care social workers consistently demonstrate skills in care integration as well as skills in community development approaches to population health.

Butler (2005) noted a similar experience in the development of community-based mental health services in the 1970s, where psychiatric social workers were identified as fundamental to the interdisciplinary approach in mental health service provision but without a clearly defined role. Butler (2005) explains that, in this instance, social workers negotiated roles that 'represented a compromise between what they would ideally like to do and what colleagues, particularly psychiatrists, expected them to do'.

Butler (2005) further noted that, as the 1970s developed and social work as a profession began to acquire full and undisputed responsibility for child protection and welfare, the momentum within the health system for community-based psychiatric social workers became lost. He further notes the 'difficulties and impossibilities' that social workers have come to acknowledge as a result of having 'primary responsibility' for 'child protection and welfare'. However, at the time, the attraction was the 'undisputed nature of the turf', so social workers became an 'undisputed authority for child welfare'. This, according to Butler (2005), seemed preferable to 'haggling over roles and responsibilities which characterised social work in mental health settings'.

Indeed, primary care social work continues to negotiate a role for itself against the back-drop of both traditional social work in the community (child protection and welfare) and traditional expectations of what primary care social workers do. Lee and Carroll (2005) suggest that 'the potential for community work to complement and enhance social work has not been fully realised'.

The challenge for primary care social work, and indeed the responsibility for primary care social workers, is to ensure that we challenge these traditional and pre-conceived notions of our role and become more explicit about the full extent of what we do and demonstrate the potential for what we can do combining 'less traditional' forms of social work. For example, the University of Michigan School of Social Work identifies that social workers bring a broader set of competencies to primary care settings (Siefert and Henk, 2001):

- Conduct risk/strength assessments of individuals, families, groups, organisations and communities along a continuum of care;
- Plan and deliver culturally-competent, gender-specific individual, family, group, organisational, programmatic and community-based capacity-building interventions:
    o For the purposes of health promotion and disease prevention; and
    o For treatment and rehabilitation or continuing care, including self-help and mutual aid, support for caregivers, and brief interventions;
- Practice effectively as a professional social worker in health organisations:
    o Participate as an interdisciplinary team member, engage in case advocacy and co-ordination, and engage in case conferencing and collaboration;
    o Assess, implement, and maintain cultural competence in programmes and organisations; and
    o Apply knowledge of management and organisational theories and practices to address selected issues facing social work in health settings, such as restructuring, work design, teambuilding, continuous quality improvement, and social marketing;

- Work effectively within communities and larger systems:
  - o Build partnerships with key neighbourhood and community organisations and institutions for the purposes of health promotion and disease prevention; and
  - o Engage in advocacy, community organising, social action, and legislative policy and regulatory approaches to promote health and prevent disease and to overcome poverty, discrimination and other barriers to equity, access and quality of care;
- Incorporate social work values and ethical principles in planning, developing and implementing interventions along the continuum of care.

Research indicates that the care co-ordination/case management role of social work in primary care settings 'improves patient health and mental health outcomes among community-dwelling older adults' (Firth *et al.*, 2003). Sommers *et al.* (2000) also noted a reduction in both the use of acute services and primary care visits among older adults where primary care social workers are involved in care co-ordination.

Further, Keefe and Enguidanos (2009) conclude that, within a future of increasing health costs for health care, fragmentation in the system and pressure to treat adults on an outpatient basis, there is a pressing need to address the multiple chronic illnesses and psychosocial needs of older adults in an urgent and cost-effective manner. They further suggest that the integration of primary care social workers in primary care settings, not only to address psychosocial issues but also to provide ancillary services such as care co-ordination and care management, has the potential to improve health outcomes for older patients.

In particular, theories of social work are the guiding principles that underpin the type of practice that may be needed in a particular context. Systems perspectives, for example, have had considerable influence upon the formal base of social work. Social work theorists have argued that a systematic perspective is what distinguishes social work from other human service professions. Systemic analyses focus on interactions within and across multiple social systems. These systems include family and friendship ties, neighbourhood systems, organisational systems, social policy systems and social structural systems. In particular, systems theory emphasises the role of these systems in contributing to individual and community wellbeing (Healy, 2005).

In the changing landscape of health service provision, social workers are called upon increasingly to outline their specific value in social service provision (Healy, 2005). Indeed, in a health system that begins to recognise the socio-economic determinants of health but which is constrained by statutory responsibilities in child protection and welfare, social workers in primary care have been, and continue to be, subject to the same pressures.

As 'systems specialists', social workers in primary care have that unique ability to provide forms of assessment at individual, group, community and organisational levels that promote systemic understanding and sustainable systemic change (Healy, 2005).

Further, in the context of integrated care, social workers begin to demonstrate their ability to navigate through systems within their role as advocate on behalf of service users but also with respect to integrated service provision within the multidisciplinary team. The systemic approach of social work is most valuable in achieving better interaction between primary and secondary care. While the health system continues to struggle to address fragmentation between services, social work as a profession has the potential to use these abilities and become proficient in care co-ordination and integration.

INTEGRATED CARE

Integration is at the heart of systems theory and, therefore, central to organisational design and performance. All organisations (and systems) are, to some extent, hierarchical structures comprising separate, but interconnected, components. These components are supposed to play *complementary* roles in order to accomplish their joint tasks (Kodner and Spreeuwenberg, 2002).

The authors above note that the lack of conceptual clarity stands as a major barrier to promoting integrated care in both theory and practice. Integrated care, they suggest, has many meanings: in the UK, integrated care is taken to mean 'shared care'; in the US, it is taken to mean 'managed care'; in other areas, it is taken to mean 'comprehensive care or disease management'. Whatever we take 'integrated care' to mean, Kodner and Spreeuwenberg (2002) suggest that the fulfilment of system aims necessitates co-operation and collaboration among and between the various parts of that system. In this regard, integration is the 'glue' that bonds the system together, enabling the achievement of common goals and optimal results.

Kodner and Spreeuwenberg (2002) further note that health systems and health care institutions are among the most complex and interdependent entities known to society. The authors note that, historically, many factors have worked to divide various types of health care institutions and services on the one hand and administrators, physicians, nurses and allied health professionals on the other – for example *via*:

- Differing rules (community *versus* hospital);
- Intersectoral boundaries (primary care team boundary *versus* mental health services boundary);
- Funding streams (GP private practice *versus* publicly-funded PCT);
- Institutional and professional cultures (medical model *versus* social determinants/community development model).

What a primary health care approach recognises and attempts to address is the reality that we now face, which is that, where there is no integration at various levels, health care performance suffers, patients get lost, much needed services are not delivered or are delayed, patient satisfaction declines and the potential for cost-effectiveness diminishes (Kodner and Spreeuwenberg, 2002).

As a method for examining levels of integration in health services, Suter *et al.* (2009) outline 10 key elements of a successfully-integrated health system. According to the authors, such a system:

- Has centralised planning and co-ordination of all services for the population group served;
- Places the patient and their experience at the centre of the integration effort;
- Provides services for an identified patient group in a geographic area;
- Standardises care by interprofessional teams using shared protocols, defined roles and responsibilities and efficient communication channels;
- Has protocols and procedures to measure care processes and outcomes for continuous quality improvement;
- Uses shared electronic records;
- Bridges organisational cultures with visionary leadership;
- Overcomes physician resistance through financial incentives and improvements to the quality of their working life;
- Uses governance structures that promote co-ordination, flatter organisational structures and community representation;
- Recognises that integration processes may increase costs before they provide savings.

Using these 10 key principles and applying them to the Irish context, health services in Ireland appear to have much to do before achieving integrated care both within services and between services.

As a starting point, primary care services development has been the subject of much examination. In particular, the report of the CAG (2010) makes the following observations:

- A considerable amount of work needs to be done to achieve cohesive functioning and to establish new relationships between primary health care providers and allied health professionals;
- 27% of professionals surveyed reported that the local population had been consulted in the development of the PCT;
- 15% reported that a community health needs assessment had been completed prior to the PCT's first clinical meeting and 7% indicated that a community health needs assessment was carried out after the first clinical team meeting;
- 18% of PCT staff who replied to the survey indicated that integration with local secondary care had improved since the PCT was established;
- 71% of teams considered that they had received adequate briefing sessions on the operation of the team, prior to the commencement of work in the PCT;
- 31% of teams considered that they had received adequate training on working in the multidisciplinary context, prior to the commencement of the first clinical team meeting (CAG, 2010).

Bearing in mind all of the shortfalls noted by the CAG, it is easy to conclude that trying to achieve cohesiveness and integration at the first level of health services (primary care) at best is complicated and at worst impracticable under current systemic constraints.

In terms of GP involvement as a core team member but also as the gate-keeper of access to most secondary services, the HSE estimated that approximately 100 GPs have declined to join a PCT. Reasons stated included lack of time, funding and lack of access to IT communication (CAG, 2010). The CAG's report also noted that a number of HSE staff operate as a team in the absence of GPs: in December 2010, there were 31 teams holding clinical team meetings without GP involvement.

Primary care team developments since the publication of the *Primary Care Strategy* (DoHC, 2001) can be said to have been a casualty of the Irish health system's own complex and multifaceted composition. As outlined previously in this chapter, the *Primary Care Strategy* is one of aspiration, which locates the responsibility for care management firmly in the domain of the primary care interdisciplinary team. It also recognised the often overlooked position that illness and ill-health are exacerbated by psychosocial factors and, in response to this, placed social workers as core team members. However, at the time of publication, Ireland could not have foreseen the difficult economic landscape that it would now be facing.

In the intervening years, what we have seen, despite the valuable contribution of primary care social workers in local primary care initiatives, is the adjournment of a commitment to deal with the management and causes of ill-health in a multidimensional way.

In 2011, the ICGP produced a report, *Primary Care Teams: A GP Perspective,* following research among its own members (ICGP, 2011). One of the advantages of PCTs noted by GPs in this report was the links with primary care social workers. GPs noted that primary care social workers (as distinct from child protection social workers) 'had protected time to meet the needs of patients in the community' (ICGP, 2011).

Despite this, the number of primary care social workers as per the IASW Special Interest Group stands at 78 whole time equivalents. With a target of 518 operational PCTs nationwide, this places one social worker for every 6.64 primary care teams. According to the CAG's report (2010), for the purposes of planning norms set in 2008, social work posts were set at one per team. The report further noted, following a review of the figures in December 2010, that the proportion of social workers working in primary care stood only at 22% of the original target. This begs the question: how can primary care social workers sustain and support the primary health care approach and commit to care management as well as care co-ordination if they are not core team members?

The above figures effectively place primary care social workers as members of the HSCNs that are designed to support PCTs. They also ensure that the systems approach that underpins much social work practice in primary care becomes further away from the patient who, it appears, is the last to be considered when decisions about where to direct resources are made.

As 'systems specialists', social workers in primary care have the opportunity to be the 'glue' that bonds primary and secondary services with the common aim of integrated care. However, the opportunities for this become curtailed under these circumstances.

Indeed, this is not a phenomenon that is confined to the social work profession. The CAG's report (2010) noted that the assignment of staff to teams has not been fully progressed. As yet, there does not appear to be sufficient resources assigned to teams, especially in the areas of occupational therapy, speech therapy, social work and in administration.

According to the CAG's report (2010), central to the successful establishment of a PCT would be:

- Teambuilding activities and joint planning involving PCT members to develop partnerships, team identity and a shared understanding of roles and boundaries;

- Engagement with communities, involving them in development proposals for their area;

- Awareness of their community's health needs;

- Adequate team briefing sessions on how the PCT should operate;

- Co-ordination and integration between primary and secondary care services.

In terms of integration of primary care services, the CAG's report (2010) states that linkages need to be established between GPs and other members of the PCT and between PCTs and HSCNs, hospital services, out-of-hours services and community intervention teams.

The report further noted that a major obstacle to information sharing was the absence of an IT infrastructure between GPs and other team members. Communication between hospitals and PCT was noted also as a major obstacle to integrated care, in particular with respect to the discharge of patients back into the community.

As previously noted, much of what is identified above as 'central to the establishment of a successful primary care team' has not yet occurred at optimal levels within primary care development. Without all of these elements in place, effectively we do not have an integrated health system with a fully-supported multidisciplinary team that is holistic in its approach to care management, health promotion and disease prevention. Under these circumstances where resources are spread so thinly, we have a primary care social work service that, while providing holistic needs assessments, is curtailed in delivering population health approaches that incorporate a social determinants ethos. What we do have, however, is a primary care multidisciplinary service that struggles with a lack of resources to 'fight fires' instead of preventing them, that is re-active instead of pro-active and is always under scrutiny because the system, through an apparent lack of resources, is 'set up to fail'. Under these circumstances, the vision of the *Primary Care Strategy*, which proclaimed a 'new way' of delivering health care services to a complex and changing demographic, becomes further and further away from the reality taking place on the ground.

The CAG's report (2010) noted that considerable work remains to be done in order to ensure that primary care services are co-ordinated to improve the patient experience. Considerable work also needs to be done to ensure that integrated care pathways between primary care services and secondary care services are effective. As highlighted above, a number of conditions need to be in place to accommodate this but, in the economic reality of scarce resources and empty posts, it is pertinent to ask the question: do we have the resources to achieve the primary health care vision of integrated care? Perhaps an even more pertinent question is: can we afford not to provide the investment to ensure that we can take this approach?

CONCLUSION

The attempt by Irish health service providers to provide a 'new way' of delivering services to a changing and complex demographic has not been without its difficulties. As previously noted, health systems are one of the most complex organisational structures known to society. It is obvious that, in attempting to keep pace with international approaches to the primary health care model and to address the spiralling costs of health care, the Irish Government undertook to develop its own system for primary care services. In doing this, it placed a number of demands upon existing services working within the community, one of which was to 'embrace the change'. This has been a contentious point in the intervening years since the publication of the *Primary Care Strategy* (DoHC, 2001), as in 2010 there was still much work to be done to achieve all of the objectives of the new and integrated health system.

One of the most innovative developments in this new health system was the introduction of social workers who would be attached to PCTs. Primary care social workers have been, and continue to be, one of the more positive aspects of primary care developments (ICGP, 2011). The introduction of social workers to community health services has not been without its difficulties, the most notable of which is the expectation of its own profession to adhere to traditional models of social work practice as well as trying to develop services for care groups outside of the 'children and families' system. Social workers in primary care are under continuous scrutiny to 'prove their worth' in a health system that is stretched for resources.

In adhering to the principles of primary health care and the 'social determinants ethos', social workers bring a broad set of skills to the primary care setting which includes the skills of assessment, case management, empowerment and advocacy, but also the less common 'clinically' accepted principles of community engagement and community development. Thus, social workers in PCTs have a responsibility to be champions of these approaches.

Social workers in their more traditional form have proven their worth in health systems in hospitals – for example, as the mediator between the needs of patients and the needs of the system to discharge the patient home. Indeed, Horne and O'Connor (2005) note that social workers in hospitals 'work at the interface between hospital and community to ensure appropriate supports following discharge from hospital'. Conversely, social workers in primary care who are located within community supports can ensure ease of transition and integration between community and hospital services.

Potentially more beneficial to the system, primary care social workers, if we can champion more diverse approaches to community health needs as a fundamental aspect of the profession, can work with individuals, communities and service providers to help build the capacity at individual and community level to help prevent hospital admission in the first instance. This will become evident in the number of community projects that primary care social workers are involved in – for example, the management of chronic diseases.

Changes to take place in the coming years within the health services include the introduction of the new 'seven speciality-specific directorates', which will focus on hospital care, primary care, mental health, children and family services, social care, public health and corporate services (O'Cionnaith, 2011). This move will separate funding streams and will designate funding for each speciality area. We watch with anticipation the effect this will have for primary care social workers who are currently managed within the children and families system but whose roles were intended for primary care.

Finally, the new HSE integrated care model, introduced in 2010, is intended to deliver services across integrated service areas (ISAs), where one person will be responsible for all hospital and community services.

The new HSE service delivery model puts the patient at the centre of the process – with PCTs at level I, community HSCNs at level II, ISAs (including secondary care hospitals) at level III and tertiary acute services at level IV (McCallion, 2010). In this new model, it is suggested that clinicians have been given a much stronger voice through the development of clinical leadership, PCTs would serve populations of 7,000 to 10,000, and 531 PCT multidisciplinary teams were mapped out around the country. HSCNs also will be established and more specialised services will be delivered through the PCTs or HSCNs. For example, Community Mental Health Teams will work with a number of PCTs at a network level (Browne, 2010).

While this new model incorporates all of the aspects required to integrate care between services and to keep the patient at the centre of care delivery, it remains to be seen how long it will take to develop pathways for implementing this particular plan in this multi-faceted health system, in particular in an economic environment such as ours. One would hope that the €20 million funding made available to 'fill vacancies in primary care' (HSE, 2012) will assist in the effective implementation of this new integrated services plan which currently remains very much in its infancy.

REFERENCES

Butler, S. (2005). 'Mental Health Social Work in Ireland: Missed Opportunities?', in Kearney, N. and Skehill, C. (eds.), *Social Work in Ireland: Historical Perspectives*, Dublin: Institute of Public Administration.

Canadian Association of Social Workers (2003). *Preparing for Change: Social Work in Primary Health Care*, Ottawa: Canadian Association of Social Workers.

Carroll, M. and Lee, A. (2005). 'Community Work: A Specialism of Social Work', in Kearney, N. and Skehill, C. (eds.), *Social Work in Ireland: Historical Perspectives*, Dublin: Institute of Public Administration.

Claiborne, N. and Vandenburgh, H. (2001). 'Social Work Role in Disease Management', *Health and Social Work*, 26(4): 217-225, cited in Canadian Association of Social Workers (2003), *Preparing for Change: Social Work in Primary Health Care*, Ottawa: Canadian Association of Social Workers.

Comptroller and Auditor General (CAG) (2010). *Report of the Comptroller and Auditor General 2010*, Dublin: Stationery Office.

Department of Health (DoH) (1985). *Report of the Committee on Social Work*, Dublin: Stationery Office, cited in Butler, S. (2005). 'Mental Health Social Work in Ireland: Missed Opportunities?', in Kearney, N. and Skehill, C. (eds.), *Social Work in Ireland: Historical Perspectives*, Dublin: Institute of Public Administration.

Department of Health and Children (DoHC) (2001). *Primary Care: A New Direction*, Dublin: Stationery Office.

Dimitrov, B.D. and Fahey, T. (2010). 'Primary Health Care Models and Suitability for Provision of E-services: An Overview', in proceedings of *Enabling Citizens' Participation, Social Inclusion and Democracy through Electronic Systems and Processes*, 18-19 March, Brunel University, London.

Firth, M., Dyer, M., Marsden, H. and Savage, D. (2003). 'Developing a Social Perspective in Mental Health Services in Primary Care', *Journal of Interpersonal Care*, 17(3): 251-262, cited in Keefe, B. and Enguidanos, S. (2009), 'Integrating

Social Workers into Primary Care: Physician and Nurse Perception of Roles, Benefits and Challenges', *Social Work in Health Care*, 48: 579-596.

Halfden, M. (1981). 'The Meaning of Health for All by the Year 2000', *World Health Forum*, 2(1).

Health Service Executive (HSE) (2007). *Transformation Programme 2007-2010*, available http://www.hse.ie/eng/services/publications/corporate/transformation.pdf, accessed April 2012.

Health Service Executive (HSE) (2012). *National Service Plan 2012: Executive Summary*, available http://www.hse.ie/eng/services/publications/corporate/nspexecutivesummary2012.pdf.

Healy, K. (2005). *Three Waves of Systems Theory: Social Work Theory in Context Creating Frameworks for Practice*, New York: Palgrave Macmillan.

Horne, M. and O'Connor, E. (2005). 'An Overview of the Development of Health-related Social Work in Ireland', in Kearney, N. and Skehill, C. (eds.), *Social Work in Ireland: Historical Perspectives*, Dublin: Institute of Public Administration.

Irish College of General Practitioners (ICGP) (2011). *Primary Care Teams: A GP Perspective*, Dublin: ICGP.

Kearney, N. and Skehill, C. (eds.). (2005). *Social Work in Ireland: Historical Perspectives*, Dublin: Institute of Public Administration.

Keefe, B. and Enguidanos, S. (2009), 'Integrating Social Workers into Primary Care: Physician and Nurse Perception of Roles, Benefits and Challenges', *Social Work in Health Care*, 48: 579-596.

Keleher, H. (2004). 'Why Primary Health Care Offers a More Comprehensive Approach to Tackling Health Inequities than Primary Care', *Australian Journal of Primary Health Care*, 7: 57-61, cited in Martin, C.M. and Sturmberg, J.P. (2005), 'General Practice – Chaos, Complexity and Innovation', *Medical Journal of Australia*, 183(2): 106.

Kodner, D.L. and Spreeuwenberg, C. (2002). 'Integrated Care: Meaning, Logic, Applications and Implementations: A Discussion Paper', *International Journal of Integrated Care*, 2(14): 1-6.

Kuzel, A. (2006). 'Variation in the Design and Performance of Primary Care: International Perspectives', *Annals of Family Medicine*, 4: 375-376, doi: 10.1370/afm.605, cited in Dimitrov, B.D. and Fahey, T. (2010), 'Primary Health Care Models and Suitability for Provision of E-services: An Overview', in proceedings of *Enabling Citizens' Participation, Social Inclusion and Democracy through Electronic Systems and Processes*, 18-19 March, Brunel University, London.

Lee, A. and Carroll, M. (2005). 'Community Work: A Specialism of Social Work', in Kearney, N. and Skehill, C. (eds.), *Social Work in Ireland: Historical Perspectives*, Dublin: Institute of Public Administration.

Lesser, J. (2000). 'Clinical Social Work and Family Medicine: A Partnership in Community Service', *Health and Social Work*, 25(2): 119-126, cited in Canadian Association of Social Workers (2003), *Preparing for Change: Social Work in Primary Health Care*, Ottawa: Canadian Association of Social Workers.

Levin, R. and Herbert, M. (2001). 'Delivering Health Care Services in the Community: A Multi-disciplinary Perspective', *Social Work in Health Care*, 34(1/2): 89-99, cited in Canadian Association of Social Workers (2003),

Preparing for Change: Social Work in Primary Health Care, Ottawa: Canadian Association of Social Workers.

Loudon, I.S. (1983). 'The Origin of the General Practitioner', *Journal of the Royal College of General Practitioners*, 33: 13-18, cited in Martin, C.M. and Sturmberg, J.P. (2005), 'General Practice – Chaos, Complexity and Innovation', *Medical Journal of Australia*, 183(2): p.106.

Marmot, M. and Wilkinson, R. (eds.) (2003). *Social Determinants of Health: The Solid Facts*, 2nd edition, Geneva: World Health Organisation.

Martin, C.M. and Sturmberg, J.P. (2005), *General Practice – Chaos, Complexity and Innovation, Medical Journal of Australia*, 183(2): 106-109.

McCallion, D. (2010). *Integrated Services Programme – Integrating Hospital and Community Services: Overview*, Irish Pharmaceutical Healthcare Association, cited in Browne, M., *Journal of the Health Management Institute of Ireland*, July, www.journal.hmi.ie.

O'Cionnaith, F. (2011). 'Overhaul Will See Seven Specialised Units Replace the HSE', *Irish Examiner*, 21 December, www.irishexaminer.com.

Rock, B.D. and Cooper, M. (2000). 'Social Work in Primary Care: A Demonstration Student Unit Utilising Action Research', *Social Work in Health Care*, 31(1): 1-17, cited in Canadian Association of Social Workers (2003), *Preparing for Change: Social Work in Primary Health Care*, Ottawa: Canadian Association of Social Workers.

Salvatore, E.P. (1988). 'Issues in Collaboration and Team Work: A Sociological Perspective on the Role Definition of Social Work Primary Health Care', *Research in Sociology of Health Care*, 7: 199-239, cited in Canadian Association of Social Workers (2003), *Preparing for Change: Social Work in Primary Health Care*, Ottawa: Canadian Association of Social Workers.

Schmidt, G., Westhues, A., Lafrance, J. and Knowles, A. (2001). 'Social Work in Canada: Results from the National Sector Study', *Canadian Social Work*, 3(2): 83-92, cited in Canadian Association of Social Workers (2003), *Preparing for Change: Social Work in Primary Health Care*, Ottawa: Canadian Association of Social Workers.

Seifert, K. and Henk, M. (2001). *Social Work in Primary Health Care*, monograph series, Philadelphia: Society for Social Work Leadership in Health Care, cited in Canadian Association of Social Workers (2003), *Preparing for Change: Social Work in Primary Health Care*, Ottawa: Canadian Association of Social Workers.

Sommers, L., Marton, K., Barbaccia, J. and Randolf, J. (2000). 'Physician, Nurse and Social Workers Collaboration in Primary Care for Chronically Ill Seniors', *Archives of Internal Medicine*, 160: 1825-1833, in Keefe, B. and Enguidanos, S. (2009), 'Integrating Social Workers into Primary Care: Physician and Nurse Perception of Roles, Benefits and Challenges', *Social Work in Health Care*, 48: 579-596.

Suter, E., Oelke, N., Adair, C. and Armitage, G. (2009). 'Ten Key Principles for Successful Health Systems Integration', *Health Care Quarterly*, 13(Special): 16-23.

Thomas, P. and Graver, L. (1997). 'The Liverpool Intervention to Promote Teamwork in General Practice: An Action Research Approach', in Pearson, P. and Spencer, J. (1997) (eds.), *Promoting Teamwork in Primary Care: A Research-based Approach*, London: Arnold.

Trotter, K. (2008). 'Primary Care Models: A Review of the Literature', in *Second Invitational Continuing Education* conference, Antigua, cited in Dimitrov, B.D. and Fahey, T. (2010). 'Primary Health Care Models and Suitability for Provision of E-services: An Overview', in proceedings of *Enabling Citizens' Participation, Social Inclusion and Democracy through Electronic Systems and Processes*, 18-19 March, Brunel University, London.

Wharf, B. (1992). *Communities and Social Policy in Canada*, Toronto: McLelland Stewart, 151-181, cited in Canadian Association of Social Workers (2003), *Preparing for Change: Social Work in Primary Health Care*, Ottawa: Canadian Association of Social Workers.

World Health Organization (WHO) (1946). 'Definition of Social Determinants of Health', www.who.int/bulletin/archives/80(12)981.pdf, Preamble to the *Constitution* of the World Health Organization as adopted by the International Health Conference, New York, 9-22 June, signed on 22 July 1946 by representatives of 61 states (official records at the WHO, No.2, p.100) and entered into force 7 April 1948.

World Health Organization (WHO) (1978). *Declaration of Alma Ata*, adopted at the International Conference on Primary Health Care, Alma Ata, USSR, 6-12 September.

12: PRIMARY CARE TEAMS IN IRELAND FROM THE PERSPECTIVE OF GENERAL PRACTICE

Margaret O'Riordan and Claire Collins

INTRODUCTION

General practice/family medicine in Ireland is delivered by *circa* 2,500 general practitioners (GPs) operating in approximately 1,500 practices, each operating as an independent unit, with an estimated 30% of GPs working in single-handed practices (Darker *et al.*, 2011). While the State finances 30% of the population's primary care, this is done by granting GPs a single annual capitation fee for each public patient on their list, rather than on a visit-by-visit basis. Private patients are not required to register with a GP and may attend more than one GP.

It is predicted that there will be 13.4 million visits *per annum* to general practice in Ireland by 2015 and 14.8 million by 2021 (Layte *et al.*, 2009). The average number of GP visits per year for a person aged 16+ years was 3.3 in 2001, ranging from 1.4 in men aged 16 to 20 years to 7.8 in women aged 81+years (Layte *et al.*, 2009).

The number of health problems has been shown to be a major predictor of frequency of GP attendances. However, an Australian study (Knox and Britt, 2004) demonstrated that specific chronic disorders had differential effects on visit frequency with anxiety, back complaints, and depression having the greatest effects on increasing patient annual visits to a GP. Regression models in this study also revealed that the visit rates of patients with diabetes, asthma, ischaemic heart disease, osteoarthritis, oesophageal disease and hypertension were mostly explained by the overall level of health problems experienced by the patient rather than to any increased demand for health care related to the specific morbidity (Knox and Britt, 2004). Similar results have been shown in Ireland with significantly higher GP and practice nurse utilisation rates and medication use among those with multimorbidity (O'Kelly *et al.*, 2011).

PRIMARY CARE TEAMS – EVIDENCE AND ESTABLISHMENT IN IRELAND

GPs have an integral role in assessing the needs of their local populations and providing services to meet these needs (Pearson *et al.*, 1996). They are responsible for assessing the majority of acutely ill patients, with up to two-thirds of primary care contacts being for acute problems; the consultations for which are "often more complex than the presentation and treatment of a single episode might suggest" (Jones *et al.*, 2010). It has been estimated to take 7.4 hours per working day to provide all recommended preventive care to a panel of 2,500 patients, plus 10.6 hours to manage all chronic conditions adequately (Yarnall *et al.*, 2003; Ostbye *et al.*, 2005). There is evidence to support primary care teams (PCTs) as a better means of delivering effective care to patients (King's Fund, 2011), in particular for managing those with long-term chronic conditions (Khan *et al.*, 2008; Coleman *et al.*, 2009; Nolte *et al.*, 2009; Goodwin *et al.*, 2010; Jenkins and Kirk, 2010; Kithas and Supiano, 2010) and in terms of cost-effectively enhancing health outcomes (Stock *et al.*, 2010).

Chronic diseases form the greatest threat to the health of populations worldwide today. The global prevalence of all leading chronic diseases is continuously increasing. In 2008, 63% of deaths were attributed to chronic diseases, with an expected increase of 15% globally between 2010 and 2020 (World Health Organization (WHO), 2011). The WHO *Global Strategy* document predicted that morbidity and disability attributable to the major non-communicable diseases (chronic disease) was expected to rise to 60% by 2020 (WHO, 2004). This poses great challenges for health care systems in Europe in providing high quality care for the chronically ill, without causing tremendous economic burdens on the community. General practice's cornerstone is continuity of care and in the US, it is considered that:

> Better continuity of care allows practitioners to use more watchful waiting and employ health care resources more judiciously (Forrest and Whelan, 2000: 2082).

The complexity of health care is increasing, associated with several factors including ageing populations and expanding co-morbidities. Most of the care of chronic disease in Ireland takes place in primary care (Department of Health and Children (DoHC), 2009). Chronic disease accounts for a significant proportion of the disease burden and an increasing workload for GPs, accounting for up to 60% of visits by patients 45 years and older (Britt *et al.*, 2009). Available Irish data indicates that 51% of Irish adults have visited a medical doctor or hospital in the previous 12 months, and that nearly one-third of these are on long-term medication for conditions such as blood pressure, arthritis, asthma, diabetes, heart disease and cancer (Irish Patient Association, 2004). Significant health inequalities between socio-economic groups also have been shown in terms of death rates and experience of illness, with double the proportion of people who are consistently poor reporting having a chronic illness in Ireland compared to the general population (Farrell *et al.*, 2008). Patients with multiple chronic diseases experience unfavourable health outcomes and give rise to challenges in patient care and medical costs (Parekh and Barton, 2010). A systematic review of chronic disease management has reported that care delivered in a primary care or community care setting improved patient outcomes with diabetes and hypertension, although the evidence is less clear for arthritis, COPD and asthma (Dennis *et al.*, 2008). In a recent Irish study, the main barriers to delivering chronic care were found to be an increased workload and a lack of appropriate funding for chronic disease management (Darker *et al.*, 2011).

In 2001, the Irish government set out to establish up to 1,000 primary care teams (PCTs) to deliver enhanced primary care services. According to the 2001 *Primary Care Strategy*, the members of the team would include GPs, nurses, physiotherapists, occupational therapists, social workers, home helps and administrators. Each team would in turn be supported by a wider network of primary care professionals, including speech and language therapists, dieticians, pharmacists, community welfare officers, chiropodists and psychologists (Department of Health and Children (DoHC), 2001). At the time of writing, the Irish Health Service Executive (HSE) reported 408 PCTs in place at the end of June 2012 and proposed that "there will be 485 PCTs in operation by end of 2012, each serving a population of approximately 8,000 to 12,000" (HSE, 2012). However, Minister Dr. James Reilly TD has said he did not accept the reported HSE figures and noted that, even if a GP had expressed an interest in becoming part of a team, this could subsequently be interpreted that a functioning team was in existence (Donnellan, 2011).

This commitment to primary care reform has been reiterated in the Department of Health (DoH) strategy document for the period 2012 to 2015, which states:

> ... the vision for primary care which the government is committed to implementing is one where: no one must pay fees for GP care; GPs work in teams with other primary care professionals; the focus is on

the prevention of illness and structured care for people with chronic conditions; primary care teams work from dedicated facilities; and staffing and resourcing of primary care is allocated rationally to meet regularly assessed needs. (DoH, 2012: 30)

The Irish College of General Practitioners (ICGP), the professional body for GPs in Ireland, has been supportive of the theoretical basis for PCTs as the optimum model for delivery of primary care services to patients. In a 2010 ICGP survey completed by 423 members (response rate *circa* 17%), 41.6% of GPs indicated that they were not part of a PCT while 10.1% indicated they would be joining a PCT in the near future. These figures are disappointing but, even worse, of the 195 GPs who reported being part of a PCT, 64.6% reported that this was poorly functioning (Meagan, 2012). The results of the survey are endorsed by a national survey by Trinity College Dublin, where only 36% of respondents indicated that their practice was functioning as a part of a PCT (Darker *et al.*, 2011). Furthermore, only 44% of respondents indicated that they believed PCTs would enhance their ability to deliver chronic disease management within their practice (Darker *et al.*, 2011). A report in 2011 by the Comptroller and Auditor General (CAG) highlighted that the number of functioning teams (as described by the HSE) was overestimated, as only 54% of PCTs reported regular GP representation at meetings and that, even if GPs had ceased to attend, teams were still reported as operating. At a fundamental level:

There has not yet been a change at the level of control and management that would put PCTs at the centre of primary care delivery (CAG, 2011: 581).

THE GENERAL PRACTICE PERSPECTIVE

In an effort to address apparent inconsistencies in reports and to capture the GP perspective on PCTs in Ireland, the ICGP carried out a review in 2011 by consulting with its members from large and small, rural and urban practices throughout the country. The review aimed to answer the following questions from a GP perspective:

- What is the definition of a successful PCT?

- What are the advantages of PCTs and what are the perceived barriers to GP involvement?

- What can be done to encourage more GPs to participate in these teams?

The first challenge was to define what is meant by a successful PCT. A consensus approach led to the following definition:

> A successful primary care team is where a patient receives a better standard of care from interacting with the team than they would receive from dealing with individual health professionals. In essence teamwork leads to the sum being greater than the parts in relation to improved quality of service for the patient (ICGP, 2011, 4).

Where GPs were actively involved in a PCT, they perceived a number of advantages from this participation. The most significant of these was improved quality of service for patients, particularly where teams were co-located in the same building. Team members, including GPs, develop a better understanding of roles, thus ensuring appropriate referrals and better use of resources. Several members of the team make house calls, which may reduce the number of visits that a GP has to undertake and enhance the service for the patient. Interreferral between GPs promotes services at primary care level and reduces referrals to secondary care. Where direct access to diagnostics (for example, radiology) is provided, it greatly enhances the ability to provide care for patients in the community and facilitates appropriate referral.

GPs also describe enhancement of clinical management and new approaches to patient care as a result of team participation. The role of the home help in particular was clearly valued by GPs. Links with the mental health team traditionally have been poor in the community but the advent of PCTs has enhanced communications and understanding in some parts of the country. The role of the primary care Mental Health Liaison Nurse, where they have been established, has been welcomed by GPs. A model for direct access by GPs to counselling services in the North East has been particularly successful in this regard. There are plans to expand this service nationwide. Links with primary care social workers have been very positively received by the GPs – as these social workers are distinct from the child protection social workers, they have protected time to meet the needs of patients in the community.

Where teams have been successful, a key person in this success has been the local primary care manager. GPs highly value managers who are pro-active, flexible, open communicators, showing a willingness to engage in a positive manner with them and thus encouraging participation and belief in the team concept. Naturally, this has led also to improved GP-HSE communications on all aspects of local service delivery.

A number of PCTs have tried to adapt and change their model of work to tailor for different patient groups – for example, single mothers with anxiety/depression in an area of deprivation (Chan *et al.*, 2011). There is a potential for a population-based approach to prevention with all team members involved – for example, team members running a Well Man or Well Woman evening for patients, suicide prevention talks, school visits.

Barriers to GP involvement in PCTs could be summarised under a number of headings, including management approach, organisation of meetings, disintegration of services, confidentiality issues, patient eligibility for services, information technology and communication and infrastructure limitations. Where teams were not successful, there was a perception of a top-down approach by HSE management with poor engagement with GPs at local level. When an initial approach to team involvement was not managed appropriately, subsequent attempts were rebuffed by GPs due to prior experience and perceptions. Only 15% of PCTs carried out a community needs assessment prior to their first clinical meeting (CAG, 2011). Frustration has built up where a PCT is formed in an area involving a number of general practices and neighbouring practices are excluded. GPs may be assigned to a number of different PCTs/meetings – as patients are assigned to teams based on their geographical location rather than general practice registration. This is a fundamental flaw in the methodology employed to define a PCT. From a GP perspective, the logical starting point appears to be the patients registered with a given general practice and then to add a number of practices together to form the foundation of the team. The concept of catchment areas – a long-established practice in community psychiatric services – has caused problems for patient access to services. A patient may be attending a GP in a health centre, for example, but may not be eligible to be seen by a physiotherapist working in the same centre based on their home address. Replicating this approach is not to be recommended. Issues related to clinical governance structures were highlighted with lack of clarity with regard to final clinical responsibility for team decisions. Furthermore, the goals/aims of PCTs were not clearly defined, in many instances leading to lack of buy-in as to the perceived advantage of participation. This was exacerbated by team members reporting to multiple managers. This silo effect where team members are reporting to largely hospital-based discipline managers is not conducive to team cohesion and productivity. Clerical support is essential – otherwise team members can spend up to 50% of their clinical time doing administrative tasks such as arranging appointments rather than seeing patients.

GPs expressed frustration at the importance placed on attending meetings, in particular where having a meeting was portrayed as equating to a successful team. GPs have to travel to meetings and do not receive expenses to do so while other team members are paid to attend and receive time in lieu if it is held out-of-hours or during lunchtime. Furthermore, when travel time is taken into account, a meeting may take up to two hours out of a busy day. Doctors who have patients in four or five PCTs cannot be expected to devote 16 to 20 hours each month to meetings. Timing and frequency of meetings were also an issue. In some instances, multiplicity of meetings in relation to PCTs was a problem – clinical meetings, business meetings, local implementation group meetings, regional implementation group meetings, etc.

Despite the appointment of additional staff, many services (for example, physiotherapy) have unacceptable waiting times for services (partially offset by the fact that close working relationships enhances identification of patients requiring urgent care and all services can be mobilised quickly – for example, care of a patient with a terminal illness). Where waiting lists exist for PCTs, patients may repeatedly not attend for appointments – a system for managing this as per hospital outpatient departments may be necessary.

In the case of successful teams, the services they currently provide are starting to disintegrate due to:

• Waiting list for access to services in the community;

• Jobs embargo.

Disintegration of services discourages GPs from joining PCTs as they perceive no benefit for their patients and a lack of true commitment on behalf of the HSE/DoH to primary care development.

Many GPs have expressed concerns in relation to patient confidentiality, especially sharing patient records. Concern in relation to consent and informed consent from patients to discuss their medical information at team meetings is an important issue for many GPs. In rural areas in particular, the presence of non-health professionals at team meetings raised the possibility of inadvertent involvement of patients' relatives/friends. GPs also expressed concern at the perceived low level of feedback provided to the patient of the outcome from the meeting.

Access for patients to PCT services was not seen as equitable throughout the country. Nursing home patients in most instances are not eligible for PCT care – this is a particular source of frustration for GPs as it seems to be based on the premise that nursing home patients are private patients at a time when large numbers are only eligible through the Fair

Deal scheme and clearly cannot afford services such as private physiotherapy. In some cases, no private patients are seen by PCTs; in other areas, a quota system seems to be in operation where a limited number can be seen per year.

Access for GPs to PCTs seems to vary from area to area. There is a wide variation in access to ancillary services both within and outside PCTs, which can be frustrating for GPs and hinders quality of patient care. Access to diagnostics and secondary care services varies with area. This should be a top priority for development in a health service that seeks to be primary care-led and mindful of resources. GPs are the only professionals available out-of-hours thereby limiting the availability of other team members, particularly when urgent situations arise. It is reported that 11% of team members have extended their working hours since the establishment of PCTs, with 3% working at weekends (CAG, 2011).

The majority of GPs use computerised medical records and have done so for a considerable period of time. Other PCT members in general have limited access to IT support and use paper records. Secure email is not available for PCT members and sending patient-identifiable clinical information by normal email breaches data protection law. The lack of a unique patient identifier hinders registration with general practice and PCTs and inhibits service provision and development. The lack of IT infrastructure has been highlighted as a major block to team communications (CAG, 2011). There is little communication between established PCTs, therefore potential opportunities to learn from each other are lost.

If projects were completed on time, it was estimated that the proportion of fully co-located PCTs would increase from 8% to 29% by the end of 2011 (CAG, 2011) – an update on which was not available at the time of writing. The preferred option for further development by the HSE is for leasing arrangements with the private sector. However, the CAG (2011) has criticised the appraisal methodology employed to reach this conclusion. The uncertainty surrounding support for development of practice premises, linked to universal reduction in GP practice income, is hindering the ability of GPs to be more pro-active in infrastructure development. One size does not fit all and a flexible approach to the ideal infrastructural developments – taking cognisance of what is already in existence – is needed.

Having analysed successful teams and perceived barriers to GP participation in teams, a number of issues need to be considered. In the first instance, successful PCTs need to be encouraged to share their experiences with others. GPs in particular should be more vocal in terms of the advantages where they perceive improved quality of care for their patients.

The following emerged from this review:

- Management:
  - o Accept that one size does not fit all;
  - o Develop a variety of PCT models based on successful teams to date – promote innovation and flexibility in approach;
  - o Focus on meeting the needs of the community and PCT members, including GPs, at a local level;
  - o Define clear goals and aims for individual teams;
  - o Provide direct access to diagnostics for GPs;
  - o Define the role of GPs and practice nurses in the context of health service reform;
  - o Develop clear lines of management for team members in a unified manner. The CAG (2011) report outlines the absence of a single manager for PCT members. The HSE plans to introduce one manager for three to five PCTs – the number and role of these managers needs careful consideration;
  - o Provide administrative support to the nursing and allied health professionals in the team and local network, including booking clinic rooms, booking appointments, recording referrals, maintaining databases, recordkeeping, typing, organising and taking minutes at PCT meetings. This facilitates health professionals to see more patients.
- Meetings:
  - o Teleconference facilities could be provided to reduce the time commitment for GPs;
  - o Alternate meeting venue to minimise travel for individuals;
  - o Flexibility in setting meeting times – for example, alternate early morning and lunchtimes;
  - o The resource implications for GPs attending meetings should be acknowledged and supported.
- Disintegration of services:
  - o If PCTs are regarded as the linchpin to develop primary care services, then they should be prioritised for development and maintenance of staff levels;
  - o Waiting lists for PCT services should be kept to an absolute minimum;

- o If PCTs are truly seen as the centre of primary health care provision, then resources must be ring-fenced for both primary care and general practice.
- Confidentiality:
  - o Issues such as sharing of records and consent need to be addressed by guidelines at national level and sharing the practical experience of implementing them on the ground could be used to encourage more GPs to participate in PCTs. Although HSE *Information Sharing Guidelines* were produced in the initial stages of establishing teams they do not appear to be in use. These guidelines could be revised and implemented.
- Access and eligibility:
  - o Access and eligibility issues need to be addressed through national guidelines and implemented uniformly throughout the country;
  - o Out-of-hours health professional availability needs to be addressed.
- Information technology and communications:
  - o Secure email for PCTs would be a major step forward;
  - o Communication *via* a local (not HSE) intranet has been used also to enhance communication between team members;
  - o Local directories of services need to be developed, disseminated and maintained;
  - o Sharing of good practice between PCTs should be encouraged.
- Infrastructure:
  - o A variety of approaches to infrastructure development should be available related to local health service needs;
  - o Clarity in terms of primary care development and the role of general practice is needed to encourage GPs to participate in infrastructural development;
  - o Innovative approaches to funding and resourcing infrastructure need to be considered.

CONCLUSION

The *Primary Care Strategy* (DoHC, 2001) promoted the concept of primary care being delivered through PCTs and this approach has been reiterated recently (DoH, 2012). The implementation of this strategy has been piecemeal at best. There are examples of PCTs that work effectively in delivering improved quality of care to patients. These teams need to be supported and their experience shared. Perceived barriers to participation need to be addressed in order to encourage further participation by GPs.

If it can be clearly demonstrated that Irish patients receive better care and health outcomes from PCT participation, this would be the best way of encouraging GPs to take an active part in team activity. The focus on holding meetings is not the right approach and does not equate to a functioning team. One size does not fit all and national approaches that do not take cognisance of local needs are doomed to fail.

In order to support GPs to maximise their potential to improve the quality of service to patients and optimise the overall use of health service funding, the following actions need to be taken as a matter of urgency:

- If PCTs are truly seen as the linchpin to support the health service, then resources must be ring-fenced for both primary care and general practice development;
- As there are finite resources available for the health service, ring-fenced resources need to move from secondary to primary care and specifically to general practice if chronic disease management is to be optimised;
- Research and monitoring to demonstrate concrete outcomes and measures of success for PCTs needs to be undertaken;
- Issues related to patient consent and confidentiality should be clearly addressed and safeguards agreed;
- Access to diagnostics for GPs will enhance services for patients, save money for the health service and support appropriate hospital referrals;
- Engagement at local level in planning and developing services needs to be undertaken and it must be acknowledged that one size does not fit all;
- PCTs should be practice population-based rather than geographical;
- Access and eligibility issues for PCTs need to be addressed;
- Investment in ICT and in particular the creation of a unique patient identifier coupled with secure email should be a priority for the health services;
- Clarity around support for infrastructural developments needs to be provided.

Creating and nurturing successful PCTs has proven to be difficult elsewhere also (Bodenheimer, 2007) and challenges exist in changing the culture to a team-based approach (Markova *et al.*, 2012). Sources of team conflict identified included scope of practice, accountability (Brown *et al.*, 2011) and role boundary issues (Ghaye, 2006; Brown *et al.*, 2011).

The King's Fund in the UK (2011) noted that delivering high-quality care requires effective teamworking and Samuelson *et al.* concluded that:

> ... the increasingly complex health needs of the population and individual patients in a changing society can only be met by promoting interprofessional collaboration within primary care teams (Samuelson *et al.*, 2012, 303).

A thematic analysis of the literature revealed that two overarching themes had an impact on interprofessional teamworking: team structure and team processes. Within these two themes, six categories were identified: team premises; team size and composition; organisational support; team meetings; clear goals and objectives; and audit (Xyrichis and Lowton, 2008). However, Howard *et al.* (2011) found that culture, leadership, and electronic medical records functionality, rather than organisational composition of the teams were the most important factors in predicting climate in PCTs.

Canadian data demonstrates that the PCT must truly function as a team and activate key processes to have a positive effect on confidence in the health care system (Khan *et al.*, 2008). Markova *et al.* (2012) have suggested that effective and sustainable teams require the setting of clear performance expectations (including role definition) and the training of leaders to use non-authoritarian techniques. Additionally, recognition that teams require work and understanding, respecting team members' roles (Sargeant *et al.*, 2008; Heslin and Ryan, 2010), clear goals with measurable outcomes (Poulton and West, 1999; Grumback and Bodenheimer, 2004; Heslin and Ryan, 2010), clinical and administrative systems (Grumback and Bodenheimer, 2004) and good communication (Grumback and Bodenheimer, 2004; Sargeant *et al.*, 2008; Heslin and Ryan, 2010) have been identified as essential factors.

It has been recommended that the GP should be empowered to take on a more expert advisory role and that stronger incentives are needed to support general practice to work in collaboration with other providers:

> ... not only to improve health, but to rise to the challenge of providing better value and more efficiency in the current context of growing demand in a period of financial austerity (King's Fund, 2011: 132).

REFERENCES

Bodenheimer, T. (2007). *Building Teams in Primary Care: Lessons from 15 Case Studies*, Oakland, CA: California Health Care Foundation.

Britt, E., Miller, G.C., Charles, J., Henderson, J., Bayram, C., Harrison, C., Valenti, L., Fahridin, S., Pan, Y. and O'Halloran, F. (2009). *General Practice Activity in Australia 1998–99 to 2007–08: 10-year Data Tables, General Practice Series Number 26*, Canberra: Australian Institute of Health and Welfare and the University of Sydney.

Brown, J., Lewis, L., Ellis, K., Stewart, M., Freeman, T.R. and Kasperski, M.J. (2011). 'Conflict on Interprofessional Primary Health Care Teams – Can It Be Resolved?', *Journal of Interprofessional Care*, 25(1): 4-10. PMID:20795830.

Chan, W.S., Whitford, D., Conroy, R., Gibney, D. and Hollywood, B. (2011). 'A Multidisciplinary Primary Care Team Consultation in a Socio-economically Deprived Community: An Exploratory Randomised Controlled Trial', *BMC Health Service Research*, 11:15.

Coleman, K., Austin, B.T., Brach, C. and Wagner, E.H. (2009). 'Evidence on the Chronic Care Model in the New Millennium', *Health Affairs*, 28(1): 75.

Comptroller and Auditor General (CAG) (2011). *Report of the Controller and Auditor General 2010*, Dublin: Stationery Office.

Darker, C., Martin, C., O'Dowd, T., O'Kelly, F., O'Kelly, M. and O'Shea, B. (2011). *A National Survey of Chronic Disease Management in Irish General Practice*, Dublin: Irish College of General Practitioners.

Dennis, S.M., Zwar, N., Griffiths, R., Roland, M., Hasan, I., Powell Davies, G. and Harris, M. (2008). 'Chronic Disease Management in Primary Care: From Evidence to Policy', *Medical Journal of Australia*, 188: S53–S56.

Department of Health (DoH) (2012). *Future Health: A Strategic Framework for Reform of the Health Service 2012 – 2015*, Dublin: Stationery Office.

Department of Health and Children (DoHC) (2001). *Primary Care: A New Direction*, Dublin: Stationery Office.

Department of Health and Children (DoHC) (2009). *Health in Ireland: Key Trends 2009*, Dublin: Stationery Office.

Donnellan, E. (2011). 'Minister "Does Not Accept" HSE Claims on Number of Primary Care Teams, *The Irish Times*, 9 May.

Farrell, C., McAvoy, H., Wilde, J. and Combat Poverty Agency (2008). *Tackling Health Inequalities – An All-Ireland Approach to Social Determinants*, Dublin: Combat Poverty Agency/Institute of Public Health in Ireland.

Forrest, C.B. and Whelan, E.M. (2000). 'Primary Care Safety-net Delivery Sites in the United States: A Comparison of Community Health Centers, Hospital Outpatient Departments and Physicians' Offices', *Journal of the American Medical Association*, Oct. 25, 284(16): 2077-83.

Ghaye, T. (2006). *Developing the Reflective Healthcare Team*, Chichester: Wiley-Blackwell.

Goodwin, N., Curry, N., Naylor, C., Ross, S. and Duldig, W. (2010). *Managing People With Long-term Conditions*, London: The King's Fund, available at: www.kingsfund.org.uk/current_projects/gp_inquiry/dimensions_of_care/the_management_of_1.html (accessed 16 November 2012).

Grumbach, K. and Bodenheimer, T. (2004). 'Can Health Care Teams Improve Primary Care Practice?', *Journal of the American Medical Association*, March 10, 291(10): 1246-51. PMID:15010447.

Health Service Executive (HSE) (2012). *Primary Care Services*, available at http://www.hse.ie/eng/services/Find_a_Service/PrimaryCare/, accessed 16 November 2012.

Heslin, C. and Ryan, A. (2010). *Improving Team Working: A Guidance Document*, Dublin: Health Service Executive.

Howard, M., Brazil, K., Akhtar-Danesh, N. and Agarwal, G. (2011). 'Self-reported Teamwork in Family Health Team Practices in Ontario: Organizational and Cultural Predictors of Team Climate', *Canadian Family Physician*, May, 57(5): e185-91. PMID:21571706.

Irish College of General Practitioners (ICGP) (2011). *Primary Care Teams: A GP Perspective*, Dublin: ICGP.

Irish Patient Association and Landsdowne Market Research (2004). *Patient Attitudes*, Dublin: Irish Patient Association and Landsdowne Market Research.

Jenkins, K. and Kirk, M. (2010). 'Heart Failure and Chronic Kidney Disease: An Integrated Care Approach', *Journal of Renal Care*, 36:127-135.

Jones, R., White, P., Armstrong, D., Ashworth, M. and Peters, M. (2010). *Managing Acute Illness: An Inquiry into the Quality of General Practice in England*, London: The King's Fund.

Khan, S., McIntosh, C., Sanmartin, C., Watson, D. and Leeb, K. (2008). *Health Research Working Paper Series: Primary Health Care Teams and Their Impact on Processes and Outcomes of Care*, Ottawa: Health Information and Research Division, Statistics Canada.

King's Fund, The (2011). *Improving the Quality of Care in General Practice*, London: The King's Fund.

Kithas, P.A. and Supiano, M.A. (2010). 'Hypertension and Chronic Kidney Disease in the Elderly', *Advances in Chronic Kidney Disease*, 17(4): 341.

Knox, S.A. and Britt, H. (2004). 'The Contribution of Demographic and Morbidity Factors to Self-reported Visit Frequency of Patients: A Cross-sectional Study of General Practice Patients in Australia', *BMC Family Practice*, 5: 17. doi: 10.1186/1471-2296-5-17.

Layte, R., Barry, M., Bennett, K., Brick, A., Morgenroth, E., Normand, C., O'Reilly, J., Thomas, J., Tilson, L., Wiley, M. and Wren, M.-A. (2009). *Projecting the Impact of Demographic Change on the Demand for and the Delivery of Health Care in Ireland*, Research Series No. 13, Dublin: Economic and Social Research Institute.

Markova, T., Mateo, M. and Roth, L.M. (2012). 'Implementing Teams in a Patient-centered Medical Home Residency Practice: Lessons Learned', *Journal of the American Board of Family Medicine*, 25: 224 –31.

Meagan, G. (2012). 'Keeping in Tune with Members', *FORUM*, 10-12.

Nolte, E., Knai, C. and McKee, M. (2009). *Managing Chronic Conditions: Experience in Eight Countries*, Copenhagen: World Health Organization on behalf of European Observatory on Health Systems and Policies.

O'Kelly, S., Smith, S.M., Lane, S., Telieur, C. and O'Dowd, T. (2011). 'Chronic Respiratory Disease and Multimorbidity: Prevalence and Impact in a General Practice Setting', *Respiratory Medicine*, February, 105(2): 236-42.

Ostbye, T., Yarnall, K.S., Krause, K.M., Pollak, K.I., Gradison, M. and Michener, J.L. (2005). 'Is There Time for Management of Patients with Chronic Diseases in Primary Care?', *Annals of Family Medicine*, 3(3): 209-214.

Parekh, A.K. and Barton, M.B. (2010). 'The Challenge of Multiple Co-morbidity for the US Health Care System, *Journal of the American Medical Association*, 303(13): 1303-1304.

Pearson, N., O'Brien, J., Thomas, H., Ewings, P., Gallier, L. and Bussey, A. (1996). 'Collecting Morbidity Data in General Practice: The Somerset Morbidity Project', *British Medical Journal*, 312: 1517-1520.

Poulton, B.C. and West, M.A. (1999). 'The Determinants of Effectiveness in Primary Health Care Teams', *Journal of Interprofessional Care*, 13(1): 7-18.

Samuelson, M., Tedeschi, P., Aarendonk, D., de la Cuesta, C. and Groenewegen, P. (2012). 'Improving Interprofessional Collaboration in Primary Care: Position Paper of the European Forum for Primary Care', *Quality in Primary Care*, 20(4): 303-12. PMID:23113915.

Sargeant, J., Loney, E. and Murphy, G. (2008). 'Effective Interprofessional Teams: "Contact Is Not Enough" to Build a Team', *Journal of Continuing Education in the Health Professions*, Fall, 28(4): 228-34. PMID:19058243.

Stock, S., Drabik, A., Büsher, G., Graf, C., Ullrich, W., Gerber, A., Lauterbach, K.W. and Lüngen, M. (2010). 'German Diabetes Management Programs Improve Quality of Care and Curb Costs', *Health Affairs*, 29(12): 2197-205.

World Health Organization (WHO) (2004). *Global Strategy on Diet, Physical Activity and Health*, WHA57.17, April, available http://www.who.int/dietphysicalactivity/strategy/eb11344/en/index.html, accessed 16 November 2012.

World Health Organization (WHO) (2011). *Global Status Report on Non-communicable Diseases 2010*, Geneva: World Health Organization.

Xyrichis, A. and Lowton, K. (2008). 'What Fosters or Prevents Interprofessional Team Working in Primary and Community Care? A Literature Review', *International Journal of Nursing Studies*, January, 45(1): 140-53. PMID:17383655.

Yarnall, K.S., Pollak, K.I., Ostbye, T., Krause, K.M. and Michener, J.L. (2003). 'Primary Care: Is There Enough Time for Prevention?', *American Journal of Public Health*, 93(4): 635-641.

SECTION IV: INTEGRATED CARE, THE OLDER PERSON AND DEMENTIA

13: HEALTH SERVICE INTEGRATION FOR THE ELDERLY: AN UNEVEN JOURNEY IN CANADA

Margaret MacAdam

INTRODUCTION

For some time, Canadian health policy-makers and some providers have been concerned with two related issues: poor quality of care for those with chronic conditions and the continued sustainability of the publicly-funded health care system. These issues are related because those with chronic conditions are the most frequent users of health care services, and inefficient use of resources in the treatment of chronic conditions contributes to higher health care spending. Those over the age of 65 (seniors) are much more likely to have chronic conditions than those younger than 65. With a rapidly-growing elderly population in many countries, the challenge of adjusting health delivery systems to improve care for those with chronic conditions is the primary focus of many reform efforts.

Among the challenges of improving care for those with chronic conditions is the need to provide care across a long period of time, using a variety of service interventions that cross traditional boundaries of commonly-understood 'health' services. Improved service co-ordination and/or integration are cited frequently as mechanisms to reduce wasted resources, fragmented care and patient dissatisfaction while improving cost-effectiveness. Reforming the delivery of care for those with chronic conditions represents a complex shift in health care systems that are currently well-structured to provide episodic care within traditional 'health' frameworks.

THE CANADIAN CONTEXT

There are 10 provinces and three territories in Canada. The provinces are the home of the vast majority of Canadians, have their own constitutional authority, and are much more developed than the territories, which are all located in the sparsely-settled North. The development of integrated care in the provinces is the focus of this chapter.

In Canada, government is structured as a confederation with significant constitutional responsibilities for social and health policy, organisation, and delivery being the responsibility of the 10 provincial governments and three territories. The provinces rely on the federal government to assist with the financing of health care. The key piece of federal legislation governing federal financial participation in health is the *Canada Health Act*, which sets out two categories of service: insured services (primary medical care and acute care) and extended health services (such as residential long-term care, home care, and ambulatory health). Only the insured services are covered by the five principles of the *Act* (universality, accessibility, public administration, portability and comprehensiveness) and restrictions on user fees and extra billing. Supportive social services such as adult day care are funded through another piece of federal legislation, the *Canada Health and Social Transfer Act*. Provinces pay from their own revenues the majority of all publicly-funded health care costs. Because funding for health services, broadly speaking, comes from different sources with differing requirements, and the social, economic, and political context in each province differs, each province has developed its own terms and conditions under which services will be provided. In spite of differing provincial circumstances, all provinces, like many countries in the developed world, are struggling to reform their health care systems to achieve better patient outcomes while managing both public expectations and public health care costs.

CONCEPTUAL AND PRACTICAL UNDERSTANDING ABOUT INTEGRATED CARE

Canadian researchers have been quite active in conducting studies of integrated care services for the elderly (Leatt *et al.*, 2000; Hébert *et al.*, 2003; Hébert *et al.*, 2010; Béland *et al.*, 2006; Suter *et al.*, 2011; Hollander and Prince, 2001; 2008; MacAdam, 2008; 2009; 2011). Their work has added to the literature on frameworks of care (Hollander and Prince, 2008), features of successful integration models (Suter *et al.*, 2011; MacAdam, 2008) and implementing and evaluating integrated care projects (Hébert *et al.*, 2010; Béland *et al.*, 2006). A recent paper by Béland and Hollander (2011), containing the results of an international review of integrated systems of care for the frail elderly, found that there were basically two types of models: a smaller community-based model and a large scale model that could be applied at the regional level. In this chapter, we describe changes in Canada at the large scale (provincial) level.

Using the framework developed by Hollander and Prince (2008), shown below in **Figure 12.1**, provincial information was gathered in 2008 about progress in developing integrated care for the elderly.

Figure 12.1: The Hollander and Prince Framework

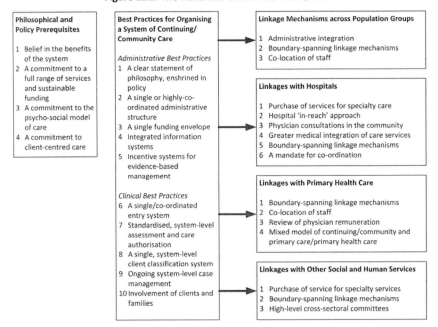

Source: Hollander and Prince, 2008.

The items of the Hollander and Prince (2008) framework for integrated care were used as a guide for survey questions. Contextual information on the utilisation of nursing home and home care services was collected in the initial survey questions. The list of possible home care services for seniors was developed from Hollander and Prince (2008). The section of the framework on linkage mechanisms was adapted to be more specific about linkage techniques as they apply to services for seniors. Complete details about the survey can be found at MacAdam (2008; 2009; 2011).

Surveys were returned from nine of the 10 Canadian provinces. The Province of Québec did not respond to the survey; to obtain data from

Québec, the questionnaire was sent to the Regional Health Authority (RHA) in the Eastern Townships (L'Estrie RHA). In the case of Manitoba, the provincial response was incomplete because some aspects of the survey were felt to be the responsibility of the RHAs. A survey was sent to the Winnipeg RHA, which provided information.

In an effort to reduce the burden on respondents, some pieces of background information were collected from Statistics Canada and other publicly-available reliable sources.

THE CONTINUING CARE CONTEXT IN CANADA

Nursing Home[5] Bed Supply and Utilisation

Table 12.1: Nursing Home Bed Supply

	BC[6]	AB	SK	MB	ON	QC/RHA[7]	NB	NS	PEI	NL
No. of seniors[8] (000s)	617.8	361.9	148.3	160.8	1,685.7	47.9	108.6	138.4	20.1	70.6
No. of nursing home beds (000s)	29.6	14.0	8.6	9.8	75.9	1.5	4.4	5.9	1.0	2.7
Beds per 1000 (65+ pop.)	47.9	38.7	58.0	60.9	45.0	31.3	40.5	42.6	50.0	38.2
Planning to build more nursing home beds	Yes	Yes	Yes	Yes	No	Yes	Yes	Yes	Yes	Yes

There are about 151,979 nursing home beds in the nine provinces responding to the survey.[9] Manitoba appears to have a larger supply of

---

[5] The provinces use a variety of terms to describe their residential long-term care services. In this survey, the term 'nursing home' is used to refer to licensed regulated facilities that provide medical, nursing and personal care services in addition to meals, housekeeping, laundry, social, spiritual and other services. Some provinces (British Columbia and Alberta, for example) provide public support for a residential option that includes supportive services for seniors who do not need the more intensive care provided by nursing homes (assisted living); others, such as Ontario, also have a more intensive level of care called a 'chronic disease hospital'. This survey does not capture the availability of other residential care options such as assisted living or chronic disease hospitals.

[6] BC = British Columbia, AB = Alberta, SK = Saskatchewan, MAN = Manitoba, ON = Ontario, QC = Québec, NB = New Brunswick, NS = Nova Scotia, PEI = Prince Edward Island, NL = Newfoundland and Labrador.

[7] Québec RHA response.

[8] Statistics Canada (2007).

nursing home beds per senior (aged 65 and over) than other provinces. All provinces, except Ontario, reported that they are increasing their nursing home bed supply (**Table 12.1**).

Home Care Services

Some provinces (British Columbia, Newfoundland and Labrador, Nova Scotia and Prince Edward Island) serve less than 10% of their 65-plus population in their home care programmes, while Ontario and New Brunswick serve about 18.4% of those aged 65 and above (**Table 12.2**).

Table 12.2: Home Care Utilisation

	BC	AB	SK	MB	ON	QC/RHA[10]	NB	NS	PEI	NL
No. of seniors[11] (000s)	617.8	361.9	148.3	160.8	1,685.7	47.9	108.6	138.4	20.1	70.6
No. of seniors served by home care services[12]	54,600	56,000	25,745[13]	27,227	310,486[14]	6,204	20,000	11,759	1,200	NA
% of seniors 65+ served by home care program	8.8%	15.5%	17.4	16.8%	18.4%	12.9%	18.4%	8.4%	5.9%	NA

---

[9] This figure does not include beds in other types of residential facilities such as chronic disease hospitals, assisted living facilities or mental health facilities or any data from Québec. Statistics Canada (2007) reports that there were 207,274 beds in residential facilities that primarily serve the aged in Canada. This figure includes Québec.

[10] Québec RHA response.

[11] Statistics Canada (2007).

[12] Some provinces reported the total number of home care clients rather than the number of seniors (65+). In those cases, the figure was compared with data in *Portraits of Home Care in Canada: 2008* (Canadian Home Care Association, 2008), which usually presented the total home care population by age and by province. Using that information, it was possible to calculate the number of seniors being served by each province.

[13] 60+.

[14] Ontario survey information was adjusted to subtract the clients served by the placement co-ordination units in order to make the Ontario figures comparable with those from other provinces.

Among the list of home care services that the literature indicates should be part of the basket of services, all provinces offer nursing, personal support, respite care and palliative care. Most also offer rehabilitation services, equipment and supplies, day programmes, home-making/housekeeping, meals, and self-directed care. Few offer transportation or supportive housing as part of the home care programme. Every province indicated that there were waiting lists for one or more home care services.

No province charges fees for the more medically-oriented home care services such as nursing, rehabilitation, palliative care, and equipment and supplies. Six provinces charge fees for personal support. There is a great deal of variation among the provinces regarding fees for other home care services. Manitoba and Ontario are the two provinces least likely to charge fees for home care services.

Provincial Progress in Implementing Integrated Care

The survey assessed the extent to which provinces are implementing the features of the Hollander and Prince (2008) framework. It also asked questions about how important each of the framework features are to provincial decision-makers.

The framework contains three basic sections: philosophical and policy prerequisites; administrative and clinical best practices; and linkage mechanisms across population groups, with hospitals, with primary care and with other social and human services. The results indicate:

- **Philosophical and policy prerequisites:** Provincial governments are supportive of the philosophical and policy requisites;

- **Administrative best practices:** Almost every province agreed that most of the administrative best practices are very important but no province has implemented all of the administrative features. For example, one of the key features of integrated care systems is the availability of integrated information systems (Kodner and Spreeuwenberg, 2002). Although all provinces report that this feature is either very or somewhat important, none reports having a fully-integrated information system. Most provinces do not have a single funding envelope for care for seniors, but those with RHAs have a single funding envelope for health services for their populations. None has an incentive system for evidence-based decision-making (but only four provinces think this feature is very important). Only five provinces report that they have a single administrative structure for continuing care services. These results seem to indicate that most provinces have yet to align their administrative structures, enablers and incentives to support a more effective care system;

- **Clinical best practices:** Provinces have been somewhat more successful in implementing clinical best practice features. Seven provinces indicate that they have a single or co-ordinated entry system to care; almost all (nine) have province-wide assessment and care authorisation instruments; seven have system-level client classification systems; six have ongoing system-level case management; and they all have mechanisms for communicating with families;

- **Linkage mechanisms:** The provinces are far less developed with regard to the boundary-spanning or linkage mechanisms of integrated care health systems. For example:

  o *Administrative linkage mechanisms across population groups:* Half of the provinces do not think that this feature of the framework is important. Only two report that they have this feature, although four report that they have staff whose job description includes acting as access points across other service sectors, such as linkages to the mental health system for seniors with mental health problems;

  o *Linkages with hospitals:* Eight provinces have implemented co-location of home care case managers in hospitals. Half report that they have physicians who make home visits to frail elders to avoid hospitalisations. Only the RHA in Québec reported that the home care system is responsible for paying for hospital Alternate Level of Care (ALC) days. This is becoming a common feature of some European systems, which view ALC days as a failure of the residential and community care system;

  o *Linkages with primary care:* Five provinces report that physician remuneration is appropriate for care of the frail elderly and four provinces indicate that physicians are adequately remunerated for home visits. Ontario reported that home care case managers are located in primary care offices, but only in some parts of the province. The Québec RHA and Prince Edward Island reported that there are physicians associated with the home care programme to co-ordinate with primary care physicians;

  o *Linkages with other social and human services:* Half of the provinces have an organised approach to eligibility for various levels of housing with supportive services. Surprisingly, only six report having a system for high-level planning of service supply for seniors needing co-ordinated care. Given the importance of effective linkages across hospitals, primary care and other human services, it appears that this is an area for greater attention by provinces.

At a high level, **Table 12.3** indicates areas of strength and weakness in provincial implementation of best practice features of continuing care.

Table 12.3: Areas of Strengths and Weaknesses

Best Practice Area	Provincial Progress	Comment
Philosophical and policy requisites	Strong	Provinces generally support the requisites
Administrative features	Mixed	
Clinical features	Quite Strong	
Linkages across population groups	Weak	
Linkages with primary care	Weak	
Linkages with hospitals	Weak	
Linkages with other health and social service providers	Mixed	

The final survey question asked respondents to describe the single most important next step that the province/RHA could take to improve integrated care for seniors. The answers to this question provide insights into the specific issues or opportunities in each province:

- In the two provinces (New Brunswick and Prince Edward Island) with two different ministries responsible for health services (hospital and medical) and social care services (long-term care homes, home care and other community services), respondents reported that the most important step they could take is to develop joint action plans between the two administrative entities;
- In Nova Scotia, which has not devolved its home care and long-term care services to the RHAs, the next step was the transfer of home and continuing care services to the RHAs. This transfer has since been accomplished;
- Newfoundland and Labrador and Saskatchewan indicated a need to develop a strategy for seniors' services that can provide a template for implementation steps;
- The Québec RHA indicated that the most important step would be to obtain additional funding;

- Ontario was in the process of implementing a $700-million investment over three years for the development of an integrated community care service system for seniors, the Aging at Home Strategy;

- The Manitoba RHA indicated that the most important next step would be to improve the integration of family physicians with community services;

- British Columbia reported that the implementation of pilot projects, called Integrated Health Networks (IHNs), and efforts to expand the use of technology (for example, tele-monitoring and shared information systems), are the most important next steps.

In summary, some of the provinces are quite far ahead in their implementation of the best practice features of integrated care systems. However, in the areas of administrative best practices and linkages with other sectors, there has been slower progress. Only the Québec RHA seems to have made significant strides in implementing integrated information systems. No province had incentives for evidence-based decision-making. The area of weakest implementation is the development of linkage mechanisms across service sectors.

Additionally, the results of the survey indicated that, while all provinces are making progress, it is uneven across the provinces and sometimes within provinces.

EXAMPLES OF INTEGRATION ACTIVITIES IN CANADA

The Integrated Health Network (IHN) Pilot Projects in British Columbia

In British Columbia, about 34% of the population who have one or more chronic conditions are responsible for 80% of total public health care costs. Providing a better health care experience for this population is the goal of 26 IHNs, pilot projects that have been implemented in the province. The specific goal the projects hope to improve is the linkage between the community care system and primary care sectors. Twenty projects are targeting patients with complex chronic health conditions, three are focused on seniors at risk, two on marginalised patients, and one is providing integrated care to those with chronic mental health conditions. If each project enrols its target population, over 42,000 patients and 586 general practitioners will be involved in the networks. Generally, projects are located in the southern part of the province but some are in rural and remote northern communities. There are five outcome areas of interest: improving patient access to primary health care; improving patient health outcomes through quality improvement; improving patient confidence and experience with the health care system; improving provider confidence with the health care system; and last, decreasing the average annual cost per patient. The evaluation results are not available but already the province is thinking about how to move from the lessons of the pilot projects to system improvements. The areas for system change include system alignment, funding models, and infrastructure support.

The British Columbia IHNs are designed to strengthen one of the weaker areas found in the survey of the provinces, which was poor models of co-ordination with primary care practitioners.

The PRISMA Project in Québec

In the Eastern Townships of Québec, there has been an organised approach to implementing improved care for frail seniors on a system level for almost 10 years. The Program of Research to Integrate the Services for the Maintenance of Autonomy (PRISMA) is a collaborative interagency model that has a number of best practice features: co-ordination among service providers; single point of entry; case management; individualised service plans; use of a unique assessment tool and case mix classification system; and a computerised clinical chart. PRISMA services are targeted to those over 65, with moderate to severe disabilities, who show good potential for staying at home and who need two or more health and social services. Based on the positive results of an initial pilot project, the model is being implemented in Sherbrooke (urban), Granit and Coaticook (rural areas). Today, the implementation rate ranges from 70% to 85% among participating agencies.

Compared to seniors living in similar communities in other parts of Québec, seniors participating in the PRISMA project are less functionally impaired, have fewer unmet needs, have higher satisfaction with services, and feel more empowered. Over time, there have been fewer visits to the Emergency Room, and fewer new hospitalisations, compared to the comparison group. To date, there have been no significant effects on re-hospitalisations, use of home care services, consultations with health professionals or use of geriatric services. By year 4, these outcomes had been achieved at no additional cost to the health care system (Hébert *et al.*, 2010).

This project implemented most of the best practice indicators of the Hollander and Prince (2008) model. Several years ago, the Ministry of Health in Québec asked all the RHAs to develop integrated care systems.

To support the RHAs, the Ministry mandated structural integration by enacting legislation requiring the merger of local hospitals, rehabilitation centres, home and community care centres and long-term care homes into one organisation (Centre for Health and Social Services). Ninety-five new organisations have been created, each one serving the residents of a designated geographic area. While it is unclear what effect the merger will have on PRISMA results, the PRISMA model does not require mergers of key provider agencies.

These examples of different approaches being taken by provinces underscore the organisational and structural variations inherent in integrated care models. They also indicate that the best practice features of the Hollander and Prince framework remain the cornerstone of health system reform for those with chronic conditions.

ONGOING NATIONAL INITIATIVES

Changing any health care system for those with chronic conditions to improve the quality of care and to reduce wasted resources is a major project, involving clinicians and administrators, organisations, funders, and policy-makers. It is always a work in progress and takes place over a long period of time. In addition to the types of service initiatives described above, there are a number of other national projects that are occurring in Canada that will contribute to the success of integrating care. One of them is to develop electronic health records that will facilitate information flow among and across providers. Quality information systems are considered to be critical to the implementation and management of integrated care systems (MacAdam, 2010; Suter *et al.*, 2007).

A major project in Canada has been to implement electronic health records. Created in 2001, Canada Health Infoway is a non-profit corporation created to foster the implementation of a pan-Canadian electronic health record network. As of 2011, the core elements of an electronic health record had been created for just over 50% of Canadians (Canada Health Infoway, 2011). To date, the emphasis for development has been in such areas as drug information systems, and digital diagnostic imaging. Going forward, Canada Health Infoway will be investing in a wider range of information and communication technologies. These include clinical systems, tele-health projects and electronic medical record systems. As these projects develop, they will be an enormous help in improving the efficiency and accountability of integrated care projects (Canada Health Infoway, 2011).

It has been suggested that effective client targeting of integrated and/or highly co-ordinated care needs to be implemented in order to prevent rapid increases in cost without achieving the policy goal of improving quality of care for those most at risk of poor outcomes (Leutz, 1999). All provinces have implemented and/or tested the InterRAI suite of assessment instruments (Hirdes, 2007). Seven of the 10 provinces are using the Home Care Assessment instrument to collect uniform reliable data about home care clients. These data are used for care planning at the clinical level but they also allow policy-makers to group home care clients by risk level, map service plans against the supply of local services, and develop performance accountability measures.

A third major pan-Canadian effort is to reform the delivery of primary care. As noted in our survey, one of the areas of weakness for the provinces is linkages with primary care providers. In addition to British Columbia's Integrated Primary Care Pilot Projects, other provinces are testing new models of primary care delivery also. One such effort is the Family Health Teams (FHTs) in Ontario. FHTs are health care organisations that include a team of family physicians, nurse practitioners, registered nurses, social workers, dieticians, and other professionals who work together to provide health care for their community. They focus on chronic disease management, disease prevention and health promotion, and work with other health care organisations, such as public health units and Community Care Access Centres. As of 2011, there were 200 FHTs in Ontario serving more than 2.7 million people (Ministry of Health and Long Term Care, 2010).

In 2003, Alberta Health and Wellness, the Alberta Medical Association and Alberta's RHAs (now Alberta Health Services) established the Primary Care Initiative (PCI) to improve access to family physicians and other frontline health care providers in Alberta. The purpose of the PCI is to develop Primary Care Networks (PCNs) and to support them in meeting the objectives of the program. They call for comprehensive care to be provided for a defined population and include linkages to other services, including specialists and other types of health care providers. The PCI oversees and supports the development of PCNs, of which there are 40 operating throughout Alberta, with more in the planning stages. About 79% of eligible family physicians in Alberta are involved in either established or developing PCNs. The goal was for 80% of all Albertans to receive care from PCN teams in 2011 (Government of Alberta, 2012) .

CONCLUSION

There is Canadian evidence that supports increased investment in improving co-ordination of care for seniors because it has the potential to improve quality of care while not increasing system total costs. A key issue becomes the removal of barriers that might be preventing provinces from moving more quickly to implement key features for improved integration. These barriers include, but may not be limited to, competing pressures for funding from other health care sectors; human resource issues; privacy concerns; difficulties in implementing linkages with the primary care and hospital sectors; lack of flexibility over budget allocations across sectors; and lack of insured coverage of home and community support services under the *Canada Health Act*. Last, a key barrier also may be the lack of conclusive findings about the cost-effectiveness of integrated care models (Hofmarcher *et al.*, 2007). Very few formal evaluations of integrated care models have been undertaken at a larger scale level, although there have been many evaluations of small disease-specific integrated projects (MacAdam, 2008; Béland and Hollander, 2011).

Nonetheless, financial and quality of care issues are pushing forward efficiency measures, such as integrating care for those with disabilities, on a larger scale. Leatt *et al.* (2000) pointed out that integration is achieved through a series of incremental steps. As can be seen from this brief review of Canadian provincial delivery systems, progress is being made, slowly but surely. There is every reason to expect that five to 10 years from now a more responsive health care system will be in place.

REFERENCES

Béland, F. and Hollander, M. (2011). 'Integrated Models of Care Delivery for the Frail Elderly: International Perspectives', *Gaceta Sanitaria*, doi:10.10.1016/j.gaceta.2011.09.003.

Béland, F., Bergman, H., Lebel, P., Clarfield, A., Tousignant, P., Contrandriopoulos, A-P. and Dalliare, I. (2006). 'A System of Integrated Care for Older Persons with Disabilities in Canada: Results from a Randomized Controlled Trial', *Journals of Gerontology Series A, Biological Sciences and Medical Sciences*, 61: 367-373.

Canada Health Infoway (2011). *Toward Critical Mass: Moving from Availability to Adoption, Annual Report 2010-2011*, available www2.infoway-inforoute.ca.

Canadian Home Care Association (2008). *Portraits of Home Care in Canada: 2008*, Ottawa: Canadian Home Care Association, available www.cdnhomecare.ca.

Government of Alberta (2012). *About PCI*, available www.albertapci.ca.

Hébert, R., Durand, P., Dubuc, N., Tourigny, A. and PRISMA Group (2003). 'Frail Elderly Patients: New Model for Integrated Service Delivery', *Canadian Family Physician*, 49: 992-997.

Hébert, R., Raiche, M., Dubois, M., Gueye, N. Tousignant, A. and PRISMA Group (2010). 'Impact of PRISMA, A Co-ordination-type Integrated Service Delivery System for Frail Older People in Quebec (Canada): A Quasi-experimental Study', *Journals of Gerontology Series B, Psychological Sciences and Social Sciences*, 65B: 107-118.

Hirdes, J. (2007). *Canadian Experiences with the InterRAI Suite of Assessment Instruments*, presentation, available www.cdhb.govt.nz/conference/interai/.../Hirdes-keynote.pdf.

Hofmarcher, M., Oxley, H. and Rusticelli, E. (2007). *Improved Health System Performance through Better Care Co-ordination*, Working Paper No. 30, Paris: OECD.

Hollander, M. and Prince, M. (2001). *Analysis of Interfaces along the Continuum of Care. Final Report: 'The Third Way': A Framework for Organizing Health Related Services for Individuals with Ongoing Care Needs and Their Families*, Victoria, BC: Hollander Analytical Services Ltd, available www.hollanderanalytical.com.

Hollander, M. and Prince, M. (2008). 'Organizing Health Care Delivery Systems', *Health Care Quarterly*, 11(1): 44-54.

Kodner, D. and Spreeuwenberg, C. (2002). 'Integrated Care: Meaning, Logic, Applications and Implications – A Discussion Paper', *International Journal of Integrated Care*, 2(Oct-Dec), available www.ijic.org/.

Leatt, P., Pink, G. and Guerriere, M. (2000). 'Towards a Canadian Model of Integrated Health Care', *Health Care Papers*, 1(2): 13-35.

Leutz, W. (1999). 'Five Laws for Integrating Medical and Social Services: Lessons from the United States and the United Kingdom', *Milbank Quarterly*, 77(1): 77-110.

MacAdam, M. (2008). *Frameworks of Integrated Care for the Elderly: A Systematic Review*, CPRN Research Report, Ottawa: Canadian Policy Research Networks, available www.cprn.org.

MacAdam, M. (2009). *Moving Toward Health System Integration: Provincial Progress in System Change for Seniors, Progress Report*, Ottawa: Canadian Health Policy Research Network, available www.ijic.org/.

MacAdam, M. (2011). 'Progress toward Integrating Care for Seniors in Canada', *International Journal of Integrated Care*, 11(26), April, Special Anniversary Edition.

Ministry of Health and Long Term Care (Ontario) (2010). *Progress on Family Health Teams*, available www.health.gov.on.ca/transformation/fht/fht_progress.html.

Statistics Canada (2007). *Population by Sex, and Age Group, by Province and Territory (in Thousands)*, available www.statscan.ca.

Suter, E., Nelly, N., Adair, C. and Armitage, G. (2011). 'Ten Key Principles for Successful Health Systems Integration', *Health Care Quarterly*, 13: 16-23.

14: DEMENTIA AND INTEGRATED CARE: A DREAM OR REALITY?

Suzanne Cahill

CASE STUDY: MISS MARJORIE MURPHY

Miss Marjorie Murphy is a 72-year-old single lady who has dementia and currently lives in a private nursing home, where she was admitted some three months ago. She has no next-of-kin and, since her late teens, she worked as a live-in housekeeper for a well-to-do family in South County Dublin. She essentially reared this couple's three children, the youngest of whom, Kevin, now aged 52, is a bachelor and continues to live at home. When Kevin took early retirement in 2010, he began to notice that Miss Murphy was doing strange things around the house, moving furniture around, forgetting to relay important telephone messages and leaving food in the fridge without realising that it had gone off. Once, he noticed her unpacking the groceries and putting tomatoes in the cutlery drawer. On another occasion, she got lost coming home from the supermarket and was finally found about three miles from where she lived and worked all her life. For the last 12 months, Kevin has been Captain in his local golf club. He has had little time to pay attention to Miss Murphy's changed behaviour or to arrange an appointment for her to see the GP. He was of the firm view that she had just been getting a bit 'doddery' and that this was a normal part of ageing.

Six months ago, Miss Murphy fell in the back garden as she was hanging clothes on the line. The fall resulted in her fracturing her hip and she suffered other facial and leg injuries. Because of the fall, she was admitted to the nearest hospital and initially spent four days on a trolley in A&E. During this time, she had no visitors. She became frightened and agitated and kept pleading with the staff to go home. After some time, she was admitted to a hospital ward and later was offered rehabilitation, including intensive physiotherapy. The hospital team found her to be an unpleasant, difficult patient in every way. In particular, she was said to be a 'real nuisance' at night, as she was prone to becoming very disruptive and agitated, keeping other patients awake. She was prescribed tranquillisers and, during the next four weeks, developed a methicillin-resistant *staphylococcus aureus* (MRSA) 'superbug'. Her condition deteriorated rapidly, to the point where she lost the ability to perform activities of daily living (ADLs) independently. She was seen by the medical social worker and it was noted that she had no next-of-kin and no home. Eight weeks later, she was discharged to a local nursing home. At no stage did she have a cognitive assessment undertaken, nor was any attempt made to discuss her discharge planning with Kevin or trial her at home. On admission to the nursing home, she was labelled as 'aggressive'. She was abusive to staff and became withdrawn and apathetic when placed in a two-bedded room. The local Psychiatry of Later Life team now has been called in to investigate her condition.

This case study reflects the need for integrated care, particularly for older people with dementia (PwD). It shows that, in Ireland, the absence of integrated care means that some people with mild to moderate dementia may end up being prematurely and unnecessarily admitted to long-term care. Had Miss Murphy been referred to a general practitioner (GP) when her earlier unusual/bizarre behaviour was first noted and had a key informant accompanied her to this appointment, the likelihood is that she may have been diagnosed with dementia and offered appropriate treatments and services. In fact, in some European and overseas countries, she would have been offered a key worker or case manager, who would then help her negotiate her way through community care services. The progression of her condition, including the challenging behaviours associated with her dementia, may have been delayed and the current situation could have been averted.

The following chapter discusses the need for integration in dementia care in Ireland. It opens with an overview of Alzheimer's disease and the related dementias and presents facts and figures about current and future prevalence rates in Ireland and the cost of dementia care. It then progresses to discuss the policy context for dementia care services in Ireland and argues that, despite the Government's alleged commitment to integrated health and social care services as embedded in policy documents, the reality is enormously different.

In progressing this argument and marshalling the case that dementia services in Ireland are totally under-resourced, findings from a recent extensive research review on dementia care in Ireland are reported. These findings point towards the need for major service development and for more extensive integration between different service sectors and different information systems in the area of dementia. The chapter draws on examples of best practice from Europe and overseas and concludes with recommendations about how, in the future, dementia care services can be more realistically integrated. Integration will mean more than political will and improved lines of communication; it will mean adequate resources being set aside and a ring-fenced budget allocated to dementia services.

INTRODUCTION

The term 'dementia' refers to a collection of illnesses caused by disorders affecting the brain and most frequently found in people over the age of 65 years. The most common cause of dementia is Alzheimer's disease. However, there are many other dementia sub-types caused by diseases, some few of which are reversible. Dementia is an invidious and complex illness that is often said to creep up on the individual: one day, the person may be calm and rational, the next he/she may be forgetful, agitated and withdrawn. The misfortune for all those involved is in attempting to make sense of behaviour that can no longer be thought of as rational or systematic.

Dementia affects memory, thinking, cognition, behaviour, personality and the ability to perform everyday tasks including ADLs. It has no single cause and there are several known and unknown, modifiable and non-modifiable, environmental and genetic risk factors that can influence the age of onset and the progression of the illness. As the illness advances, the symptoms become more apparent as the decline in memory, cognition and functional ability begin to impact on normal work, everyday and social life. Most dementia sub-types are progressive and terminal.

Nowadays, an early diagnosis of dementia is more relevant than ever before, due to the increasing numbers of pharmacological and non-pharmacological interventions available for Alzheimer's disease and the other related dementia (Geldmacher *et al.*, 2003) and due to the growing awareness of the benefits of early interventions (Iliffe *et al.*, 2009). GPs are in a strategic position to recognise dementia and, by virtue of the large numbers presenting in primary care, to play a key role in its diagnosis. However, diagnosing dementia (including differentiating normal age-related changes in memory and cognition from the more pathological symptoms of dementia), can pose serious challenges to GPs, since dementia is a complex illness, mimicked and/or sometimes superimposed by other age-related conditions. The diagnosis of dementia requires considerable time and expertise. This, along with the progressive nature of the illness, makes it difficult to determine the time of onset and difficult to estimate incidence rates for the illness (Phillips *et al.*, 2011).

Not all cases of dementia are visible because onset usually occurs gradually, with mild symptoms often attributed to other causes (Cahill and Shapiro, 1997). The hidden or invisible nature of dementia may arise also because the individual or family member may deny/disguise the symptoms or because the illness may cause a lack of insight so that the person affected may not be aware of the problem. In Ireland, like in other countries (Vernooij-Dassen *et al.*, 2005), stigma acts as a major barrier to dementia diagnosis (Moore and Cahill, 2013). In Ireland, it has been argued also that early diagnosis – and sometimes, any diagnosis – is the exception rather than the rule.

Currently, there are over 42,000 Irish PwD (Pierce *et al.*, 2013) and this figure (in line with population ageing) is set to rise to somewhere between 140,000 and 147,000 by 2041. In fact, the prevalence of dementia almost doubles every 20 years. Today, most Irish people who have dementia (26,000) live at home and in the community; about 14,000 are living in long-term care (Cahill *et al.*, 2012); and much smaller numbers are found in hospitals and in psychiatric settings. Many, including those in long-term care, are not known to service providers (Cahill *et al.*, 2010) nor indeed have had the advantage of having a diagnosis, never mind a differential diagnosis.

Although the risk of getting dementia increases with age, it must be remembered that dementia is not a normal part of ageing and early onset (dementia in those aged less than 65 years) affects about 4,000 people in Ireland, many of whom are male. Some of these people with early onset (about 700) have Down's Syndrome and dementia. These younger people are especially vulnerable, as dementia is not widely recognised as a chronic condition that can affect those other than aging adults. There are no dedicated dementia services for this particular age group, many of whom face unique and complex challenges attempting to avail of service systems and structures not designed for their age group.

Dementia is not widely known as a chronic illness that, in some cases, could be avoided or at least deferred, were the public better informed about risk factor modification and about the importance of primary prevention. For example, by addressing modifiable risk factors, including taking physical and mental activity, enjoying a healthy diet, drinking alcohol in moderation, managing blood pressure, cholesterol, blood sugar and weight, protecting the head from injury and not smoking, some cases of dementia could be avoided or at least delayed. By delaying the onset of dementia by two years, prevalence rates could be reduced by 20% and, by delaying it by five years, prevalence rates could be halved (Brodaty *et al.*, 2005). Ireland has been slow to develop risk reduction dementia programmes and Irish people by and large are not cognisant of the fact that they have the opportunity to optimise their health and to minimise the risk of acquiring a dementia or to delay its progression by engaging in healthy lifestyles.

Dementia is a costly illness – in Ireland, the economic cost of dementia estimated for the year 2010 was €1.69 billion. Informal care accounted for the largest proportion of these costs and was estimated to be €807 million; residential care was the next highest cost at €731 million; and formal health and social services came in at €88 million. The average cost of care was estimated at €40,500 per person *per annum* (Connolly *et al.*, 2012). Broadly speaking, these costs are in line with cost estimates derived in other countries. Of course, the financial cost of dementia care is only one component of the overall cost of care, which includes social, emotional and psychological costs. It is these hidden costs that are a lot more difficult to identify and it is these same costs that cause family members much frustration, distress and hardship.

THE POLICY CONTEXT FOR DEMENTIA CARE IN IRELAND: THE NEED FOR INTEGRATED CARE

Public policy for dementia care in Ireland has been slow to evolve and, unlike other European and overseas countries, Ireland as yet has no national dementia strategy although strident efforts are currently underway to produce a strategy by 2013. This is at a time when, across Europe, other countries are developing second and third iterations of their dementia plans/strategies. The care of PwD in Ireland therefore is largely determined by public policy designed for older people in general and by community and residential care policies. There is as yet no ring-fenced funding set aside for dementia care services. Indeed at the time of writing, it is impossible to ascertain what proportion of the Irish health budget is spent on dementia services. The stated and over-arching objective of Government policy for older people, including those with dementia, is to maintain their independent living by keeping them at home for as long as possible. Yet in practice, the financing of care for PwD is biased towards institutional care (Pierce *et al.*, 2013) and the reality in

Ireland is that the main bulk of community care services for those with dementia are provided free of charge by family caregivers.

Integrated care (that is, care services that are consumer-driven, well-planned and organised, and which provide a seamless pathway (Kodner and Spreeuwenberg, 2002)), although now firmly embedded in public policy in Ireland (Doocey and Reddy, 2010), is more of a dream than a reality, it could be argued, for the majority of families who have a relative experiencing dementia. Indeed, those few dementia services that are available are often the responsibility of several different Local Health Offices (LHOs) and Government departments (including the Department of Health, Department of the Environment, Community and Local Government and the Department of Social Protection) and the remit of many different health service professionals including GPs, old age psychiatrists, geriatricians, neurologists, memory clinics specialists and public health nurses, each attached to the public, private, and voluntary sectors.

There is no single point of entry to health and social care services for a person with symptoms of dementia and the situation for those with early onset dementia is even more complicated. Indeed, it has long been noted that PwD in Ireland fall between the cracks of disability services, services for older people, and mental health services (O'Shea and O'Reilly, 1999). Dementia support, training and advocacy services are also the remit of several different voluntary and statutory organisations, including the Alzheimer Society of Ireland (ASI), the Dementia Services Information and Development Centre (DSIDC), the Western Alzheimer's Association, the Cork Alzheimer's Society, the Carers Association, and Age Action Ireland.[15]

The various components of the health system, whether based in the home, community, acute care, or institutional care settings, work alongside separate funding streams and budgets. There is also limited liaison between the different service sectors and limited connectivity between hospital services, community and residential care sectors. This disparate and patchwork-quilt approach to dementia services in Ireland, it could be argued, results in poor quality of care and contributes to important health and psychosocial needs remaining unmet. The approach is also partly responsible (as the case study at the opening of this chapter illustrates) for the unnecessary hospitalisation and premature

---

[15] The Carers Association and Age Action Ireland are non-governmental organisations (NGOs) dedicated to services for older people in general and do not offer dementia-specific services. They are included here since their services extend to those families where a person has dementia.

institutionalisation of people with dementia and for the high economic cost of dementia care.

FURTHER EVIDENCE OF THE NEED FOR INTEGRATED SERVICE DELIVERY SYSTEMS IN IRELAND — THE POLICY PARADOX

Despite the rhetoric of integrated care (see Health Service Executive (HSE), 2001; HSE, 2007) as noted earlier, the Irish dementia care landscape is fragmented and inequitable with little evidence of real or appropriate service integration (Cahill *et al.*, 2012). A recent research review on dementia services commissioned by the Government has shown that health and social care services are poorly co-ordinated across the country and it is not uncommon for PwD to come into contact with health and social services only when a serious crisis arises (Cahill *et al.*, 2012). The review has pointed also to major gaps in service delivery for PwD, lack of co-ordination of services, poor transition between care settings, insufficient information available, systems failures, a deficiency of valid and reliable data on dementia and a total absence of clearly defined pathways through care. It is interesting and ironic that these same findings were published in 2012, some five years after the HSE's national programme of transformation – a programme that supposedly focused on the delivery of integrated care.

The same research review has highlighted the need for more integrated services and has called for a case management approach to dementia care services – an approach long adopted in several European and overseas countries. There is a need for adequate referral systems to guide PwD to the right place at the right time, as well as adequate communication between professionals, including between primary and secondary care service providers. There is a need for dementia advisors in the community and dementia champions in hospital settings. There is a need for a transfer of knowledge, so that the day-to-day care of PwD is undertaken by those with training and expertise and who are realistically paid. There is a need to promote continuity of care, so that the individual can go from service to service without being subjected to repeated and, at times, demoralising and tiresome multiple assessments. There is a need for what one Swedish dementia expert argues is a 'first class ticket' in the individual's journey through dementia.

This review of dementia services represents the first phase in a wider process leading to the development of a national dementia strategy in Ireland. The second phase of strategy development will involve public consultation and the setting up of an advisory committee. Already a call for submissions has been made by the Government and several written submissions have been received from the main dementia organisations, some of which are available online. A perusal of some of these submissions yields further evidence of the absence of integrated dementia care services. In the ASI's submission, for example, it is recommended that a "system of integrated care pathways supported by a case manager" be introduced to enable service providers and supports for PwD to work in a joined-up and consistent way. DSIDC likewise calls for the dementia strategy to instigate the development of a dementia care pathway and to outline the resources needed to put this in place. Communication protocols, regionally-based memory clinics and access to services and supports not based on age or geographical location should support this pathway.

As mentioned earlier, this absence and need for a more co-ordinated integrated approach to dementia services is all the more curious given the abolition of the former Health Boards in 2005 and their replacement by a unified HSE structure, which was allegedly (amongst other reasons) undertaken to ensure that integrated care services would be developed across Ireland. In fact, service integration was formally recognised in the HSE's *Corporate Plan 2008-2011*: "The integration of services across the service spectrum from disease prevention through primary and community care to hospital care, to allow the service user to be managed at the most appropriate level for their care needs" (HSE, 2008), yet in the HSE's *National Service Plans*, including its 2012 Plan, which identifies key priorities, no reference whatsoever is made to dementia services and, indeed, there has been little evidence of any real integration in dementia services (HSE, 2012). The new restructuring of services and funding in the Department of Health, resulting in the appointment of seven directors responsible for (i) hospital care, (ii) primary care, (iii) mental health, (iv) children and family services, (v) social care, (vi) public health and (vii) corporate/shared services may further threaten or undermine any ideological or practical attempts to fully integrate dementia services.

BEST PRACTICE IN INTEGRATED CARE OVERSEAS

Managing dementia well in primary care, including ensuring that primary care team members are trained to detect the early signs and symptoms of dementia, whilst not guaranteeing integrated care, would constitute the first stage in the individual's 'first class train ticket' on his/her journey through dementia. However, considerable evidence to date suggests that GPs in Ireland prefer not to get involved in this area (Cahill *et al.*, 2006; Cahill *et al.*, 2008; Moore and Cahill, 2013). A recent cross-national study (Ireland and Sweden) has shown that, whilst Irish GPs believed that early ·diagnosis of dementia was important, they themselves were not pro-active in this area and for a variety of reasons refrained from getting involved (Moore and Cahill, 2013). In the UK, for example, under the Quality Outcomes Framework (QOF), financial incentives exist for GPs to diagnose dementia. Under the same scheme, GPs are required also to offer service users with dementia a face-to-face review of their care annually. Such face-to-face consultations also include an independent consideration of the needs of the family caregiver.

The Scottish Government has produced very helpful standards for integrated care pathways for mental health, including a dementia care standard. This dementia standard acknowledges the fact that service users with dementia and their carers will have different needs at different stages in the course of the illness and that there is a need for close working relationships to be developed with all key stakeholders delivering dementia care services (National Health Service, 2007). The same standard points to the need to assist PwD to understand and manage the illness and support any retained ability. There is a need to ·assist family caregivers to continue to care for as long as possible, to recognise the special needs of younger PwD and to anticipate the care and support PwDs that need later in the course of the illness and to help service users and informal carers plan ahead.

CURRENT PRACTICE IN THE DIAGNOSIS OF PEOPLE WITH DEMENTIA IN IRELAND

Returning to the topic of primary care, it could be argued that enhanced primary care is at the heart of integrated care especially in the context of dementia. As mentioned in the introduction of this chapter, the prevalence of dementia is set to rise very significantly in future years and enhanced primary care services will need to be ratcheted up in order to deal with the increasing numbers of people likely to present with dementia and to provide treatments and other non-pharmacological interventions. Despite a very significant increase in primary care services across Ireland, there is as yet no emerging evidence that dementia care is being better managed or indeed that health and social care services for those coping with dementia are integrated (Moore and Cahill, 2013).

Early diagnosis in primary care brings with it certain advantages. Research has shown that early diagnosis and intervention improves quality of life for PwD and their caregivers (Banerjee *et al.*, 2009) and that carer support and counselling at diagnosis can reduce the need for long-term care (Mittleman *et al.*, 2007).

As stated earlier, GPs are well-positioned to diagnose dementia early, since the GP is normally the first person with whom the individual or family member will consult when worried about the signs and symptoms of memory or cognitive problems. The advent of primary care practices in Ireland, of which there are now over 400 (and an additional up to 50 new services emerging), means that other multidisciplinary team members also are well-placed to be on the alert for possible cases of dementia in the community. However, unlike other illnesses, there are no simple tests to diagnose dementia. Dementia requires clinical judgment based on observation and information, including a collateral history obtained from the patient and family members, along with the use of screening tests and, in some cases referral to a geriatrician, old age psychiatrist, neurologist or memory clinic.

Barriers to integrated care for primary care staff include a deficiency in the numbers of memory clinics across Ireland. Memory clinics or memory assessment centres could offer primary care practitioners specialist help with differential diagnosis and expertise (as is the case in other countries) and specialist support in interventions for more complicated cases of dementia. Yet there are insufficient memory clinics (only 14 across the country) to cater for the some 26,000 people known to have this illness. The West of Ireland, which carries the highest share of dementia, has no memory clinic. Several of the extant memory clinics offer only very patchy services and several fail to employ a full complement of staff but rather co-opt in staff employed in other sectors.

Norway, a country with a population similar in size to Ireland (4.8 million people), has 20 memory clinics and, in France and the UK, memory clinics are in evidence throughout the country. Indeed, one of the goals of the UK's *Dementia Strategy* was to ensure that memory clinics would be located in every town across the UK over a five-year period (Department of Health (UK), 2009: 21). In Ireland, even where memory clinic services exist, lengthy delays are often experienced by GPs attempting to access such diagnostic services (Cahill *et al.*, 2008). For instance, the current waiting time for accessing the National Memory Clinic at St. James's Hospital, Dublin is approximately nine months (Matthew Gibb, personal communication, September 2012).

Access to diagnostic services, including MRI and CAT scans, in Ireland is also a key problem and acts as a barrier to integrated dementia care. An Irish study conducted some years ago showed that GPs, particularly those living in rural areas, experienced considerable delays accessing diagnostic services such as CAT and MRI scans (Cahill *et al.*, 2008). Many of the GPs surveyed reported they lacked confidence in diagnosing dementia. Most had never undergone dementia-specific training and the majority (83%) expressed a desire to be upskilled in dementia. In terms of disclosure, most showed a reluctance to share the news of dementia with their patients. Reasons included their perceptions of the patient's ability to understand information and the impact the disclosure might have on the individual because of stigma.

Diagnosing dementia in primary care takes time. Disclosure patterns vary but best practice suggests that disclosure should take place over a prolonged period of time (Phillips *et al.*, 2011). Making the diagnosis well therefore requires time and resources. Yet unlike other countries such as the UK and Scotland, in Ireland there are no financial incentives for GPs to get involved in this area and there are no agreed targets for improvement in early diagnosis. There is a need to support the development of shared care protocols between GPs and secondary care services and to support GPs in the ongoing management of PwD in the community. In Scotland, the concern about the under-diagnosis of dementia by GPs has led National Health Service Boards there to establish agreed targets for improvements in early diagnosis and for service response to PwD. The resulting outcome has been positive.

GUIDELINES FOR DEMENTIA DIAGNOSIS

Guidelines that foster the development of integrated care pathways for PwD through primary care have been produced in other countries but as yet are not available in Ireland. The New Zealand guidelines, first produced in 1997, have undergone a second iteration and, since 2003, are available online (Ministry of Health (NZ), 1997). They provide a useful template for practitioners who may be unsure of what to do with complicated cases of dementia. These guidelines also assist GPs to decide which patients should be referred to which services – rehabilitation, mental health or aged care. Canada has consensus guidelines originally developed in 1999 (Chertkow, 2008) and several guidelines from the USA, including from the US Preventive Services Task Force (USPSTF, n.d.), have been developed in recent years.

The Australian guidelines for dementia in primary care, *Care of People with Dementia in General Practice Guidelines* (Royal Australian College of General Practitioners (RACGP), 2006) are highly prescriptive and encourage GPs to engage in case finding. These guidelines recommend that when dementia is suspected, the GP should obtain a full clinical history, interview the patient and family both together and separately and assess the patient's ability to undertake daily activities. The instrumental ADL scale should be used and a home visit should be undertaken by the GP or member of the primary care team in order to assess the quality and safety of the home environment.

The Australian guidelines (RACGP, 2006) also highlight the GP's role in driving assessment, medication compliance, legal capacity and other legal matters, including the making of advance directives and enduring powers of attorney. The guidelines recommend a complete physical examination, directed towards assessing known and possible co-morbidities as well as addressing possible reversible causes of memory loss. They reinforce the view that the detection and diagnosis of dementia is a lengthy and challenging process that usually involves third parties, including the carer, the specialist and, most importantly, the person experiencing the symptoms. Ireland needs to develop similar guidelines for GPs to assist them diagnose dementia in primary care.

Current Practice in the Care of People with Dementia in the Community

Apart from ratcheting up primary care services, a carefully planned and co-ordinated approach to community care, with clear referral pathways between primary and secondary care service providers, also lies at the heart of integrated dementia care services. Yet, as argued earlier in this chapter, community care services for PwD in Ireland are difficult to access and the type of service received depends largely on luck, on the voice and perseverance of the next of kin (or advocate) and on where the individual lives. Family caregivers are the linchpin to the success of community care, yet only a small proportion receives the critical services needed to sustain this form of care. We cannot assume that, in the future, family members will be available to, or will want to, provide care services free of charge. The burgeoning numbers of older people who, in the future, are likely to have dementia will place huge pressure on these family members unless community care services are expanded to meet the new reality. The time for action is therefore now.

In Ireland, unlike the UK, Australia and the Scandinavian countries, there are no aged care assessment teams based in the community and no dementia-specific teams offering home and community services, thereby providing the necessary linkages into other more specialist services, such as memory clinics, acute hospital care and residential care. France, for example, as part of its Dementia Plan has large numbers of interdisciplinary teams providing home and community care services to people living at home with dementia. Norway and Sweden have specialist dementia teams in the community that liaise with primary and acute care staff. Preliminary evidence suggests that, where families in Ireland have the good fortune to be brought into contact with public health nurses because of a relative's dementia, access to other community care services may arise more rapidly. However, there is also research showing that, in Ireland, only a small proportion of those families where a relative has a dementia are known to service providers (Begley, 2009). In countries like Australia, dedicated home care packages exist for PwD living in the community, enabling services to be flexible and individualised to peoples' unique and complex needs. In Ireland, the more long-term care packages that would be more suited to PwD are not well-resourced and not all health care professionals accept those who may require overnight care or 24-hour supervision.

Services such as day care, public health nursing, home care packages and respite are fragmented, inequitable and under-developed and no set criteria are currently in place to assess client eligibility for services. Despite evidence showing that the West of Ireland carries the highest proportion of PwD – counties such as Roscommon, Mayo, Galway and Sligo known to have (relatively speaking) a large proportion of their population with dementia – this region has no dedicated day care or home care packages. Despite a number of HSE data sets now available on community services, including day care, home care and old age psychiatry, it is next to impossible to extrapolate useful information on dementia. It is as if dementia also remains invisible or hidden in the community.

Residential Care

Good residential care, where a diverse range of long-term care options are available (DeLange *et al.*, 2011) to PwD, from 'group living' to 'clustered houses' to 'nursing home dwellings' to 'specialist care units' (as is the case in The Netherlands) and where ideally PwD can be helped to maintain linkages and connections back to their former community (for example, allowed continue to attend day care, despite being resident in a nursing home, or be enabled to access end-of-life care, including palliative care services within the same facility) is another important component of integrated care services for PwD. Yet in Ireland, long-term care continues to be medicalised, with limited alternate care options, besides the traditional nursing home model (Cahill *et al.*, 2012). There is very little flexibility within long-term care settings to enable other pre-existing service supports such as those described here.

The result is that many older people in Ireland fear admission to a nursing home, aware that entrance will mean their being disconnected and isolated from their former community and lifestyle (Cahill and Diaz-Ponce, 2011) and referred on to unfamiliar service providers such as GPs or visiting old age psychiatrists or community mental health teams. Today in Ireland, about two-thirds of all people in long-stay care probably have dementia and there is emerging evidence to suggest that the transition from community to residential care is often rushed and not well-managed (Bobersky, 2010) and that services are not well integrated. In other countries such as Australia and the UK, residential respite care is used as an entrée into long-term care and key workers or case managers are available in countries such as The Netherlands or Australia to assist families deal with this important transition. No such services exist in Ireland.

Integrated care in the context of long-term care for PwD does not merely refer to integrated services but also integrated systems (Nies and Berman, 2004). Here in Ireland, we are not good at integrating systems in relation to older people's services and we are even less well accomplished at integrating systems for dementia care. For example, the HSE's national register of public and voluntary units and beds is one of two systems currently in place for collecting data on long-stay beds in public and voluntary settings and is updated monthly. Nursing Homes Ireland (NHI) also collects data on long-stay beds in the private sector but the methods used by NHI to collect information differ from the HSE's national register. NHI, for example, uses the 10 former Health Board areas as the basis for disaggregating data to regional level whilst the national register uses HSE LHO area. However, NHI does not collect data on units and beds in the private and most voluntary long-stay care settings.

HOPE FOR THE FUTURE: SOME EMERGING TRENDS TOWARDS INTEGRATION

The recent HSE and Atlantic Philanthropies jointly-funded Genio initiatives for dementia care services in Ireland have real potential to demonstrate elements of integrated care, provided true collaboration occurs between each of the key stakeholders and between each of the four sites in which these pilot projects will emerge and provided learning and information is shared. The Genio projects present an alternative 'activity-led' response to the needs of PwD. They involve a group of stakeholders that have designed services and supports relevant to particular community needs. One of the key values of these pilot projects in terms of integration is that systems will be put in place for shared learning. A national co-ordinator has been appointed and the project will be evaluated by a group of external experts.

Likewise, the HSE's forthcoming Single Assessment Tool (SAT) for older people, including those with dementia, when rolled out, will form a core part of supporting the development of an integrated care pathway approach. Through SAT, PwD and the family caregiver will undergo a needs assessment which should trigger an integrated response to meeting needs and identifying what locally-based services and supports are available. As noted by Haggerty *et al*. (2003), in developing well-linked, co-ordinated or fully integrated services, continuity is the key priority and service planners need to consider integration not as a static but rather as a dynamic process constantly in a state of flux and change.

THE GOLD STANDARD OF APPROPRIATE CARE IN DEMENTIA SERVICES

In conclusion, this chapter has argued that, despite public policy allegedly promoting integrated care services for older people, including those with dementia, much evidence continues to exist demonstrating that the baseline profile of dementia services in Ireland is low, services are poorly resourced and fragmented and integration is aspirational and not a reality. A key argument marshalled in the chapter is that enhanced primary care is at the heart of integrated care and there is a need for guidelines for dementia in primary care to be developed and for more incentives, resources and supports to be made available to primary care staff to support them in the early diagnosis of dementia. There is a need for a key worker or case management approach to be adopted in dementia care.

An integrated care model for dementia is one that would take on board the individual's entire journey through dementia, from initial assessment and diagnosis, to medical treatments and social care interventions, to long-term care and end-of-life care, including palliative care treatments. It would guarantee a 'first class ticket' for the individual in his/her journey through dementia, with a single point of access for health and social care services. Guidelines would be set down for those working in primary care practices that would help ensure early diagnosis. More memory assessment services would be available around the country to provide counselling services to the 'worried well' and to support primary care practitioners diagnose dementia. These memory services would serve also as centres of excellence. They would have an educative role, promoting primary prevention and risk reduction and educating the public about modifiable risk factors for dementia.

An integrated care pathway in dementia care ideally would mean community-based dementia teams, working in tandem with primary care teams and trained to conduct assessment and diagnostic services in peoples' homes and to help families come to terms with transitions into long-term care and into hospices. Flexible, around-the-clock, individualised services, underpinned by person-centred principles, would be organised around service users, in response to their individual needs. Clients would receive seamless continuous services and would not have to undergo degrading and repeated assessments. They would not be aware of any boundaries existing between services. Packages of care would be arranged and delivered in a dialogue between users, carers and providers with evidence of true partnerships in care. As is the case in some overseas countries, the interests and needs of carers would be viewed in their own right.

All primary and secondary care services and all allied health professionals would be integrated into an organised care pathway that would be clearly visible to the user, along with the family caregiver and other service providers. This is particular necessary for younger PwD and for other sub-populations who may be at heightened risk, including people from the Travelling community and people with Down's Syndrome. Efforts would be made also to moderate or harmonise data collection approaches used by various organisations and the tools and procedures used in various regional units so that direct information could be aggregated and regional comparisons made. A national register for dementia and other neurodegenerative diseases would be established, enabling the monitoring and measurement of the impact of dementia.

In conclusion, we are now at an important juncture in Ireland in relation to the development and expansion of dementia services. A national strategy on dementia is soon to be produced, which will involve wider consultation with all of the main stakeholder groups, including PwD themselves and their family caregivers. We must ensure that a focused, sustained and strategic coalition exists between the main advocacy foci and the professional groups for dementia care (Cahill *et al.*,

2010). This consultation also will include the direct involvement of the government through the Department of Health. Developing this strategy is an important first step, which hopefully will generate resources for dementia. For PwD and their caregivers, this strategy promises much, provided a ring-fenced budget to dementia services is set aside. We must seize the opportunity available now to enhance and improve services for this very vulnerable group of people. We must ensure that any new models of care for dementia reflect truly integrated services.

REFERENCES

Banerjee, S., Samsi, K., Petrie, C.D., Alvir, J., Treglia, M., Schwam, E.M. and del Valle, M. (2009). 'What Do We Know About Quality of Life in Dementia? A Review of the Emerging Evidence on the Predictive and Explanatory Value of Disease-specific Measures of Health-related Quality of Life in People with Dementia', *International Journal of Geriatric Psychiatry*, 24: 15-25.

Begley, E. (2009). *"I know what it is but how bad does it get?" Insights into the Lived Experiences and Services: Needs of People with Early-State Dementia*, PhD thesis, Trinity College Dublin.

Bobersky, A. (2010). 'Relocating People with Dementia to Specialist Care Units: The Experiences and Views of Family Caregivers', paper to the *Annual Research Day*, Department of Medical Gerontology and Mercer's Institute for Research on Ageing, Trinity College Dublin, 7 May.

Brodaty, H., Sachdev, P. and Anderson, T.M. (2005). 'Dementia: New Projections and Time for an Updated Response', *Australian and New Zealand Journal of Psychiatry*, 39(11/12): 955-958.

Cahill, S. (2010). 'Developing a National Dementia Strategy for Ireland', *International Journal of Geriatric Psychiatry*, 25: 912-916.

Cahill, S. and Diaz-Ponce, A. (2011). '"I hate having nobody here, I'd like to know where they all are": Can Qualitative Research Detect Differences in Quality of Life among Nursing Home Residents with Different Levels of Cognitive Impairment?', *Aging and Mental Health*, 15(5): 562-72.

Cahill, S. and Shapiro, M. (1997). '"At first I thought it was age", Family Carers' Detection of and General Practitioners' Diagnosis of Early Stage Dementia', *New Doctor*, 67.

Cahill, S., Clark, M., O'Connell, H., Lawlor, B., Coen, R.F. and Walsh, C. (2008). 'The Attitudes and Practices of General Practitioners regarding Dementia Diagnosis in Ireland', *International Journal of Geriatric Psychiatry*, 23(7): 663-669.

Cahill, S., Clark, M., Walsh, C., O'Connell, H. and Lawlor, B. (2006). 'Dementia in Primary Care: The First Survey of General Practitioners', *International Journal of Geriatric Psychiatry*, 21: 319-324.

Cahill, S., Diaz-Ponce, A., Coen, R.F. and Walsh, C. (2010). 'The Under-detection of Cognitive Impairment in Nursing Homes in the Dublin Area: The Need for On-going Cognitive Assessment', *Age and Ageing*, 38(1): 128-130.

Cahill, S., O'Shea, E. and Pierce, M. (2012). *Creating Excellence in Dementia Care: A Research Review to Inform Ireland's National Dementia Strategy*, Dublin and

Galway: Living with Dementia Research Programme, Trinity College and Irish Centre for Social Gerontology, National University of Ireland Galway.

Chertkow, H. (2008). 'Diagnosis and Treatment of Dementia. Introduction - Introducing a Series Based on the Third Canadian Consensus Conference on the Diagnosis and Treatment of Dementia', *Canadian Medical Association Journal*, 178(3): 1273-1285.

Connolly, S., Gillespie, P., O'Shea, E., Cahill, S. and Pierce, M. (2012). 'Estimating the Economic and Social Costs of Dementia in Ireland', *Dementia: The International Journal of Social Research and Practice*. doi: 10.1177/1471301212442453.

DeLange, J., Willemse, B., Smit, D. and Pot, A.M. (2011). 'Housing with Care for People with Dementia in The Netherlands', paper to *Workshop on Housing with Care for People with Dementia*, Trinity College Dublin, 11 November.

Department of Health (UK) (2009). *Dementia Strategy*, London: HMSO.

Doocey, A. and Reddy, W. (2010). 'Integrated Care Pathways: The Touchstone of an Integrated Service Delivery Model for Ireland', *International Journal of Care Pathways*, 14(1): 27-29.

Geldmacher, D., Provenzano, G., McRae, T., Mastey, V. and Ieni, J. (2003). 'Donepezil is Associated with Delayed Nursing Home Placement in Patients with Alzheimer's Disease', *Journal of the American Geriatrics Society*, 51: 937-994.

Haggerty, J., Reid, R., Freeman, G., Starfield, B., Adair, C. and McKendry, R. (2003). 'Continuity of Care: A Multidisciplinary Review', *British Medical Journal*, 327(7425): 1219-1221.

Health Service Executive (HSE) (2001). *Primary Care: A New Direction*, Dublin: Stationery Office.

Health Service Executive (HSE) (2007). *Transformation Programme 2007-2010*, Dublin: Stationery Office.

Health Service Executive (HSE) (2008). *Corporate Plan 2008-2011*, Dublin: Stationery Office.

Health Service Executive (HSE) (2012). *National Service Plan 2012*, Dublin: Stationery Office.

Iliffe, S., Jain, P. and Wilcock, J. (2009). 'Recognition and Response to Dementia in Primary Care: Part 1', *InnovatAit*, 2(4): 230-236.

Kodner, D. and Spreeuwenberg, C. (2002). 'Integrated Care: Meaning, Logic, Applications and Implications: A Discussion Paper', *International Journal of Integrated Care*, 2(14): 1-6.

Ministry of Health (NZ) (1997). *Guidelines for the Support and Management of People with Dementia*, Wellington, New Zealand: Ministry of Health.

Mittelman, M.S., Roth, D.L., Clay, O.J. and Haley, W.E. (2007). 'Preserving Health of Alzheimer Caregivers: Impact of a Spouse Caregiver Intervention', *American Journal Geriatric Psychiatry*, 15: 780-789.

Moore, V. and Cahill, S. (2013). 'Diagnosis and Disclosure of Dementia – A Comparative Qualitative Study of Irish and Swedish General Practitioners', *Ageing and Mental Health*, 17(1): 77-84.

National Health Service (2007). *Report on Standards for Integrated Care Pathways for Mental Health*, London: NHS Quality Improvement, in partnership with The Scottish Government.

Nies, H. and Berman, P.C. (2004). *Integrated Services for Older People*, Dublin: European Health Management Association.

O'Shea, E. and O'Reilly, S. (1999). *The Action Plan on Dementia*, Dublin: National Council on Ageing and Older People.

Personal Communication with Matthew Gibb, Senior Social Worker, National Memory Clinic, St. James's hospital, September 2011.

Phillips, J., Pond, D. and Goode, S. (2011). 'Timely Diagnosis of Dementia: Can We Do Better? A Report for Alzheimer's Australia', paper, 24.

Pierce, M., Cahill, S. and O'Shea, E. (2013). 'Planning Dementia Services: New Estimates of Current and Future Prevalence Rates of Dementia for Ireland', *Irish Journal of Psychological Medicine*, 30(1): 13-20, available at http://doi.org/10.1017/ipm.2013.3.

Royal Australian College of General Practice (RACGP) (2006). *Care of People with Dementia in General Practice Guidelines*, accessible at http://www.racgp.org.au/ Content/NavigationMenu/ClinicalResources/RACGPGuidelines/CareofPatientswithDementia/20060413dementiaguidelines.pdf.

US Preventive Services Task Force (USPSTF) (*not dated*). *Guidelines*, available http://www.ahrq.gov/clinic/uspstfix.htm.

Vernooij-Dassen, F., oniz-Cook, E., Woods, R., DeLepeleire, J., Leuschner, A., Zanetti, O. and Iliffe, S. (2005). 'Factors Affecting Timely Recognition and Diagnosis of Dementia across Europe: From Awareness to Stigma', *International Journal of Geriatric Psychiatry*, 20: 377-386.

15: INTEGRATED CARE FOR OLDER PEOPLE IN IRELAND: PERHAPS JAM TOMORROW?

Desmond O'Neill

INTRODUCTION

When the celebrated American conductor Kent Nagano took the helm of the Hallé Orchestra in Manchester at a low ebb in its fortunes, an interviewer in an English paper questioned him why he was taking up the post. The reply, to the effect that when you buy into the stock market, you don't buy high, is a suitable analogy for the level of integration of health and social services for older people in Ireland. There are the beginnings of the development of frameworks of care and common tools for the assessment of older people, but at the time of writing the situation is that integration in a mixed public and private health system (O'Neill and O'Keeffe, 2003) is patchy at best, and takes place in a context of a reluctance by many groupings of health care professionals to adequately age-attune the undergraduate education and postgraduate training of their members. For example, a 2009 publication by the Irish Nursing Board on nursing older people (the first of its kind) completely failed to mention gerontological nursing (An Bord Altranais, 2009): it is hard to imagine that a similar guidance on nursing of children, or of patients in the emergency department or coronary care unit, would have failed to mention the relevant specialism in nursing.

That this matters can be clearly seen by a survey of referral patterns of older people discharged from hospital to their public health nurses – in one study from an Irish teaching hospital, the rate of referral of older people to the public health nurse was lamentably low, but was running at over 80% from the department of geriatric medicine (Murphy, 2002). Nested within this finding is a ray of hope: if, as has been the case, the Irish State continues to invest in specialist health care for older people –

geriatric medicine, gerontological nursing, old age psychiatry – then this may lead to an increased integration of care, as an elemental part of gerontological training is to plan transfers of care and to work in a joined-up fashion. A 2011 decision that at least one-third of consultant physicians to the Acute Medicine Programme in Ireland must be trained in geriatric medicine is encouraging in this regard (O'Neill *et al.*, 2012).

The problems associated with integrated care for older people (and other demographic groups) stem from a range of issues, including a lack of clarity on eligibility/entitlements, failure to provide universal training in gerontology to health and social care workers, multiple service providers, and the absence or extreme paucity of some services (such as speech and language therapy, clinical nutrition and social work) in the community (Hickey *et al.*, 2012). And even where such services arise, ageist practices may occur: in my own area of practice, even in the second decade of the 21st century, a new community service in speech and language therapy rationed access on the basis of only seeing patients under 65 rather than on need.

EXPERIENCES OF OLDER IRISH PEOPLE WITH HEALTH AND SOCIAL SERVICES

In terms of older people's own views on health services, the first longitudinal study on ageing in Ireland (HeSSOP-2) gave a helpful perspective of experiences of older Irish people with the health and social services (O'Hanlon *et al.*, 2005). It confirmed that access to services varied significantly with location, with those in the east of the country receiving more services than in the west of the country. The take-up of a wide range of services was low in European terms, although it was not clear from the data whether this was due to a lack of their availability or restrictive eligibility criteria. The general practitioner (GP) and public health nurse (PHN) are the key elements of the primary care system. The GP is a pivotal health professional contact for older people, with 93% having consulted their GP in the previous year. The PHN has a less prominent profile, with 15% having been visited by a PHN in the past year. Use of other services was very limited, with many older people stating that they would like to use them, but were deterred by lack of information and barriers to access including cost, availability, stigma and transport. This is a major challenge, as more than one-third of older people in the community found to be 'severely impaired' in carrying out activities of daily living (ADLs) had not received any home services in the past year. One in 10 people experiencing extreme disruption to their lives through illness had not received any of the home or community-based services studied (O'Hanlon *et al.*, 2005).

About half of those using physiotherapy or podiatry services paid for them, clarifying that older people are not just passive recipients of care (O'Neill and McGee, 2007), one of the most telling findings related to the benefits of universal access to health care. Between the two waves of the study, free medical access to primary care was granted to all those over the age 70, regardless of income: the rate of vaccination against influenza doubled in the eastern region of Ireland in the second wave, and by 50% in the western region.

So what happens to older people in the Republic of Ireland with complex care needs who, for example, are discharged from hospital? A large study of older people discharged from an Irish university hospital indicated that patients over the age of 80 felt moderately less ready for discharge than those under the age of 80 but had higher expectations of support on discharge: however, over 80% had no support in place at the time of discharge (Coffey and McCarthy, 2012). By six weeks after discharge, there were increases in informal support, with an increase in support with medication management (12%), followed by support with household activities (10%), ADLs (9%) and transport (4%). In addition, a higher percentage of respondents aged 80 and over received all forms of informal support in comparison with those aged 65 to 80. The increase in formal support (home helps predominantly) occurred mostly in those who were using the home help service prior to admission. Significant relationships existed between lower perception of readiness at discharge and increased use of informal and formal support post-discharge. These findings are consistent with an earlier qualitative study of experiences of older Irish people discharged from hospital (McKeown, 2007). A troubling aspect of this pattern is that much of the support therefore seems to depend on the availability of family, friends and neighbours: those without such supports, whether through social isolation/exclusion, family circumstances or mental health issues, may add poor access to services as an additional burden to their already high level of vulnerability.

In the absence of discernible mechanisms to assess need or to attend to the older patient's perception of discharge readiness, it is not surprising that almost one-quarter had been re-admitted to hospital within six weeks, a telling argument for better assessment of, and provision for, care needs and their delivery in a better integrated manner. An intimation of the challenge of matching measured need and service provision can be gleaned from a 2007 study that showed increased nursing time, but not home help provision, with increased dependency and complexity of needs (Byrne *et al.*, 2007).

For those in nursing homes, the provision of integrated care is also inadequate, as evidenced by a study examining the therapy support for stroke survivors discharged to nursing homes with significant and complex disability (Horgan *et al.*, 2011). The provision of these important aspects was raised at many public preparatory meetings for the Nursing Home Subvention Scheme (the so-called 'Fair Deal') but all such questions were stone-walled by both the Health Service Executive (HSE) and the Department of Health and Children (DoHC), a worrying portent of the low political priority of comprehensive, integrated care for older people at that time.

FUTURE PROMISE?

So, if the past and the present are unpromising in terms of integrated care for older people, does the future hold more promise? While some of the auguries at a central government level have not been promising – it took the Irish government almost a decade to respond to the United Nations plan for ageing: *The Madrid International Plan for Action on Ageing* (United Nations Economic and Social Council, 2007), and the National Positive Ageing Strategy remains in suspended animation – at least two initiatives are of some note.

The first is the HSE's National Clinical Programme for Older People (NCPOP), in association with the Royal College of Physicians in Ireland (**www.hse.ie/eng/about/Who/clinical/natclinprog/OlderPeople.html**), one of a series of similar programmes commenced in 2010 that represent possibly the first time that the health services in Ireland have engaged in a constructive and systematic fashion with the medical profession in developing medical services in Ireland.

Under the capable leadership of a geriatrician, Dr. Diarmuid O'Shea, the NCPOP has developed blueprints for care of older people in a range of settings, as well as providing a focus for age-attuned care in the other clinical programmes. The programme is beginning to develop a portfolio of responses that recognises the complexity of care of older people, and provides appropriate responses. An early change arising from the programme is the stipulation that at least one-third of appointments of consultant physicians to the emerging Acute Medicine Programme are qualified in geriatric medicine, a recognition of the striking efficacy of geriatric medicine in reducing death and disability among older people. One of the aspects of the programme has been to promote the development of a SAT to measure the care needs of older people: it has become clear that the Irish system needs a unified system for assessing disability and vulnerability among older people who are accessing services, whether community, hospital or nursing home.

In this, it builds on the findings of the first formal review of a nursing home scandal in Ireland, the Leas Cross review (O'Neill, 2006) (and many decades of activity and concern by Irish geriatricians and their allies (O'Neill *et al.*, 2001)). The Leas Cross review recommended, and the HSE and the DoHC accepted, that the Minimum Data Set (MDS) should be implemented in Irish nursing homes. In this and other settings, we have known for some time that practitioners in all sectors have been failing to detect functional loss, and this is an important time in Ireland when there is a possibility for establishing widely-recognised measures of functional loss and disability. Of equal importance is that any scale should be internationally used so that we can benchmark quality of care, service developments and the degree to which services are 'older-friendly'. Finally, there is also the imperative of high-quality, comparable data for research, a point brought home to the author personally when trying to establish disability data for nursing home populations (Falconer and O'Neill, 2007).

USING A MINIMUM DATA SET

In this, Ireland trails behind North America and much of the rest of Europe, where for over 20 years determined efforts have been made to validate assessment processes for older people that are relevant, concise and valid. The main contender is the InterRAI/MDS family (**www.interrai.org**, North America and many European countries) in its Nursing Home, Acute Care, Home Care versions.

The RAI/MDS set has a long pedigree, and the series of assessment instruments comprise an integrated health information system because they have consistent terminology, common core items, and a common conceptual basis in a clinical approach that emphasises the identification of functional problems. There is vast experience with this instrument, largely arising out of the mandatory requirement in the USA that all nursing home residents have the instrument administered on admission and quarterly thereafter. It has also significant academic investment by geriatricians and gerontologists in Europe and North America, and of most importance, is subject to constant renewal, as the emerging science of gerontology and geriatric medicine changes our understanding of disability and effective management of complex care needs of older people (Bernabei *et al.*, 2008). There are more than 400 papers on Medline (the major biomedical repository of scientific papers) on this family of instruments, and many more on CINAHL and other scientific databases.

The MMDS, as a part of the Resident Assessment Instrument (RAI), was developed by the Health Care Financing Administration (HCFA) to assist US nursing homes in developing a comprehensive care plan for each resident, following the realisation of scandalously low levels of care by the Institute of Medicine (IOM). The IOM report in 1986 identified uniform resident assessment as essential to improvement in the quality of care delivered to residents and reform of the survey process (IOM, 1986).

When the *Omnibus Budget Reconciliation Act of 1987* (OBRA 87) became law in 1987, HCFA began a process of public comment leading to a final rule implementing the law. The process was completed on 22 December 1997 and includes the requirement to electronically encode and transmit all MDSs to the State in which each facility is licensed: the equivalent in Ireland would be the HSE. The MDS is a standardised assessment instrument specified by HCFA and optionally supplemented by States (with approval from HCFA), which collects administrative and clinical information about residents. The MDS is a very complete and well-designed assessment which, when used with the Resident Assessment Protocols and professional judgment, is a comprehensive assessment and care planning tool.

The MDS collects assessment information on each resident's characteristics, ADLs, medical needs, mental status, therapy use, and other things involved in comprehensive planning for resident care. The MDS is used to assess every resident in state-licensed facilities on admission, with a quarterly review and annual re-assessment. Significant change in a resident's condition causes a new comprehensive MDS (including review of the care plan) to be completed to ensure the resident receives appropriate care. The MDS can serve as the primary clinical assessment tool for all residents within nursing facilities, as it is a comprehensive yet reasonably brief assessment. The MDS (with additional triggered assessments) is sufficient for most care settings.

The MDS also can be used to generate Resource Utilization Groups (RUG-III), effectively a case mix system that sets levels of dependency for a resident based on the functional support requirement and medical needs of each resident. Using the MDS, a computer programme first calculates an ADL score, a depression index, and a cognitive performance score. It then identifies each of the major groupings for which the resident is qualified. The ADL index, depression index and cognitive performance scales are also very useful clinically. They can help to identify residents with depression and to guide the care planning to help the resident cope or resolve the depression. The cognitive performance scale can assist during care planning to set realistic goals for residents, as well as to identify changes in cognition that could be reversed or treated.

So the MDS is clinically useful, reasonably brief, computerised, and fulfils four goals: it supports individual care plans; it can help generate dependency levels (through RUGS); it assists regulatory authorities; and it allows for the collection of meaningful statistics nationwide. Overall, it has been deemed to be successful by both nursing home staff and regulators (Marek *et al.*, 1996) and is now used widely through the developed world (Jorgensen *et al.*, 1997; Morris *et al.*, 1997; Topinkova *et al.*, 1997; Carpenter *et al.*, 1999; Jensdottir *et al.*, 2003). It is perhaps unique in its robust ability to support improved standards and research in nursing homes (Mor, 2004), although it will not do so on its own, and needs to be implemented in a context that recognises the importance of appropriate philosophies of care, staff training and resourcing.

The Acute Care module has been assessed by several groups (Carpenter *et al.*, 2001), with supportive clinical studies (Gray *et al.*, 2008; Jonsson *et al.*, 2006), and the Home Care module also has been extensively validated – of particular interest for those involved with the Elder Abuse National Implementation Group, there is also the potential for identifying those at risk of elder abuse (Shugarman *et al.*, 2003). The Home Care assessment starts with a single page screening questionnaire – if this reveals little by way of problems, then the process stops at that point. If problems are detected, the full assessment protocol is used.

In 2012, a working group of the HSE selected the InterRAI as the single assessment tool of choice, after outlining the parameters of an effective assessment tool, and through a rigorous assessment process looking at specifications such as validity, reliability, international comparability and the degree to which the tool is regularly updated. Although clearly there will need to be a significant investment in training and information technology to support the implementation of this process, this development of a common language of the often complex care needs of older people has enormous potential to support better provision, targeting and integration of care in each of the sectors of health care: community, hospital and nursing home. In addition, it will facilitate the communication of such care needs in transitions between these sectors which occur with increasing frequency as we age (Kelman and Thomas, 1990).

REFERENCES

An Bord Altranais (Irish Nursing Board) (2009). *Professional Guidance for Nurses Working with Older People*, Dublin, An Bord Altranais.

Bernabei, R., Landi, F., Onder, G., Liperoti, R. and Gambassi, G. (2008). 'Second and Third Generation Assessment Instruments: The Birth of Standardization in Geriatric Care', *Journals of Gerontology Series A, Biological Sciences and Medical Sciences*, 63(3): 308-313.

Byrne, G., Brady, A.M., Horan, P., Macgregor, C. and Begley, C. (2007). 'Assessment of Dependency Levels of Older People in the Community and Measurement of Nursing Workload', *Journal of Advanced Nursing*, 60(1): 39-49.

Carpenter, G.I., Hirdes, J.P., Ribbe, M.W., Ikegami, N., Challis, D., Steel, K., Bernabei, R. and Fries, B. (1999). 'Targeting and Quality of Nursing Home Care. A Five-nation Study', *Aging* (Milano), 11(2): 83-89.

Carpenter, G.I., Teare, G.F., Steel, K., Berg, K., Murphy K., Bjornson, J., Jonsson, P.V. and Hirdes, J.P. (2001). 'A New Assessment for Elders Admitted to Acute Care: Reliability of the MDS-AC', *Aging* (Milano), 13(4): 316-330.

Coffey, A. and McCarthy, G.M. (2012). 'Older People's Perception of their Readiness for Discharge and Postdischarge Use of Community Support and Services', *International Journal of Older People Nursing*, doi: 10.111/j.1748-3743.2012.00316.x.

Falconer, M. and O'Neill, D. (2007). 'Profiling Disability within Nursing Homes: A Census-based Approach', *Age Ageing*, 36(2): 209-213.

Gray, L.C., Bernabei, R., Berg., K., Finne-Soveri, H., Fries, B.E., Hirdes, J.P., Jonsson, P.V., Morris, J.N., Steel, K. and Arino-Blanco, S. (2008). 'Standardizing Assessment of Elderly People in Acute Care: The InterRAI Acute Care Instrument', *Journal of the American Geriatric Society*, 56(3): 536-541.

Hickey, A., Horgan, F., O'Neill, D., McGee, H. and Inasc, O.B. (2012). 'Community-based Post-stroke Service Provision and Challenges: A National Survey of Managers and Interdisciplinary Healthcare Staff in Ireland', *BMC Health Service Research*, 12(1): 111.

Horgan, F., McGee, H., Hickey, A., Whitford, D.L., Murphy, S., Royston, M., Cowman, S., Shelley, E., Conroy, R.M., Wiley, M. and O'Neill, D. (2011). 'From Prevention to Nursing Home Care: A Comprehensive National Audit of Stroke Care', *Cerebrovascular Disease*, 32(4): 385-392.

Institute of Medicine (IOM) (1986). *Improving the Quality of Care in Nursing Homes*, Washington DC: IOM.

Jensdottir, A.B., Rantz, M., Hjaltadottir, I., Gudmundsdottir, H., Rook, M. and Grando, V. (2003). 'International Comparison of Quality Indicators in United States, Icelandic and Canadian Nursing Facilities', *International Nursing Review*, 50(2): 79-84.

Jonsson, P.V., Finne-Soveri, H., Jensdottir, A.B., Ljunggren, G., Bucht, G., Grue, E.V., Noro, A., Bjornson, J., Jonsen, E. and Schroll, M. (2006). 'Co-morbidity and Functional Limitation in Older Patients Underreported in Medical Records in Nordic Acute Care Hospitals when Compared with the MDS-AC Instrument', *Age Ageing*, 35(4): 434-438.

Jorgensen, L.M., el Kholy, K., Damkjaer, K., Deis, A. and Schroll, M. (1997). 'RAI - An International System for Assessment of Nursing Home Residents', *Ugeskr Laeger*, 159(43): 6371-6376.

Kelman, H.R. and Thomas, C. (1990). 'Transitions between Community and Nursing Home Residence in an Urban Elderly Population', *Journal of Community Health*, 15(2): 105-122.

Marek, K.D., Rantz, M.J., Fagin, C.M. and Krejci, J.W. (1996). 'OBRA '87: Has It Resulted in Better Quality of Care?', *Journal of Gerontological Nursing*, 22(10): 28-36.

McKeown, F. (2007). 'The Experiences of Older People on Discharge from Hospital following Assessment by the Public Health Nurse', *Journal of Clinical Nursing*, 16(3): 469-476.

Mor, V. (2004). 'A Comprehensive Clinical Assessment Tool to Inform Policy and Practice: Applications of the Minimum Data Set', *Medical Care*, 42(4(Suppl.)): III 50-59.

Morris, J.N., Fries, B.E., Steel, K., Ikegami, N., Bernabei, R., Carpenter, G.I., Gilgen, R., Hirdes, J.P. and Topinkova, E. (1997). 'Comprehensive Clinical Assessment in Community Setting: Applicability of the MDS-HC', *Journal of the American Geriatric Society*, 45(8): 1017-1024.

Murphy, C. (2002). 'Liaison between Hospital Nurses and Public Health Nurses on the Discharge of Elderly Patients from Hospital to Home', *All Ireland Journal of Nursing and Midwifery*, 2: 33-37.

O'Neill, D. (2006). *A Review of the Deaths at Leas Cross Nursing Home 2002-2005*, Dublin: Health Service Executive.

O'Neill, D., Andersen-Ranberg, K., Cherubini, A., Strandberg, T., Petermans, J. and Michel, J.P. (2012). 'Must Be Trained in Geriatric Medicine', *British Medical Journal*, 344: e2909.

O'Neill, D., Gibbon, J. and Mulpeter, K. (2001). 'Responding to Care Needs in Long-term Care: A Position Paper by the Irish Society of Physicians in Geriatric Medicine', *Irish Medical Journal*, 94(3): 72.

O'Neill, D. and McGee, H. (2007). 'Oldest Old Are Not Just Passive Recipients of Care', *British Medical Journal*, 334(7595): 651.

O'Neill, D. and O'Keeffe, S. (2003). 'Health Care for Older People in Ireland', *Journal of the American Geriatric Society*, 51(9): 1280-1286.

O'Hanlon, A., McGee, H., Barker, A., Garavan, R., Hickey, A., Conroy, R. and O'Neill, D. (2005). *Health and Social Services for Older People II (HeSSOP II): Changing Profiles from 2000 to 2004*, Dublin: National Council on Ageing and Older People.

Shugarman, L.R., Fries, B.E., Wolf, R.S. and Morris, J.N. (2003). 'Identifying Older People at Risk of Abuse during Routine Screening Practices', *Journal of the American Geriatric Society*, 51(1): 24-31.

Topinkova, E., Sgadari, A. and Haas, T. (1997). 'Urinary Incontinence in Patients in Long-term Institutional Care: Results of an International Study in 8 Countries', *Cas Lek Cesk*, 136(18): 555-558.

United Nations Economic and Social Council (2007). *First Review and Appraisal of the Madrid International Plan of Action on Ageing: Preliminary Assessment*, New York: United Nations.

16: INTEGRATED CARE PATHWAYS FOR PEOPLE WITH DEMENTIA: EXPLORING THE POTENTIAL FOR IRELAND AND THE FORTHCOMING NATIONAL DEMENTIA STRATEGY

Kate Irving, Lisa McGarrigle, Grainne McGettrick and Maurice O'Connell

INTRODUCTION

Internationally, dementia strategies provide a clear guide to the content of high-quality health and social care services for people with dementia. In addition to specific strategy documents, many countries also have more detailed localised pathways intended to be a more comprehensive clinical guideline for health professionals.

This paper presents an analysis of integrated care pathways (ICPs) for people with dementia, defining what they are, how they operate in practice and the implications for dementia care policy in Ireland and, in particular, for the forthcoming National Dementia Strategy.

There is an appetite for change in dementia care. Research suggests that the current level of care provision is uneven throughout the country, with major deficiencies being identified in the standard of care of people with dementia in both acute hospital and long-stay facilities (Cahill *et al.*, 2012). The development of a National Dementia Strategy for Ireland represents a unique and important opportunity for creativity in terms of providing a much clearer pathway, more positive outcomes and a smoother journey for the person with dementia and their families, along with better use of existing resources and cost savings for carers.

There are some significant differences between countries in terms of emphasis on stages of the care pathway. For example, there is a clear focus on risk reduction in the dementia services in Australia, along with primary care, access to counselling and community support (Brodaty and Cumming, 2010). These aspects play a much less central role in, for example, dementia services in the UK, where there is an emphasis on timely diagnosis and public and professional attitudes to dementia (Banerjee, 2010). These key differences between emphases of service provision pose important questions about what priorities should be emphasised within the Irish health and social care system.

Dementia often is defined as a chronic condition characterised by symptoms such as disturbed memory, orientation problems, behavioural changes and comprehension. There are several different forms of dementia, of which Alzheimer's disease is probably the most common. These definitions stem from an illness-orientated understanding of dementia and can lead to excess disability (Drossel and Fisher, 2006).

More recently, there has been a move to define dementia from the perspective of the person with dementia and as a disability (Gilliard *et al.*, 2005). Viewing dementia as a psychological and social disability allows for a more holistic understanding of the condition (Cahill *et al.*, 2012). This shift in perspective, away from a medicalised model, is to be welcomed as it holds potential for emphasis to be placed on the quality of life of the person living with dementia. From this perspective, given the right enablement and supports, there is better hope that a person may draw meaning and joy from life and continue to contribute to society and the wider community despite their disability.

However, currently dementia is associated with an increase in the use of medical services and can pose a challenge with regard to caregiving. Many hospitals are not designed to care for people with cognitive impairment and this may prove challenging in terms of caring for the individual's personhood in addition to the acute problem for which they were admitted (Moyle *et al.*, 2008). The needs of individuals with dementia are often complex and frequently require services from a number of organisations (Rees *et al.*, 2004).

UNDERSTANDING INTEGRATED CARE PATHWAYS

ICPs are instruments designed to map out the direction of clinical and administrative activities for all care professionals for a diagnosis-specific group. Essentially, ICPs chronologically pinpoint the key steps to be taken throughout the person's care journey (Rees *et al.*, 2004). Instead of re-active or crisis care, ICPs are designed to provide an improved service for both patients and carers through a more pro-active care planning approach (Scottish Government, 2010). The establishment of ICPs is useful in that they aim to facilitate the introduction of clinical protocols, promote change in practice through the systematic collection of clinical data for audit, and improve communication with patients by providing them with a clear summary of their expected care plan (Campbell *et al.*, 1998).

There are two essential components that characterise dementia care pathways: a service map, and a tool to audit the pathway (Saad *et al.*, 2008). The goals of integrated care are to enhance quality of care and quality of life, service user satisfaction, and system efficiency for individuals with complex needs (Kodner and Kyriacou, 2000). ICPs are specific translations of broader national policy that enable the policy in the context of local circumstances (for example, service availability, geography and population structure). Essentially, ICPs take agreed national policy and translate it into practice in a particular local context.

With Ireland's ageing population on the rise, there will be a corresponding rise in the number of adults with long-term conditions such as dementia. Those aged 65 and over in Ireland currently represent 11% of our total population. This is expected to double from approximately 0.5 million today to over 1 million by 2031 (Cahill *et al.*, 2012). A move towards more integrated working in terms of planning and service delivery could help achieve better outcomes for those with dementia and make the best use of current resources.

Integrated dementia pathways have been found to improve dementia services in terms of access to services and informing service users of the steps to be taken throughout their care journey (Saad, 2004). In the UK, a National Health Service (NHS) report on dementia services in the West Midlands outlined the core principles applicable to a good dementia pathway. These include respect for both patients and carers; adaptability and flexibility; a clear map and route-finder; taking into account transitions and adjustments between pathway parts; links to other service providers for managing co-morbidities; and maximised personal control and empowerment (Saad *et al.*, 2008).

THE PRACTICAL APPLICATION OF INTEGRATED CARE PATHWAYS

Developing a dementia pathway is a complex undertaking for a number of reasons. Dementia is an umbrella term for many different diseases, all of which have similar symptoms, but different aetiologies (that is, causes), different management strategies and different licensed treatments.

The onset of dementia generally is gradual and there is no definitive biological marker of disease onset. Regardless of the specific type of dementia, each individual experiences it very differently with different presentations of problem features, physiological changes, psychological reactions, and family and community responses, making definition of a proper response to dementia difficult.

More integrated working also can support people with long-term care needs through increased personalisation of care. Personalised care for people with dementia involves placing the individual at the centre of the care process and tailoring support to their individual needs. A person-centred approach to care can enhance service efficiency, avoid unnecessary hospital admissions (which, in turn, reduces care costs), and has been found to reduce agitation in people with dementia living in residential care (Chenoweth *et al.*, 2009; Social Care Institute for Excellence (SCIE), 2008).

A personalised approach can be applied across all stages of the disease lifecycle, including prevention, assessment, care planning, service provision and ongoing support (SCIE, 2008). An effective integrated care pathway for dementia promotes personal control and empowers both patients and carers (Saad *et al.*, 2008).

ICPs can be used in the health service as a formalising mechanism for procedures that involve multi-agency working (Currie, 1999). It has been suggested that a move from fragmented care in hospitals to anticipatory, integrated and continuous care in communities may help to promote health (Cook, 2008). This is particularly true for dementia care, where individuals tend to have multiple needs and may require skills belonging to multiple circles (Downs and Bowers, 2008). More integrated health and community support can help to build relationships between different agencies to improve the health and wellbeing of patients and to achieve efficiencies and also to reduce organisational barriers that may exist between these agencies (SCIE, 2011).

EVIDENCE OF THE BENEFITS OF INTEGRATED CARE PATHWAYS

The development of an effective ICP for dementia should incorporate a multidisciplinary specialist service team to guide the person with dementia and their caregivers as their condition progresses. An ICP is designed to be used as a guide and, where necessary, the professionals' judgement may override the advice of the tool (Dementia ICP Development Group, 2010; Hall, 2001).

It is widely recognised that the implementation of ICPs is largely supported by both service users and staff as a result of increased service efficiency (Lowe, 1998; Atwal and Caldwell, 2002; Gunstone and Robinson, 2006; Tucker, 2010; Ham *et al.*, 2011; Hean *et al.*, 2011).

The professional, organisational and patient-associated benefits of ICPs are numerous. In the UK, a qualitative study was conducted to investigate a multidisciplinary team's experience of an ICP pilot in an inpatient dementia assessment service. The team identified benefits that included the pathway's influence on care management, increased efficiency, improvements in teamworking and, most importantly, enhancement of the experience of patients and carers (Hall, 2001).

Evidence also suggests that ICPs improve documentation of care (Main *et al.*, 2006) and deepen caregivers' understanding of the sequence of medical practices for the patient (Kazui *et al.*, 2004). A systematic review conducted to examine the circumstances in which ICPs are most effective found that they are a useful tool in reducing variation in practice, improving physician agreement about treatment options and changing professional behaviours in the desired direction (Allen *et al.*, 2009).

Summary of Benefits

Individuals with dementia tend to have multiple needs and, therefore, often require multidisciplinary care. A move towards more integrated care can help to:

- Bridge gaps that may exist between different agencies;
- Place the focus on the individual needs of the person with dementia.

The current evidence-base suggests that the development of an ICP for people with dementia is beneficial for both professionals and patients in terms of:

- Increased efficiency;
- Reduced variation in practice;
- Improved interprofessional communication to help tailor support to individual patient needs.

For ICP implementation to be successful, a focus on team development and education about integration is essential. **Figure 16.1** provides a good overview of essential features of an effective ICP.

Figure 16.1: The West Midlands Darzi Dementia Care Pathway

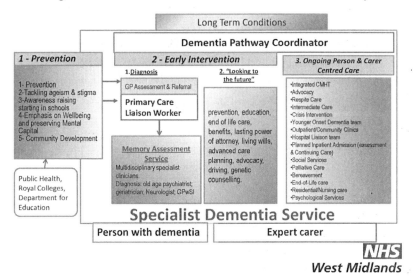

Source: Saad *et al.*, 2008.

Challenges

Although there is a strong evidence-base for the benefits of ICPs, there are several challenges that must be addressed if an ICP is to be successful. There has been some concern that ICPs deliver 'cookbook medicine', as they are characterised by pre-determined stages of care (De Luc, 2001). However, in some circumstances, this can be viewed as a strength by helping to guide the novice practitioner (Gunstone and Robinson, 2006) while more experienced practitioners, where necessary, can override the tool in favour of their clinical judgement (Hall, 2001). Any deviations from the pathway are monitored and recorded through variance reporting in order that appropriate changes can be made to the ICP (Gunstone and Robinson, 2006).

Other documented challenges – including issues such as lack of a defined common goal between members of a multidisciplinary team due to differing expectations; insufficient interprofessional communication; and diversity of practice at an organisational level – can contribute to poor outcomes in ICP implementation (Atwal and Caldwell, 2002). Change management in terms of team development and education about integration can overcome these potential difficulties and foster effective interprofessional teamworking (Rees *et al.*, 2004). Generally, there is a great deal of support for the principle of integrated care.

TWO INTEGRATED CARE PATHWAYS
CASE STUDIES

A comprehensive literature search was conducted in order to get a sense of how the principles of integrated care are being applied internationally. As evidenced from a number of national dementia strategies, including in Australia, Canada, the UK, France and The Netherlands, there is a large-scale move towards integrated systems of care.

In the UK, the National Health Service (NHS) has rolled out integrated care pilots across a number of clinical areas, including dementia. What follows is an analysis of two of these pilot programmes in order to demonstrate the key features necessary for effective integrated care. These two cases were chosen as they offered the greatest level of detail and background information and provided information across a number of areas, which made them comparable.

Case Study 1: Newquay, England

The Newquay Dementia Integrated Care Pilot (**Table 16.1**) was developed as part of a countrywide dementia programme in the UK and received two years' funding from the Department of Health. In Newquay, 361 people live with dementia out of a population of 23,000. Within the next 20 years, this number of people with dementia is expected to double. Aware of this growing need and the emerging pressures on specialist teams, the three general practitioner (GP) practices in the Newquay Practice-based Commissioning Group began to explore new ways of caring for people with dementia in terms of an ICP approach.

The ICP approach piloted in Newquay was based on clinical guidelines from the National Institute for Health and Clinical Excellence, as well as recommendations from the National Dementia Strategy, the National Carers Strategy, and the National End-of-Life Strategy. This model of care emphasises close integrated working across health and social care systems, the delivery of GP-led memory clinics in association with specialised support from community mental health teams (CMHTs), pro-active case management as well as strengthening community networks and support.

Given the specific needs of people with dementia, the aim of the pilot was to separate dementia from the traditional structure of secondary care-based 'Older People's Mental Health Services' and to place greater emphasis on treating dementia as a long-term condition, best managed through integrated and preventative case management anchored in primary care.

Table 16.1: Newquay Dementia Integrated Care Pathway Pilot

Phase 1 Diagnosis	Phase 2 Low Intensity	Phase 3 Medium Intensity	Phase 4 High Intensity	Phase 5 Specialist
Case Management	**Case Management**	**Case Management**	**Case Management**	**Case Management**
Diagnosis *via* GP GP referral to memory clinic for diagnosis	GP Memory Advisor Patient does not require CMHT input Support to GP from CMHT Memory Nurse as required	Specialist Memory Nurse Patient care delivered by CMHT Seamless access to GP, Social Care, and Community Health Services	Community Matrons District Nurses GP Care coordinated by lead clinician for major health problems Support/input from Memory Nurse as required	Consultant (Psychiatrist) Consultant (Geriatrics) GP Care coordinated by lead clinician for major health problems Support/input from CMHT
Care Needs	**Care Needs**	**Care Needs**	**Care Needs**	**Care Needs**
Dementia blood screens Physical checks Patient profile Health promotion Peer/carer support Social care provision Crisis contact	Information Advice Monitoring Carer Support	Information Advice Weekly/Monthly Contact Carer Support Access to Social Services Assessment of Risk Support with Activity of Daily Living (ADLs)	Major physical health problems requiring intensive nursing support	Acute medical conditions Acute difficult to manage behaviours with no physical cause

Phase 1 Diagnosis	Phase 2 Low Intensity	Phase 3 Medium Intensity	Phase 4 High Intensity	Phase 5 Specialist
Services	Services	Services	Services	Services
Memory service Interim care plan	Health Promotion Information and Advice Physical Health Check Cognitive Health Check Peer Support – Memory Café Carer Support/ information	Information and Advice Needs/Risk Assessment Weekly/Monthly phone call Weekly/Monthly home visit Carer Support/Informat ion Access to Respite Cognitive Stimulation Group Medication Review Access to Social Care Annual health check Peer Support – Memory Café	District Nursing Community Matron Nursing Local Hospital Admission Hospital at home Falls clinic Physiotherapy TIA clinic Specialist Nurses End of Life	Regular consultant input Hospital admission Consultant clinics Home visits

The Newquay ICP takes a person-centred approach, placing the individual with dementia and their family at the centre of service plans. Within this personalised framework, appropriately-trained staff strive to meet specific personal needs in a timely and responsive manner.

The core objectives of the pilot included increasing the number of people receiving a diagnosis of dementia, improving health and life outcomes for people with dementia and their carers, and viewing dementia as a long-term condition necessitating continuity of care from the point of diagnosis until the end-of-life.

The chosen approach involved GP-centred case management; simple pathways and overlapping services; anticipatory care to prevent, defer or reduce the number of admissions to care homes and hospitals and to reduce length of stay; and shared expertise between and across 'mainstream' and 'specialist' services.

Implementing the pilot proved challenging for individuals and organisations with regard to behaviour, systems and processes. Overall, positive changes in care, staff and the experience of patients and carers have occurred in Newquay. However, it is difficult to pinpoint exactly what outcomes are directly attributable to the work of the pilot. Changing a model of service delivery across a whole system can prove challenging and therefore requires strong project management. Fully-integrated care is not yet systemic in Newquay.

Case Study 2: Lanarkshire, Scotland

In October 2010, North Lanarkshire Community Health Partnership (CHP) was successful in a bid to become a demonstrator site for the Scottish Government's Dementia Strategy. The focus of this pilot project was to investigate the impact of a whole system redesign in relation to the dementia pathway.

The pilot takes a strategic approach to the mapping out and analysing of the entire dementia pathway in order to identify the key areas in need of improvement. The Lanarkshire Dementia ICP (**Table 16.2**) focuses particularly on improving rates of diagnosis and responding to challenging behaviour and aims to deliver clear pathway(s) for people with dementia from onset to end-of-life care (Dementia ICP Development Group, 2010). It was put together by a local development group consisting of NHS staff, service users and carers, local authorities, voluntary organisations and the independent sector.

This stepped model of care adjusts care in stages according to the lack of effect of lower intensity interventions. This model promotes a person-centred approach and a move towards positive management of individual risk, maximising choice and access to evidence-based interventions. It has been designed for any person over 16 years of age who presents with dementia. The development of this ICP is ongoing.

Table 16.2: Lanarkshire Dementia Integrated Care Pathway Pilot

Phase 1 Cognitive Impairment – Assessment and Diagnosis	Phase 2 Complex Needs - Psychological and Behavioural Symptoms	Phase 3 Long-Term Care / End-of-Life Care
MDT Intervention	MDT Intervention	MDT Intervention
Referral to memory service/outpatient clinic for assessment	Management of behavioural and psychological symptoms, including depression, psychosis, agitation and aggression	Advanced planning in relation to end of life care (reviewed at least annually)
History and examination – including carer, driving	Delivery of psychological therapies based on the principle of matched care (those referred to the service are matched to the appropriate level of treatment for the level of complexity of their difficulties)	Includes consideration of preferred place of treatment if condition worsens
Post-diagnostic support	All interventions are used by formal and informal carers working with people with dementia and for use by people with dementia	Gold Standards Framework – evidence-based approach to optimising the care for patients nearing the end of life delivered by generalist providers
Advance planning	A checklist is used to aid the review of patients who develop behavioural and psychological symptoms of dementia (BPSD) – aims to provide structured review of the BPSD and precipitating factors (physical and environmental)	Lanarkshire Palliative Care Assessment Tool (LPCAT) – to assess and manage palliative care needs
Information and support for carers		Liverpool Care Pathway (LCP) – transfers the hospice model of care into other care settings

Phase 1 Cognitive Impairment – Assessment and Diagnosis	Phase 2 Complex Needs - Psychological and Behavioural Symptoms	Phase 3 Long-Term Care / End-of-Life Care
Services	Services	Services
Dementia Cafés	Reminiscence therapy*	Care assessment
Post-diagnosis support groups	Validation therapy*	Community Care
1-1 support providing advice on planning for the future, living well with dementia, advanced statements on future treatment, anticipatory care planning and power of attorney	Non-pharmacological interventions for behaviour that challenges*	Hospital Care
Memory clinics – work closely with Alzheimer Scotland for post-diagnostic support	Cognitive Stimulation therapy*	Care homes
Dementia Awareness and Resource Pack – ensures dignity and respect and quality of care are met across all care settings	Cognitive Behaviour therapy (for depression)*	Carer support
	Caregiver interventions programmes*	
	Occupational Therapy interventions*	
	Art Therapy*	

* The availability of these interventions in Lanarkshire will be determined through the ongoing implementation of the Psychological Therapies Strategy.

Case Study Comparison: Newquay and North Lanarkshire

There are a number of similarities between the ICPs being rolled out in Newquay and North Lanarkshire. In both areas, a pro-active care planning approach is taken to diagnosis and intervention. For instance, in Newquay, focus is placed on increasing the number of people receiving a diagnosis of dementia through improved access to assessment services. In North Lanarkshire, a pro-active approach is taken also, as the ICP aims to improve rates of diagnosis and to tailor delivery of interventions across the key milestones of the journey through care.

In both ICPs, emphasis is placed on advanced planning with regard to end-of-life care. In both Newquay and Lanarkshire, dementia is viewed as a long-term condition that requires continuous care from the point of diagnosis until the end of life.

There is a strong focus on psychological interventions across both ICPs – for example, cognitive stimulation therapy and access to memory cafés. Newquay and Lanarkshire both advocate a person-centred approach to care, where the individual with dementia and their carers are placed at the centre of service plans.

Improved partnership working with CMHTs is also a key element of both ICPs. In North Lanarkshire, this is particularly evident with regard to palliative care, as the Lanarkshire Palliative Care Assessment Tool (LPCAT) is mainly used by community nurses. In terms of multidisciplinary care and team development, Newquay and Lanarkshire employ a model of care that emphasises close integrated working across health and social care systems and shared expertise between professionals.

The ICPs will be used also to produce variance data about the care and interventions provided. This data is an essential component of the ICPs as it will allow comparisons to be made between the care being provided in each locality and the care planned by the ICP. The data collected will flag areas of the ICP that are in need of modification.

There are some differences between the two care pathways in terms of management and intervention. The model of care in Newquay centres largely on the GP and includes the delivery of GP-led memory clinics in association with pro-active GP-centred case management. In North Lanarkshire, however, the central role of the GP is not as evident, since more emphasis appears to be placed on developing the skills and knowledge of the non-specialist workforce, including those in A&E and GP practices, through further training.

With regard to the development of services, both service users and carers were included in the local ICP development group in Lanarkshire. While this does not appear to be the case in Newquay, service users and their carers were invited to describe their experience of the Newquay ICP, which may be useful in highlighting areas in need of further development.

INTEGRATED CARE PATHWAYS AND THEIR RELEVANCE TO THE IRISH CONTEXT

The Irish dementia landscape is highly fragmented and inequitable in terms of access to services and supports. There are currently no defined care pathways for people with dementia in terms of home care support and day care and long-term care facilities. Services available to people with dementia are frequently inadequate, inconsistent and badly co-ordinated throughout the country (Dementia Services Information Development Centre, 2009). Community support services for people with dementia and their carers are under-developed and, often, people with dementia only come into contact with health and social services if a crisis occurs (O'Shea, 2007). A study examining family carers' experience of their relative's transition to a nursing home (Argyle *et al.*, 2010) highlighted deficiencies in formal supports. It was found that most respondents had problems with understanding and negotiating the system of formal support and, in some cases, inadequate or inaccessible domiciliary support influenced their decision to pursue nursing home care for their relative. Their confusion was exacerbated by fragmentation of services, as well as cutbacks in formal support services. In terms of accessing support for the person with dementia at the pre-admission stage, the lack of availability of advice and guidance made a lasting impression on respondents, with most feeling that improvements could be made in this area. Dementia has not yet permeated into the minds of the public or policy-makers when it comes to priority-setting and the allocation of scare public resources (Cahill *et al.*, 2012). Cahill *et al.* (2012) also highlight a number of key questions for consideration before initiating integrated care for dementia could be successfully developed in Ireland.

Questions of System Inefficiencies

It is clear that a large number of individuals and their families are marginalised by difficulties arising not just from the scarcity of service, but from difficulties in negotiating the system, and inefficiencies or lack of joined-up thinking between services. Inequities in relation to access to services are considerable, with geographical location the strongest predictor of the level of service received. For instance, those in rural areas appear to be at a particular disadvantage due to high transport costs and the length of travel time to and from centres (O'Shea and O'Reilly, 1999). There are very limited supports currently in place to help the person with dementia and their carer negotiate the complex health and social care system. According to the Health Information and Quality Authority's *National Quality Standards for Safer Better Healthcare* (2010), equity is a key aspect of high quality and safe health care. It is these issues that ICPs are designed to address. A strong service user voice in this respect, following the example of the Lanarkshire model, would seem to be best practice in terms of addressing the service user voice.

Questions of Economics

Given the evidence of fragmentation and inequality of service distribution around Ireland and the current economic climate, the need for efficient use of resources has never been greater. The evidence from this review shows some economic benefits of ICPs for dementia. However, what it also shows is the care needed towards matters of measurement. Such remodelling of services frequently results in changes to satisfaction but complexities in providing evidence of greater cost-effectiveness. Any such changes in Ireland would be wise to involve the services of a health economist and to pay close attention to the collection of robust baseline data for later comparison.

Questions of Role Clarity/Competence

A clear message from this review is that case management is required if quality care is to be realised. This leads to the question: who will do this? While some steps in the pathway can be addressed by the re-organisation of existing services (and therefore, does not necessarily entail additional resources or budget), there is also a clear need for identified case workers in dementia care to facilitate the effective delivery of services. *An Action Plan for Dementia* (O'Shea and O'Reilly, 1999) states that the most effective way of ensuring flexible and integrated care provision is through the introduction of a case management model to plan and co-ordinate services for people with dementia and their carers. Where possible, the person with dementia should play a major role in developing a personal care plan that fits their own particular preferences and circumstances.

With this in mind, a large body of very helpful work has been done (de Vries *et al.*, 2010), suggesting two key roles in dementia care that are competency-based rather than discipline-specific. The first of these roles is the primary care liaison role to address the needs of people who present at GP practices with a range of memory loss, behaviour changes and changes in cognitive functioning symptoms. This role is intended to be commissioned by a practice-based commissioning cluster of GPs, working with GP practices and lists and working with these presenting clients to signpost them into the memory assessment process so that a differential diagnosis then follows. The second role is dementia care pathway co-ordinator. This role/service starts as soon as the diagnosis has taken place and then is the key to helping the person and their family to navigate their journey through the course of dementia and to ensure they receive services to which they are entitled. ICPs offer local solutions to local problems.

THE IMPLICATIONS FOR IRISH DEMENTIA POLICY

From a health policy context, dementia policy in Ireland has received relatively little attention and remained significantly under-resourced. People with dementia remain largely invisible in the 'system', despite the growing numbers. Within the *Programme for Government* (Fine Gael/Labour, 2011), there is a commitment to developing a National Dementia Strategy by 2013. Action is required to ensure that this strategy is implemented and that it delivers on the recognised needs of people with dementia and their carers and helps to improve their experience of living with dementia. The National Dementia Strategy will be the ideal platform for the launching of new ideas and ways of working. Developing ICPs will become an essential part of the future landscape of dementia care.

Given Irish demographics and the cost of dementia care of just over €1.69 billion each year (Cahill *et al.*, 2012), Irish policy-makers will have to find suitably sustainable and cost-effective ways not only to support a good quality of life for the person with dementia but also to address the growing challenge it will present in the not-too-distant future. The population with dementia in Ireland is expected to increase from an estimated 41,447 in 2006 to 67,493 in 2021 (a 63% increase from 2006 to 2021) and to 140,580 in 2041 (a 240% increase from 2006 to 2041) (Cahill *et al.*, 2012). One such exploration should be looking at 'integrated' care and how to effect change within an existing system that is disjointed, inequitable and highly fragmented.

Some tentative conclusions to this review can be drawn. First, that there is much good practice to learn from international experience where innovation and community action, coupled with service level commitment and attention to the voice of service users, have lead to demonstrated improvements in the quality of life for people with dementia.

Second, it is clear that a one-size-fits-all approach will not 'retrofit' into the landscape of dementia care in Ireland, given the current unequal distribution of services nationally, which is further compounded by the impact of fragmented services historically. For this reason, it will be necessary to pilot an ICP in several test sites in Ireland to ensure that the model developed is sufficiently robust and transferable to be able to meet the needs of people with dementia across the country.

These test sites must develop a strong service user voice if they are to authentically represent people with dementia and their carers. Modern services should be developed in consultation with people with dementia, and, where possible, the person with dementia should play a major role in developing a care plan that reflects their own particular needs, preferences and circumstances. Notwithstanding this, one clear reason for incomplete assimilation of ICPs is not paying enough attention to embedding the approach within local services. This should be a key objective of any pilot so that previous shortfalls in planning are not replicated. This embedding will require a significant sharing of expertise between the specialist services (currently in CMHTs and memory clinics) and primary care services.

Third, while it is undoubtedly the case that significant service reform can be achieved by integrating and planning care more effectively, getting people with dementia to use mainstream services where appropriate and signposting care in a more coherent manner, it is also true to say that case management is required if integrated care is to become a reality with the potential to have a meaningful impact on the lives of those living with dementia.

The two competency-based roles described by de Vries *et al.* (2010) are the flexible response required to address inequalities that exist in service provision. Clearly, this will require training and development as such roles do not already exist formally in Ireland. Careful placement of these roles within the system will be required with attention to embedding the ICP in wider care practice and to how best to join up fragmented services.

A recent research review on dementia care in Ireland states:

> … the best way to ensure that people get the services they need is to develop a system of case management for people with dementia … In this country, very few people with dementia have been allocated a case manager … a key contact person knowledgeable about a whole range of pertinent dementia-related issues (Cahill *et al.*, 2012).

Finally, there is a need to concentrate on issues of measurement and to collect baseline data if pilot sites are to become more than mere islands of good practice. In order to present compelling evidence on cost-effectiveness in such a complex change in practice, data will have to convince policy-makers of both the efficacy and cost-effectiveness of such a system.

REFERENCES

Allen, D., Gillen, E. and Rixson, L. (2009). 'Systematic Review of the Effectiveness of Integrated Care Pathways: What Works, For Whom, In Which Circumstances?', *International Journal of Evidence-Based Healthcare*, 7: 61-74.

Argyle, E., Downs, M. and Tasker, J. (2010). *Continuing to Care for People with Dementia: Irish Family Carers' Experience of Their Relative's Transition to a Nursing Home*, Dublin: Alzheimer Society of Ireland.

Atwal, A. and Caldwell, K. (2002). 'Do Multidisciplinary Integrated Care Pathways Improve Interprofessional Collaboration?', *Scandinavian Journal of Caring Sciences*, 16(4): 360-367.

Banerjee, S. (2010). 'Living Well with Dementia: Development of the National Dementia Strategy for England', *International Journal of Geriatric Psychiatry*, 25(9): 917-922.

Brodaty, H. and Cumming, A. (2010). 'Dementia Services in Australia', *International Journal of Geriatric Psychiatry*, 25(9): 887-995.

Cahill, S., O'Shea, E. and Pierce, M. (2012). *Creating Excellence in Dementia Care: A Research Review for Ireland's National Dementia Strategy*, Dublin: Trinity College Dublin and the Irish Centre for Social Gerontology.

Campbell, H., Hotchkiss, R., Bradshaw, N. and Porteous, M. (1998). 'Integrated Care Pathways', *British Medical Journal*, 316(7125): 133-137.

Chenoweth, L., King, M.T., Jeon, Y.H., Brodaty, H., Stein-Parbury, J., Norman, R., Haas, M. and Luscombe, G. (2009). 'Caring for Aged Dementia Care Resident Study (CADRES) of Person-centred Care, Dementia-care Mapping and Usual Care in Dementia: A Cluster-randomised Trial', *Lancet Neurology*, 8(4): 317-325.

Cook, A. (2008). *Dementia and Wellbeing: Possibilities and Challenges*, Edinburgh: Dunedin Academic Press.

Currie, L. (1999). 'Researching Care Pathway Development in the United Kingdom: Stage 1', *Journal of Research in Nursing*, 4(5): 378-384.

De Luc, K. (2001). *Developing Care Pathways: The Handbook*, Oxford: Radcliffe Medical Press.

de Vries, K., Brooker, D. and Porter, T. (2010). *Workforce Development for Dementia: Development of Role Competencies and Proposed Training for Primary Care Liaison Workers to Support Pathway to Diagnosis of Dementia*, Worcester: Institute of Health and Society, University of Worcester, Association for Dementia Studies.

Dementia ICP Development Group (2010). *Dementia ICP Consultation Draft*, available http://www.nhslanarkshire.org.uk/Involved/consultation/Documents/MentalHealth ICP/Dementia-ICP-Consultation-Draft-August 2010.pdf, accessed 2010.

Dementia Services Information Development Centre (2009). *National Positive Ageing Strategy for Ireland*, available http://www.dohc.ie/issues/national_positive_ageing/DementiaServicesInformationDevelopmentCentre Submisison.pdf?direct=1, accessed 26.04.2012.

Downs, M. and Bowers, B. (2008). *Excellence in Dementia Care: Research into Practice*, Maidenhead: McGraw-Hill.

Drossel, C. and Fisher, J.E. (2006). 'Dementia: The Role of Contingencies in Excess Disability', *European Journal of Behaviour Analysis*, 7(2): 177-180.

Fine Gael/Labour (2011). *Programme for Government: National Recovery 2011-2016*, Dublin: Fine Gael/Labour.

Gilliard, J., Means, R., Beattie, A. and Daker-White, G. (2005). 'Dementia Care in England and the Social Model of Disability', *Dementia*, 4(4): 571-586.

Gunstone, S. and Robinson, J. (2006). 'Developing an Integrated Care Pathway in Dementia', *Mental Health Practice*, 10(2): 34-37.

Hall, J. (2001). 'A Qualitative Survey of Staff Responses to an Integrated Care Pathway Pilot Study in a Mental Health Care Setting', *Nursing Times Research*, 6(3): 696-705.

Ham, C., Dixon, J. and Chantler, C. (2011). 'Clinically Integrated Systems: The Future of NHS Reform in England?', *British Medical Journal*, 342(1): 905-906.

Hean, S., Nojeed, N. and Warr, J. (2011). 'Developing an Integrated Memory Assessment and Support Service for People with Dementia', *Journal of Psychiatric and Mental Health Nursing*, 18(1): 81-88.

Health Information and Quality Authority (2010). *Draft National Standards for Safer Better Healthcare: Consultation Document*, Dublin: Health Information and Quality Authority.

Kazui, H., Hashimoto, M., Nakano, Y., Matsumoto, K., Yamamura, S., Nagaoka, K., Mori, E., Endo, H., Tokunaga, H., Ikejiri, Y. and Takeda, M. (2004). 'Effectiveness of a Clinical Pathway for the Diagnosis and Treatment of Dementia and for the Education of Families', *International Journal of Geriatric Psychiatry*, 19(9): 892-897.

Kodner, D.L. and Kyriacou, C.K. (2000). 'Fully-integrated Care for Frail Elderly: Two American Models', *International Journal of Integrated Care*, 1.

Lowe, C. (1998). 'Care Pathways: Have They a Place in "the New National Health Service"?', *Journal of Nursing Management*, 6(5): 303-306.

Main, J., Whittle, C., Treml, J., Woolley, J. and Main, A. (2006). 'The Development of an Integrated Care Pathway for All Patients with Advanced Life-limiting Illness - The Supportive Care Pathway', *Journal of Nursing Management*, 14(7): 521-528.

Moyle, W., Olorenshaw, R., Wallis, M. and Borbasi, S. (2008). 'Best Practice for the Management of Older People with Dementia in the Acute Care Setting: A Review of the Literature', *International Journal of Older People Nursing*, 3(2): 121-130.

O'Shea, E. (2007). *Implementing Policy for Dementia Care in Ireland: The Time for Action is Now*, Dublin: Alzheimer Society of Ireland.

O'Shea, E. and O'Reilly, S. (1999). *An Action Plan for Dementia*, Report No. 54, Dublin: National Council for Aging and Older People.

Rees, G., Huby, G., McDade, L. and McKechnie, L. (2004). 'Joint Working in Community Mental Health Teams: Implementation of an Integrated Care Pathway', *Health and Social Care in the Community*, 12(6): 527-536.

Saad, K. (2004). 'Integrated Care Pathways for Young Onset Dementia', *Journal of Dementia Care*, 12(2): 29-31.

Saad, K., Smith, P. and Rochfort, M. (2008). *Caring for People with Dementia: It's Really Time to Do Something Now*, Birmingham: NHS West Midlands.

Scottish Government (2010). *Proactive, Planned and Co-ordinated: Care Management in Scotland*, available http://www.scotland.gov.uk/Resource/Doc/309283/0097424.pdf, accessed 23.11.2011.

Social Care Institute for Excellence (SCIE) (2008). *SCIE Report 20: Personalisation: A Rough Guide*, available http://www.scie.org.uk/publications/reports/personalisation.asp, accessed 27.04.2012.

Social Care Institute for Excellence (SCIE) (2011). *Social Care and Clinical Commissioning for People with Long-term Conditions*, available http://www.scie.org.uk/publications/ataglance/ataglance45.pdf.

Tucker, H. (2010). 'Integrating Care in Norfolk - Progress of a National Pilot', *Journal of Integrated Care*, 18(1): 31-37.

SECTION V: INTEGRATED CARE FOR MENTAL HEALTH AND DISABILITY SERVICE USERS

17: INTEGRATED CARE IN MENTAL HEALTH

John Saunders

INTRODUCTION

This chapter sets out to discuss and describe the process of integrated care in Irish mental health care services. It discusses the changes in Irish mental health care services over the years and describes the shift from segregated silo-based provision of mental health care towards a more integrated community-based model of care, which is more person-centred. The chapter discusses what is meant by the term 'mental health' and the legislative and policy changes that have taken place in Ireland since the 1960s, such as the *Mental Health Act, 2001*, *Vision for Change* (Mental Health Commission (MHC), 2006) and the National Mental Health Services Collaborative project, which is the most recent attempt at bringing about integrated care in Ireland.

Since the founding of the State, health care has been provided by statutory authorities, initially through various forms of local government – that is, county, town and borough councils. Since 1971, health care in Ireland (including mental health care) has been delivered by Regional Health Boards operating on regional boundaries. Historically, regardless of the statutory provider, it is true to say that service has been provided in a segregated way. In mental health care specifically, services traditionally were provided in custodial care settings where various professionals delivered forms of care and treatment, often without reference to each other's presence. Typically, these models of care were hierarchical and dominated by the medical profession. Thus, right up to the present, we have in Ireland a mental health service that is largely medicalised and still has many traces of the old segregated asylum model. The effect of regionalisation was to introduce largely unintended regional variations in service delivery. The Boards included local political representation and were subjected frequently to political attention. This regional autonomy resulted *inter alia* in the development of disintegrated siloed systems of service delivery, with wide variations in the quality and quantity of services.

The *Health Act, 2004* attempted to rectify this situation through the development of the Health Service Executive (HSE), a unitary body that sought to provide a national framework for the delivery of services in Ireland. A fundamental operational principle of the HSE was the development and delivery of a national health service based on equity and equality. Central to such an aspiration is the development of integrated models of service delivery.

WHAT IS MENTAL HEALTH?

The term 'mental health' is used to refer to 'a state of wellbeing in which the individual realises his/her abilities, can cope with the normal stresses of life, can work productively and fruitfully and is able to make a contribution to his/her community' (World Health Organization (WHO), 2001, p.1). Mental health is shaped by many individual, interpersonal, social and cultural factors and influenced by a person's biological make-up, emotional resilience, sense of harmony, access to resources, sense of belonging, level of social support, resistance to stress, autonomy, competence and spirituality.

The term 'mental ill-health' is used to describe the full range of mental health problems that might be encountered, from psychological distress to severe and enduring mental illness. Mental illness refers to a specific condition, such as schizophrenia, bi-polar disorder and severe depression. The WHO argues (2001) that mental health for each person is affected by individual factors and experiences, social interaction, social structures and resources and cultural values. It is influenced by experiences of everyday life, in families and schools, on the streets and at work.

We also know that those who experience poverty, disadvantage and exclusion are at an increased risk of suffering from poor mental health. There is a consistent relationship between poor mental health and social exclusion indicators, such as low income, poor education, unemployment and low social status. Those with a chronic illness have a significantly higher risk of poverty than those without chronic illness (WHO, 2001: 13).

THE INCIDENCE OF MENTAL ILL-HEALTH IN IRELAND

Irish self-report surveys have found consistently that one in 10 respondents report a personal experience of mental illness (National Office for Suicide Prevention, 2007; Mental Health Ireland, 2003; 2005).

In the most recent of these surveys, commissioned by the National Office for Suicide Prevention in 2007, this level increased to 13% for women and 8% for men. In the Mental Health Ireland surveys, of those reporting a mental illness, over two-thirds had experienced some form of depression, 3% reported eating disorders and 9% experienced anxiety disorders, phobia or panic attacks. The Central Statistics Office (2007) found that 30,500 adults aged between 15-64 years old described themselves as having a 'mental nervous emotional problem', including intellectual disability, representing 10.2% of the total with disabilities of working age in Ireland.

One in four people will experience mental ill-health at some point in their lives (WHO, 2001). This statistic also applies to Ireland (Department of Health and Children (DoHC), 2001).

The WHO estimates that at least 5% globally suffer from severe and enduring mental illness and between 5% and 20% experience broader mental ill-health. However, these statistics may underestimate how common mental illness is over the course of life, as one large American study found that half the population would experience a mental illness at some point in their lives (Kessler *et al.*, 2005).

THE HISTORICAL PERSPECTIVE OF MENTAL HEALTH SERVICES IN IRELAND

Modern mental health care services in Ireland were inherited in the 17th and 18th centuries from the British asylum model (Robins, 1986). This model essentially was one of custodial care and incarceration, usually distanced from the centres of population, and housed many people who had displayed mental health difficulties or some kind of anti-social behaviour. It is true to say that the quality of care in many of these establishments essentially was custodial and, in many cases, there was little emphasis placed on treatment interventions or indeed discharge back to the community. The asylum-based mental health care services became a long-term proposition in Irish society.

This model of treatment evolved over the 19th and 20th century and, by the middle of the 1960s, in Ireland there were 18,084 people living in long-term care in large Victorian-style asylums on the periphery of towns and cities (MHC, 2006). These asylums were total institutions, essentially self-supporting communities with their own supplies of food from their own farms or local community.

Legislative Changes

The report of the Commission of Inquiry into Mental Illness (Department of Health (DoH), 1966) was the first modern document to point the direction away from the traditional asylum model. Although a very brief document, the report did suggest that there was a need for the reduction in the number of people living in asylums and more emphasis to be placed on short-term admission and the development of community-based models.

Planning for the Future

It was not until December 1984 that a more comprehensive policy document, entitled *Psychiatric Services – Planning for the Future*, was published (DoH, 1984). This document was unique from a number of perspectives.

First, it outlined in detail the way mental health care services should be delivered and included detailed chapters on general adult mental health care services and specialist services such as children and adolescents, alcohol- and drug-related problems and care of the elderly. What is most interesting about the document is that it was the first to signal clearly the need to move from an asylum- or hospital-based delivery of service to a community-orientated one, where the emphasis would be on the provision of comprehensive psychiatric care within a community environment. The main thrust of the report's conclusions was that the psychiatric needs of the community should be met by comprehensive and integrated services made up of a number of components located in the community. A number of changes were necessary if this objective was to be achieved – in particular, there needed to be a decided shift in the patterns of care from an institutional to a community setting, with close links between psychiatry and other community services.

The report went on to discuss that these recommendations required some financial investment and that the authors were acutely aware of the financial difficulties rising from the recession of the 1980s. It pointed out, however, that the main financial consequence of the recommendations would be a diversion of current expenditure on institutional to community services rather than an increase in total expenditure. The report also pointed out that, if the recommendations were not implemented, the capital requirement in order to retain the existing structure would be much greater.

In respect of integrated service provision, *Planning for the Future* set out the model of comprehensive services whereby every person who needed it would have access to a comprehensive psychiatric intervention. A comprehensive service meant one that catered for the variety of needs of people with psychiatric illness. The components of such a service would include prevention and early identification, assessment and treatment services, inpatient care, day care, outpatient care, community-based residences and rehabilitation and training. Such a range of services should be available locally. The different services should be co-ordinated so that the patient could transfer easily from one to another. The psychiatric team should be responsible for ensuring that the services provided by them were integrated with general practitioners (GPs), community care and voluntary services. The contribution of GPs and other professionals to the primary care of the mentally ill should be supported by the psychiatric teams through the formation of effective working links. As far as is possible, there should be continuity of professional responsibility between the various services provided by the psychiatric team.

Thus was set out the early model for the delivery of integrated care in mental health care in Ireland. *Planning for the Future* went on to describe the notion of a community-orientated service. This was a range of facilities that should be developed to serve the needs of a particular community. The service should be located in the community, so it is close to where people live and work. This kind of service required some new facilities but would provide an alternative to the centralised and largely institutional models now in existence, which were planned at a time when more modern treatment methods were not available. The community-orientated service emphasises outpatient treatment and day care so that patients can continue to live in their own homes. The need for professional services to provide support for the families of patients living at home also was recognised.

Planning for the Future went on to describe the concept of a sectorised service. The provision of a comprehensive psychiatric service to a population of a known size in geographical boundaries would be an important step in developing locally-based psychiatric services. A service organised in this way is described as a sectorised service. A multidisciplinary psychiatric team would be placed in each sector with responsibility for providing the required services. The precise size of the sector would depend on local circumstances and factors such as the density of population in a particular area and existing administrative boundaries. The report recommended a population size of 25,000-30,000 in each sector. Some services would need to be developed for more than one sector. Such centralised services might include, for example, inpatient services, services for the elderly and services for the mentally ill and infirm persons.

The *Green Paper* on Mental Health

In June 1992, the Government published a *Green Paper on Mental Health* (DoH, 1992). The *Green Paper* was in two parts:

- Part 1 reviewed progress in the development of mental health care services. It outlined how these services were being developed in accordance with the recommendations with the study group on the development of psychiatric services in *Planning for the Future*;
- Part 2 contained proposals for new mental health legislation to replace the *Mental Treatment Act, 1945*.

Comments were invited on the *Green Paper*, particularly in relation to proposals for new legislation.

In 1994, the Government published a document called *Shaping a Healthier Future* (DoH, 1994), where the priorities for developing psychiatric services were included. These priorities, which were set in the context of an overall framework for development of health care services, were to:

- Promote mental health in co-operation with the voluntary mental health services bodies;
- Provide a Department of Psychiatry in general hospitals;
- Integrate mental health and primary health services and, in particular, to strengthen the role of GPs in the care of the mentally-ill;
- Provide comprehensive specialist assessments in community support services in each Health Board for people suffering from dementia, including Alzheimer's, and their carers;
- Provide appropriate facilities for the care of the mentally-ill whose behaviour is a risk to themselves and to others;
- Introduce a new *Mental Health Act* to give greater protection to the civil rights of the small number of people with a mental illness who have to be detained for treatment and to bring legislation into conformity with the *European Convention on Human Rights*.

It was the last point in the *Green Paper* on the issue of protection of civil rights that lead to the publication of the Government *White Paper* entitled *A New Mental Health Act* (DoH, 1995). Although the *White Paper* was concerned with the development of a new *Mental Health Act*, it recommended that a new Act be seen as just one of the measures to be taken to reform mental health care services. The *White Paper* noted that the overwhelming majority of people with a mental illness were cared for within the mental health care services with their consent. Only a small minority at any one time needed to be treated without their consent according to rules set out in legislation. The *White Paper* also announced the Government's intention to define in new legislation the role of Health Boards in relation to the provision of services for people who are mentally ill. It pointed out that new legislation opened the opportunity to provide a statutory framework for the development of psychiatric services as recommended in *Planning for the Future* (DoH, 1984) and to integrate further those services with mental health services in general.

The *Mental Health Act, 2001*

It was not until 2001 that a new *Mental Health Act*, which sought to give protection to people detained by involuntary admission to mental health care services, was enacted.

The Act set up the Mental Health Commission (MHC) as an independent statutory body to enable the full enactment of the *Act*. The principal function of the MHC was to promote, encourage and foster the establishment and maintenance of standards in group practices in the delivery of mental health care services and to take all reasonable steps to protect persons detained in approved centres under the Act. Furthermore, the MHC would undertake or arrange to have undertaken such activities as it deemed appropriate to foster the standards and practices referred to in the *Act*. Under the *Act*, persons who are involuntarily detained for treatment in approved centres could have that decision reviewed by a third party tribunal, which would seek to confirm or revoke the decision of involuntary detainment. Additionally, the MHC set out a number of rules and codes of conduct for best practice in the delivery of mental health care services. It also set out a quality framework for the improvement of mental health care services in Ireland.

Finally, the *Mental Health Act, 2001* set out the detail of the new post of the Inspector of Mental Health Care Services, which reports annually on the inspection of approved centres.

Since the MHC was established in 2001, much of its activity has been directed towards the development of comprehensive and integrated approaches to mental health care services. Many documents and discussion papers have been produced around the issues of quality, teamworking, development of specialist mental health care services and the development of standards of integrated care practices in Irish mental health care services. For full detail on the work of the MHC, refer to the website **www.mhcirl.ie**.

Vision for Change

In 2003, the Minister for State at the Department of Health and Children (DoHC), Tim O'Malley, announced the formation of a Mental Health Expert Group to review policy in mental health care services and to make recommendations on improvements and change. This 21-person expert group sat for three years and involved over 300 people in a process of a discussion and deliberation on the development of comprehensive modern and appropriate mental health care services.

In 2006, the Minister launched a new policy document called *Vision for Change: The Report of the Expert Group on Changes in Policy* (MHC, 2006). *Vision for Change* built on the earlier work of *Planning for the Future* (DoH, 1984) and the report of the Commission for Inquiry into Mental Illness (DoH, 1966) and was seen as a comprehensive, radical and forward-thinking document in the development of comprehensive appropriate community-based mental health care services. Its key recommendations were:

• Involvement of service users and their carers should be a feature of every aspect of service development and delivery;

• Mental health promotion should be available for all age groups, to enhance protective factors and decrease risk factors for developing mental health problems;

• Well-trained fully-staffed community-based multidisciplinary community mental health teams (CMHTs) should be put in place for all mental health services, providing mental health services across the individual's lifespan;

• To provide an effective community-based service, CMHTs should offer multidisciplinary home-based and assertive outreach care and a comprehensive range of medical, psychological and social therapies relevant to the needs of service users and their families;

• A recovery orientation should inform every aspect of service delivery and service users should be partners in their own care. Care plans should reflect the service user's particular needs, goals and potential and should address community factors that may impede or support recovery;

- Links between specialist mental health services, primary care services and voluntary groups that are supportive of mental health should be enhanced and formalised;

- The mental health services should be organised nationally in catchment areas for populations of between 250,000 and 400,000. In re-aligning catchment boundaries, consideration should be made of the current social and demographic composition of the population, and to geographical and other administrative boundaries;

- Organisation and management of local catchment mental health services should be co-ordinated locally through mental health catchment area management teams, and nationally by a Mental Health Service Directorate;

- Service provision should be prioritised and developed where there is greatest need. This should be done equitably across all service user groups;

- Services should be evaluated with meaningful performance indicators annually to assess the added value that the service is contributing to the mental health of the local catchment area population;

- A plan to bring about the closure of all mental hospitals should be drawn up and implemented. The resources released by these closures should be protected for re-investment in the mental health service;

- Mental health information systems should be developed locally. These systems should provide the national mental health minimum data set to a central mental health information system. Broadly-based mental health service research should be undertaken and funded;

- Planning and funding of education and training for mental health professionals should be centralised in the new structures to be established by the HSE;

- A multiprofessional manpower plan should be put in place, linked to projected service plans. This plan should look at the skill mix of teams and the way staff are deployed between teams and geographically, taking into account the service models recommended in this policy. This plan should be prepared by the National Mental Health Service Directorate working closely with the HSE, the DoHC and service providers;

- An implementation review committee should be established to oversee the implementation of this policy;

- Substantial extra funding is required to finance this new mental health policy. A programme of capital and non-capital investment in mental health services as recommended in this policy and adjusted in line with inflation should be implemented in a phased way over the next seven to 10 years, in parallel with the re-organisation of mental health services;

- *Vision for Change* should be accepted and implemented as a complete plan.

Implementation of *Vision for Change*

The progress on the implementation of *Vision for Change* to date has been painfully slow. In its first report (DoHC, 2007), the Independent Monitoring Group (IMG) charged with reporting on implementation noted that *Vision for Change* had been embraced by all parties as the framework for developing services for people with mental health problems and that important first steps had been taken to implement the recommendations of the report in the years since it was launched. The report went on to say that it found issues of concern, principally the lack of a systematic approach to implementation of the report and the lack of clarity around responsibility for implementation in the HSE.

Subsequent reports of the IMG year on year reported that progress was slow, inconsistent and showed wide regional variations. In its third annual report on implementation (DoHC, 2009), the IMG noted that there had been little substantial progress in the implementation of *Vision for Change*. The IMG went on to note that there was an absence of corporate leadership, a reduction in revenue allocation as envisaged in *Vision for Change* and little or no attention given to service user involvement or the fundamental recovery ethos of *Vision for Change*.

The reasons for slow implementation can be categorised as:

- The lack of a systematic framework for the implementation of the policy;

- The lack of corporate leadership in the form of a designated directorate of services with sole responsibility for implementation of the policy;

- An inability to free up existing resources trapped in old-fashioned mental health care services and a reduction in the expected allocation of new resources from Government;

- The effects of the HSE recruitment embargoes from 2007 to 2009 and the public service moratorium from 2009 to date, which have had a crippling effect on the ability of the HSE to populate community mental health teams.

Additional factors that are required to bring about significant change include changes in the operational culture of service delivery, greater flexibility on how mental health care services are delivered and a focus away from traditional methods of service delivery towards new models based on person-centeredness and underpinned by the recovery ethos.

The National Mental Health Services Collaborative

The most recent example of a pro-active approach towards the development of integrated care in Irish mental health service is the National Mental Health Service Collaborative (NMHSC).

The genesis of the NMHSC lay in the publication by the MHC of the *Quality Framework for Mental Health Services in Ireland* (MHC, 2007). This provided a very clear framework of standards that providers of mental health services were expected to meet, including as standard 1.1:

> Each service user has an individual care and treatment plan that describes the levels of support and treatment required in line with his/her needs and is co-ordinated by a designated member of the multidisciplinary team, i.e. a key worker (MHC, 2007).

The *Quality Framework* was accompanied by a draft audit toolkit to enable services to assess compliance with its standards. The Mental Health Inspectorate's findings for approved centres for 2007 demonstrated a compliance level of only 18% with article 15 of the *Regulations* (S.I. No. 551 of 2006):

> The registered provider shall ensure that each resident has an individual care plan.

This contrasted starkly with an 83.6% compliance rating returned in self-assessment for the same issue over the same period. It was clear that there was a significant gap between expectations and performance, and between subjective and objective assessments of that performance. Discussion over the following two years as to how better implementation could be achieved culminated in the November 2009 paper, *Quality Framework for Mental Health Services in Ireland. Implementation – Where to from Here?* (MHC, 2009), which laid out detailed proposals for the establishment of a NMHSC to address this issue, including its objectives, scope, structure and process.

The 11 published objectives of the NMHSC were to:

1. Carry out a knowledge review to provide an evidence-informed approach to individual care and treatment planning.

2. Involve service users and carers in all aspects of the collaborative, including steering group, reference panel, clinical lead group and project teams from the initial start-up phase of the collaborative right through to and including the evaluation phase.

3. To generate key change ideas and target improvement measures relating to individual care and treatment planning to support recovery.

4. To use/develop appropriate data collection tools.

5. To enhance the capability and capacity of the project teams for improvement.

6. To fulfil the statutory requirements of approved centres in relation to Article 15: care and treatment planning (project teams from approved centres).

7. To attain standard 1.1. of the *Quality Framework* and the relevant criteria for standards 1.2, 1.3, 1.5, 2.1, 2.2, 3.1, 3.2, 3.3, 3.4, 3.5, 4.2, 6.1, 7.3, 7.4, and 8.1.

8. To compare service user outcomes between the NMHSC sites and sites that are not part of the NMHSC.

9. To elicit service user and carer experiences of the NMHSC.

10. To evaluate the NMHSC process and to take that 'learning' to further implement mental health services quality initiatives.

11. To develop and implement a strategy for spreading individual care and treatment planning to all mental health services.

The NMHSC was established in November 2009 and originally was intended to conclude its work in April 2011, a project period of 18 months. During the project period, this was extended for three months to allow for attention to issues of sustainability and spread, with completion of the formal project period in July 2011.

The collaborative included: clinical and professional staff, administrative staff, service users and carers; HSE and independent sector services; and national organisations and local mental health services. Its structure included a steering group, a clinical lead group, local project teams (led by local project facilitators) and a national project manager. The responsibilities of the main project sponsors were set out in a formal legal agreement between the MHC, the HSE, and both St. John of God Hospital Limited and St. Patrick's University Hospital.

Summarising in my own words, the final report of an Independent Evaluation of the NMHSC set out the following recommendations:

FOR EVERYONE
Press on: it is worth it. Whilst it is important not to overclaim for the benefits of individual care planning – not every service user will be interested, or will benefit – there is comfortably enough evidence from this collaborative, as from other work on this issue, that the benefits of the approach outweigh the effort required.

FOR NATIONAL STEERING GROUP AND EVALUATION PROJECT GROUP MEMBERS
In some shape or form, maintain a national focus for service development on this issue. This does not mean extending the life of this collaborative; that would be unlikely to succeed, as the energy behind this particular set of people and activities probably has run its course. It could mean new collaboratives, with more specific focuses, and taking account of the recommendations here. At the very least, it should mean some individual or group of people taking responsibility for considering and acting on the learning from this collaborative, preparing and taking forward a clear, focused, 'next steps' plan.

Members of the National Steering Group appear highly committed to the role and, more importantly, the future of this partnership. The HSE, along with the MHC and private sector partners, need quickly to take a definitive stance on the future of the group a) to see through implementation and b) to consider other areas of focus. As things stand, we couldn't help but be left with the sense that its members considered their job to be only almost half-done.

FOR NATIONAL STEERING GROUP AND EVALUATION PROJECT GROUP MEMBERS
Continue to work on the issue of professional separatism. This will not be solved quickly, but it will not be solved at all without continuing effort and attention. Whilst we are confident that An Bord Altranais is committed to promoting multidisciplinary practice, and multidisciplinary care plans, its statement on this topic unfortunately has left room for ambiguity and can be interpreted differently by individual nurses in terms of its implications for day-to-day practice. Psychiatrists (at least as a body – there are obvious personal exceptions) are widely perceived to be poorly engaged in the process. If it were possible to work towards a simple, short, practical guide, advising local professionals as to their roles and duties in care planning; and if it were possible for this to be issued jointly by the MHC and the national leaderships of all of the relevant professions; and if individual professional leaders could be found who would be

willing to champion the approach, all of this could have a considerable impact on local practice.

FOR NATIONAL STEERING GROUP AND EVALUATION PROJECT GROUP MEMBERS, AND NATIONAL PROFESSIONAL BODIES

Announce the intention, within a feasible period (say a year), of publishing a suite of national mandatory care planning documentation, with variants for different types of service. These would not be perfect, and they would need revision in use, after a time. However, at a stroke, this would: facilitate spread of care planning; facilitate the inspection process (as it would be obvious what is being looked for); end the wasteful duplication of effort of local teams designing and redesigning documents, which ought not in any event to be the main focus of care planning work; improve opportunities for service user and carer engagement and empowerment, as they would encounter similar documentation everywhere. The templates could (and should) be made publicly available. The value of the templates would be increased if they were published alongside brief guidance and examples of what a good plan might look like. A key change idea that emerged from the February 2010 Reference Group was to standardise individual care planning across mental health services, and this would represent an important ` means of doing so.

FOR EVERYONE

By whatever means can be found, strengthen the availability of training in all the various aspects of care planning. As set out in above, the topic is complex, and professionals from all disciplines would benefit from training in their specific roles and responsibilities. Team-based multidisciplinary training would have a role here also. Training programmes need not be time-intensive – much could be achieved with programmes of single-day events, and with e-learning formats – but the key is to ensure that staff seeking to improve their skills have easy access to the means of doing so. Within this, attention needs to be given to processes that would support the transfer of training into practice, for example: supervision, informed case discussions, champions and site-based support. Attention also needs to be given to the role of managers in bringing about service change.

In May 2012, the HSE published guidance papers to support the implementation of *Vision for Change*. In the context of community mental health care service delivery, the guidance papers focus on the need to achieve integrated service delivery. In the discussion of the continuum of community care, the HSE stresses:

Where such specialist developments take place it is important that the work processes of the various teams mirror each other as closely as functionally possible to ensure minimum disruption to the service user and carer experience for those who have to navigate between them at various stages in the recovery journey (HSE, 2012).

Most recently, the DoH, in outlining its new vision for Irish health services, cites integrated care as an essential pillar for the delivery of responsive and appropriate services:

Integrated service delivery is required in order to respond to the challenges of growing numbers of people with chronic conditions and the increasing prevalence of co-morbidity in the population (DoH, 2012).

CONCLUSION

This chapter set out to give a historical overview on the move from segregated, silo-based provisions of service within mental health care towards a model that is seen as being more integrated and person-centred. Overall, that process, which was initiated back in the 1960s, has been a slow, inconsistent path, whereby changes in legislation and policy have led a top-down approach. It has to be said, however, that there are many local and regional initiatives in the delivery of mental health care services that are essentially bottom-up approaches and that seek to create change on the ground to bring about best practice in the delivery of mental health care services. The NMHSC project is described in detail as the most recent attempt to bring about integrated care in Ireland.

In conclusion, we can say that, while the target of integrated care in mental health care services has not yet been reached, we are well on the journey towards that destination. There is a requirement on Government, mental health care service providers, professionals and service user groups to work in coalition towards the achievement of a fully-integrated, person-centred, recovery-orientated mental health care service. Collaborative care planning will be successfully implemented only if the system wants it to work. The most important factor in effecting any change is the desire to change.

REFERENCES

Central Statistics Office (2007). *Vital Statistics Yearly Summary 2006, Quarterly National Household Survey*, Dublin: Stationery Office.
Department of Health (DoH) (1966). *Report of the Commission of Inquiry on Mental Illness*, Dublin: Stationery Office.

Department of Health (DoH) (1984). *Psychiatric Services – Planning for the Future*, Dublin: Stationery Office.

Department of Health (DoH) (1992). *Green Paper on Mental Health*, Dublin: Stationery Office.

Department of Health (DoH) (1994). *Shaping a Healthier Future: A Strategy for Effective Health Care in the 1990s*, Dublin: Stationery Office.

Department of Health (DoH) (1995). *White Paper: A New Mental Health Act*, Dublin: Stationery Office.

Department of Health (DoH) (2012). *Future Health - A Strategic Framework for Reform of the Health Service 2012 – 2015*, Dublin: Stationery Office.

Department of Health and Children (DoHC) (2001). *Quality and Fairness: A Health System for You*, Dublin: Stationery Office.

Department of Health and Children (DoHC) (2007). *Report of the Independent Monitoring Group on the Implementation of* Vision for Change, Dublin: Stationery Office.

Department of Health and Children (DoHC) (2009). *Report of the Independent Monitoring Group on the Implementation of* Vision for Change, Dublin: Stationery Office.

Health Service Executive (HSE). (2012). *Guidance Papers on Implementation of A Vision for Change*, Dublin: HSE.

Kessler, R.C., Berglund, P., Demler, O., Jin, R. and Walters, E.E. (2005). 'Lifetime Prevalence and Age-of-onset Distributions of SDSM-IV Disorders in the National Co-morbidity Survey Replication', *Archives of General Psychiatry*, 62: 593-602.

Mental Health Commission (MHC) (2006). *Vision for Change: Report of the Expert Group on Mental Health Policy*, Dublin: Stationery Office.

Mental Health Commission (MHC) (2007). *Quality Framework: Mental Health Services in Ireland*, Dublin: Stationery Office.

Mental Health Commission (MHC) (2009). *Quality Framework: Mental Health Services in Ireland: Implementation – Where to from Here?*, Dublin: Stationery Office.

Mental Health Ireland (2003). *Attitudes to Mental Illness*, Dublin: Mental Health Ireland.

Mental Health Ireland (2005). *Attitudes to Mental Illness*, Dublin: Mental Health Ireland.

National Office for Suicide Prevention (2007). *Mental Health Awareness and Attitudes Survey Preliminary Findings April 2001*, Dublin: National Office for Suicide Prevention.

Robins, J. (1986). *Fools and Mad – A History of the Insane in Ireland*, Dublin: Institute of Public Administration.

World Health Organization (WHO) (2001). *Mental Health: New Understanding, New Hope: World Health Report*, Geneva: World Health Organization.

18: INTEGRATED CARE PATHWAYS IN MENTAL HEALTH: RECENT DEVELOPMENTS IN SCOTLAND

Mark Fleming, Linda McKechnie and David Thomson

INTRODUCTION

The National Health Service (NHS) Scotland, in collaboration with the Scottish Government, is taking a national approach to improving the quality and safety of mental health services. It is applying national standards at local NHS Board level that support continuous quality improvements and elements of service redesign. An important aspect of this work is the development, implementation and sustainable use of integrated care pathways (ICPs) for people with mental health conditions across the whole journey of care. Emphasis should be made that introducing and using ICPs in this way is widely perceived as a long-term improvement programme.

An ICP is an agreement by a local, multidisciplinary, multi-agency group of staff and workers to provide a comprehensive service to a clinical or care group. ICPs are based on current views of good practice and any available evidence or guidelines and have mechanisms to track whether patients are receiving all aspects of the care detailed. ICPs encourage good practice and improve services for service users and carers. They also provide a structure to find out where people are not getting the care they need ('gap analysis') and help to reduce variation in care across Scotland.

This chapter offers a perspective on taking such a national approach, whilst ensuring local developments are aligned to local priorities, needs and resources. We discuss the policy context, the importance of leadership and engagement, support structures to progress developments of ICP, local implementation, developments aligned to the e-health agenda, sustainability of momentum and the need to evidence impact.

NATIONAL STANDARDS FOR INTEGRATED CARE PATHWAYS FOR MENTAL HEALTH

The Clinical Standards Board for Scotland (2001) launched a series of clinical standards to support the improvement of care for people with schizophrenia across Scotland. NHS Boards, which were for a time NHS Trusts, throughout Scotland considered how best to meet the recommendations and requirements of the standards. Due to the vast variation in demographics, geographical coverage and differing resources available within each NHS Board area, no one single approach was adopted.

An example of early developments at local level is given from NHS Ayrshire and Arran. Discussions with senior managers and clinicians in North Ayrshire led to a decision being made to explore how ICPs and a networked e-health records system could support the journey of care for patients. Initially, this was identified for patients with schizophrenia but the benefits of developing this approach for other key diagnosis areas and generically across mental health services was quickly realised.

The local community health partnerships, in conjunction with the local authority, applied for a grant from the Scottish Mental Health and Wellbeing Fund and were successful in achieving funding to take this concept forward. The project went on to develop, in conjunction with lead clinicians, an ICP for patients with schizophrenia. It also procured a networked clinical information system that would support the patient journey, collect important assessment, care planning, contact and ICP variance information and make this available 24/7 to clinicians in both community- and ward-based environments. The reporting tools associated with the electronic patient record clinical information system adopted also created variance reports, where clinicians and managers could measure how well they were doing against standards and so work with staff and key stakeholders to improve patient care.

As developments progressed across Scotland, a national report by the Clinical Standards Board for Scotland (2004), suggested that patients would receive much better care if their services were co-ordinated using an ICP approach. The report suggested that services should:

> … work together to design the journey of care for people with schizophrenia. This is known as an integrated care pathway (ICP) and provides a way of assessing a person's ongoing progress and the effectiveness of their personal care plan. ICPs make it easier for patients, carers, health care professionals and other staff to work together in the planning and delivery of care and treatment (Clinical Standards Board for Scotland, 2004).

These conclusions were echoed by the then newly-established NHS Quality Improvement Scotland in a national overview of schizophrenia services in Scotland:

> The key findings identified that mental health services sometimes lack co-ordination, do not deliver evidence-based interventions, do not record outcomes and often do not meet service user-assessed needs. To address these findings, NHS QIS published its three-year strategic work programme in 2005, *Improving the Quality of Mental Health Services, 2005-2008*. To ensure that mental health services continue to improve, three key areas were identified: care, often provided by different organisations, should be co-ordinated by means of ICPs; the success of a service should be measured by the extent to which the needs of service users are actually met; and information systems should be developed to enable assessment of the first two key areas (NHS Quality Improvement Scotland, 2004).

In 2006, the Scottish Executive Health Department (SEHD) published *Delivering for Mental Health* (SEHD, 2006), which addresses the need to set targets and commitments for the development of mental health services in Scotland. It takes forward the Millan Principles, which underpin Scotland's mental health legislation, the *Mental Health (Care and Treatment) (Scotland) Act, 2003*, and marks a national commitment to a new style of working for mental health services. Healthcare Improvement Scotland is taking this work forward in conjunction with NHS Scotland and partner organisations by developing standards for ICPs, as set out in Commitment 6:

> NHS QIS will develop the standards for ICP for schizophrenia, bipolar disorder, depression, dementia and personality disorder by the end of 2007. NHS Board areas will develop and implement ICPs and these will be accredited from 2008 onwards (SEHD, 2006).

THE SCENE IS SET: SO WHAT DO WE DO NOW?

It is often said that you should never make assumptions, this being especially relevant when you attempt to build common momentum without having a common vision and understanding of how to achieve that vision. Consideration should be given to how ICPs are understood, interpreted and intended for use. In our journey, it has become very apparent that there are many variations of interpretation influenced by factors such as profession, organisational allegiance, service user or provider and what experience and exposure to pathways of care a person has. Willingness to embrace multidisciplinary and multi-agency approaches, access to learning/education and what supports are given to participate and perform within the established pathways, all have a bearing.

In order to promote a common understanding of what we mean by ICPs and their intended use, Healthcare Improvement Scotland has included relevant information within the standards, published an online ICP Toolkit (**www.icptoolkit.org**). In addition, definitions are constantly reinforced during information and education deliveries by the national co-ordinators as part of their on-going support role.

An ICP is much more than a document of care. The ICP system of care encompasses how care is organised, co-ordinated and governed. The implementation of the ICP will improve the quality of mental health services by focusing the attention of local care providers on key steps along the journey of care. The most important aspect of ICP is the recording, analysing and acting on variances, allowing the comparison of planned care with care actually given and enabling the implementation of continuous quality improvement.

The development of the ICP in mental health services offers new opportunities for quality improvement that are under the control of local agencies, whether from NHS Scotland, local authorities or voluntary organisations. The ICP allows local services to assess their own practice and offer tools to help drive the redesign of services to meet the assessed needs of service users (and their informal carers) and to facilitate closer working in collaboration with other agencies to deliver a co-ordinated service.

Integrated care pathways for mental health standards have four main elements:

- **Process standards:** Describe the key tasks that affect how well ICPs are developed in a local area;
- **Generic care standards:** Describe the interactions and interventions that must be offered to all people who access mental health services;
- **Condition-specific care standards:** Build on the generic care standards and describe the interactions and interventions that must be offered by mental health services to people with a specific condition;
- **Service improvement standards:** Measure how ICPs are implemented and how variations from planned care are recorded and acted on.

Condition-specific Care Standards

The standards for the five conditions build on and complement the key components identified in the generic care standards. Considered alongside the process and service improvement standards, the condition-specific care standards outline a set of expectations for the local management and organisation of care in mental health services. Equally, the standards represent an ongoing commitment to improving the quality of treatment and outcomes for service users and their informal carers.

As part of a wider system of continuous quality improvement, the generic and condition-specific care standards form the care elements of the ICP.

The process standards in essence exist to ensure there are strong foundations for NHS Boards and partner agencies to develop their ICPs. These components are essential and are required to be in place, sufficiently resourced and their importance acknowledged at executive support level. We know from experience that, when the process standards are not being met, components or personnel not in place or supported *via* local governance structures, progressing ICPs can suffer in terms of pace, perceived importance and sustainability.

The Establishment of Local Infrastructures

Establishing process standards commences the journey and involves the essential aspects of engagement, identification of clinical leads and building the relationships to local governance structures. NHS Boards manage these aspects of development locally, with some choosing to have individuals (often a consultant psychiatrist) for each condition-specific set of standards. Other Boards with more limited resources choose to merge several clinical areas into a condensed number of remits. However you choose to adopt this role, consider the importance and impact of having established clinical leads. Obviously, they bring clinical expertise and guidance but additionally they influence cultural aspects of change by influencing how ICPs are perceived and received. Their involvement and commitment heightens the profile of ICPs and supports the credibility of this approach. Anecdotally, having senior clinicians in these clinical lead roles enhances executive-level awareness and support.

Key stakeholder engagement has become a 'must do' statement for many locally- and nationally-driven improvement approaches. There is no doubting the value and benefit of this, but in reality it may be more difficult at times than acknowledged. The challenges include: differing perspectives influenced by professional roles; service users' and carers' perspectives weighted by personal experience; tensions between competing resources; capacity *versus* demand; and human factors such as pessimism, negativity and fear of change. This list is not exhaustive in identifying what needs to be considered but makes the point that engagement takes consideration, planning, excellent communication and the promotion of secondary gain: the 'what's in it for you' factor.

An eclectic approach is advocated in seeking engagement, using avenues of established professional relationships and existing interdisciplinary and multi-agency connections between professions and agencies. Scoping and seeking involvement where gaps exist in representation, using service users' and carers' groups and considering the format of approach are all essential to successful progress. Getting the ICP issue on the agenda of influential groups, offering awareness and education sessions where beneficial, formal invitation *via* executive managers and welcoming those who express an interest and enthusiasm that initiate approach also are advocated.

Further advice suggests actively selecting who to involve and identifying those who have the drive for change and the willingness and flexibility to adapt. Early adopters are those who have leadership skills and who recognise the importance of being first followers, these often being the catalyst of change and momentum. Also, they recognise the important connections between those spearheading change and the masses that are needed to ensure useful implementation.

Ensuring appropriate routes of governance are in place early in the process reduces organisational risk and helps to build the credibility of ICP approaches. Consideration needs to be given to considering issues such as: what systems are required to help manage referrals; arrangements for triage and assessment processes needed; and how will variance (the differentials between planned care and what care is actually delivered), be recorded, interpreted and used, to support on-going improvements. We discourage attempting to develop ICPs without first investing the time and effort in considering the elements of process standards, but also in reflecting on what is required to constitute the essential components that need to be put in place.

Key Approaches to Building Pathways

At the earliest opportunity, process mapping should take place. Building a picture of what current service looks like provides the opportunity to identify where waste exists and what does not add value. This helps to identify where improvements can be made and how.

Process mapping can help you to:

- Identify current patterns of service delivery and available resources;
- Examine the journey of care for service users and informal carers;
- Establish the strengths and weaknesses of current service provision;

- Quantify demands on the services;
- Identify the gaps in services;
- Identify gaps in staff skills and competencies; and
- Identify how the journey of care can be improved (**www.icptoolkit.org**).

This is a multi-disciplinary agency/stakeholder approach. It encourages wide-ranging inclusion and openness. No ideas at this stage are beyond scope, no matter how 'out there' they appear. This method not only provides the seeds of improvements in context but promotes a culture of innovation, the welcoming of new ideas and the acknowledgment of contribution.

It should be noted that process mapping events do not have to be completed on the same day commenced. We tend to think of development approaches that involve consultation and people taking time out of their diaries to complete and finish events. The real value of this approach is enabling prolonged periods of exposure to the developing mapping process, allowing more people to contribute to the process at their convenience.

An example of how this can be facilitated could include leaving the charted process on the wall of a staff room, a board room, or a ward setting, with the last enabling service users and their carers to contribute at their convenience. The end result is a more informed, rounded and inclusive map of services, ensuring that an accurate picture of the current arrangements is arrived at. This map then details where improvements can be made within a partnership-based work process, and with widespread ownership of the process in mind.

Having carried out process mapping exercises, informed discussions then can take place around how best to progress developments. This may include approaches such as cost benefit analysis, local resource scoping and prioritising demands, but also including considerations about local and national drivers. All should be considered in the context of developing the pathways aligned to the national standards for ICP for mental health.

Generic and Condition-specific Standards

Although there are condition-specific standards that have focused significance for aspects of care relevant to certain diagnoses, it should be re-emphasised that all condition-specific standards are built on the content of the generic standards, which apply to all who come in to contact with mental health services. Developing approaches and implementing the generic standards, as with all other aspects, requires engagement, commitment and leadership. This has to be evident throughout all aspects of the organisation. In order that local leadership is well-informed and supported, Healthcare Improvement Scotland has constructed a combined network of support mechanisms with dedicated roles associated with driving developments locally. Examples of supports are:

- National co-ordinators;
- Local co-ordinators;
- Networking and learning events;
- Online toolkit;
- Links to other national priorities and drivers;
- Underpinning by Executive and Government support.

How does each of these support local ICP developments and implementation?

National Co-ordinator

As mentioned earlier in the chapter, delivering on national standards whilst maintaining local flexibility and autonomy, is challenging. So why have national co-ordinators? This post offers connectivity between national ambitions and local delivery. It is the co-ordinators' function to provide guidance and support to those delivering ICP. This is achieved through a variation of involvements, including the development and provision of education and training, facilitating events, providing evidence-based information and contributing to local delivery groups. Provision of expert advice and guidance to health care teams on clinical governance matters and change management, leading to the improvement of quality of care for service users, is also an essential role.

The national co-ordinators often present at local, national and international events and support several networks and forums. This promotes consistency of information to a broad spectrum of networks and gives an opportunity to ensure the pathways approach is advocated in as many ways as possible. This also has a beneficial effect on the culture of pathway working.

Local Co-ordinator

The individual or group of individuals who take local responsibility for representing the interests of ICP developments at their Board level contribute to the reporting of progress and challenges through local governance mechanisms and engage with the national framework. Local co-ordinators can have a dedicated role or an extended role to their substantive post but it should be stated that, where personnel have a dedicated role, there appears to be an improved pace of progress observed. Local co-ordinators also act as the primary identifiable link to the national supports, discussing progress, raising concerns and relaying requests for specific supports from external resources.

Network and Learning Events

A scheduled programme of network meetings attended by local and national co-ordinators ensures the opportunity for peer support, sharing of good practice and the opportunity to discuss both individual and common challenges. These meetings also afford the opportunity to share practice by way of showcase presentations, with presenters from the Boards on a rotational and voluntary basis. The benefit of this forum lies in ensuring common comprehension of developments, demands and intended plans for future progress. The format of the meetings should be reviewed regularly, in a cycle of continuous improvement.

Over a number of years, a wider network of people involved in or interested in care pathway work has been established. The Scottish Pathways Association (SPA) is an established group of NHS Boards and partner agencies from all over Scotland, that are developing, implementing and evaluating the use of ICPs in many different clinical areas. The main purpose of SPA is to provide support and training on the development, implementation and sustainable use of care pathways (**www.scottishpathways.com**).

The SPA has a national committee, which is responsible for the strategic direction and implementation of support and consists of representatives from various organisations involved in health care. It is multidisciplinary/multi-agency in its membership. Since May 2009, the SPA has been a member of the European Pathway Association (EPA) and has representation on the EPA Council. The EPA is an international not-for-profit organisation of clinical/care pathway networks, user groups, academic institutions, supporting organisations and individuals, whose aim is to support the development, implementation and evaluation of clinical/care pathways.

Sharing Information

In addition to the national network meetings, we acknowledge the importance of sharing information with the wider group of key stake-holders. Helping others to learn from your successes, as well as when things have not gone to plan, is not only extremely helpful but, we would argue, ethically essential. Sharing information with others can accelerate progress, contribute to consistency, and fundamentally reduce costs whilst improving efficiency of resources.

A series of online resources has been developed to offer opportunities of sharing information. In addition to the ICP Toolkit (**www.icptoolkit.org**) hosted by Healthcare Improvement Scotland, there is the national database of positive and innovative practice in mental health, PIRAMHIDS (**www.piramhids.com**), developed by NHS Quality Improvement Scotland and supported by the Scottish Government. Resources such as these aid quick and easy access to information when undertaking improvement work, especially when systemic review and changes are involved.

There is an establishing relationship between developments from the world of ICP and the emerging work of the Scottish Safety Patient Programme for Mental Health. This again is a good example where different national programmes of work can complement and support the continuing progress towards a safe, efficient and person-centred health service. Both of these programmes feature heavily in the newly-published *Mental Health Strategy for Scotland: 2012-2015* (Scottish Government, 2012) and will continue to support improvements that will have a positive influence on the experience of those who engage with mental health services in Scotland.

MONITORING PROGRESS

An accreditation approach was taken initially in Scotland, with the principle that NHS Boards would be able to evidence implementation of ICP in line with the standards. The foundation level accreditation required NHS Boards to have in place the key components of the process standards by September 2009. All NHS Boards were successful in achieving this.

Since then, there has been a shift in thinking away from the traditional accreditation model to one of evidence of continuous improvements. This evidence model focuses on more specific elements of the standards being implemented, including the gathering of information used to assess performance, as well as informing areas of improvements that need to be encouraged.

To assist NHS Boards in monitoring their own progress, we developed a learning, monitoring and development aid (LMDA). This is structured on a scale-based self-assessment, and encourages organisations to rate to what extent their standards of development/ implementation have been achieved. This ranges from zero, where nothing regarding the specific standard has been achieved, to mid-range ratings reflecting some progress in establishing practice within the pathway, all the way through to level 9, where the pathway has been developed, tested, rolled out and the use of variance recording in place. This assists NHS Boards' awareness of developments. It also supports planning and resource allocation. Ultimately also, it contributes to the development of organisations that offer a framework of communication fed through appropriate governance routes.

The 'So What' Factor

There is a growing culture of ensuring that health services consider the impact of their actions. This gives rise to several questions:

- If we attempt to improve something, how did we do it?
- What were the significant aspects of learning?
- And most importantly, did it improve the patient experience?

We call this the 'so what' factor. When developing and implementing ICPs in practice, it is crucial that, from the outset, consideration is given to ways of gauging performance and finding out how well our services function. As mentioned, a key aspect in achieving this is through the recognition of variance: being able to record information that tells us whether planned care is actually being delivered. When variance is evident, we need to ensure that we have the ability to analyse why this happened:

- Is there something we could have done differently?
- Is there a system in place that allows us to use this information to close the improvement loop?

NHS Boards have developed various ways of doing this: from those that have paper records systems, using weekly recording sheets and manually screening the information, to those that have invested in electronic records/systems, which allow information to be extrapolated as a by-product of clinical information input. It should be noted that, although an electronic system is not essential, we are seeing an emerging picture where Boards that have invested in an electronic record system are able to provide information and evidence of performance more easily and, to a degree, to measure impact.

The use of information within some Board areas highlights that the recording of diagnoses was much less than clinicians were aware of. Through the collection of data and the subsequent recognition of variance, improvement cycles were acted on. This in turn resulted in much-improved rates of recorded diagnoses.

A further example of the positive use of recorded variance was highlighted where completed risk assessments were judged to be at a lower level than acceptable. Again, from recording this variance, the magnitude of the problem was identified, resulting in the Board prioritising the required aspect of care, thereby delivering a very significant overall improvement in performance and care. Having an electronic record system is strongly advocated as the process of improvement is greatly aided by the efficiency of such a system. NHS Boards will be asked to produce evidence of improvements over the coming years and testing the processes involved using ICP has already begun.

Integration

It should be noted that, when considering ICP at national strategic level, one must be mindful of the number of challenges, changes and demands being placed on health providers. It is crucial that duplication of work, processes and procedures are avoided. This can be facilitated by ensuring that those involved in developing and implementing ICPs have a good awareness of all other key programmes of work and national drivers. In Scotland, this has been achieved to an extent by ensuring the ICP programme of work had a voice on other national programme groups and that invitations were extended to others to contribute to ICP groups. This inclusion, alongside the recognition of all relevant programmes of work, and the improvement in science when presenting/delivering information about ICPs, helps promote mutual awareness and improves consideration of wider approaches that involve the progression and support for joint working.

The success of this approach seems evident, as ICP approaches are represented through national product and efficiency work, such as *Releasing Time to Care* (an adaptation of the Productive Ward series developed by the National Institute of Improvement), and also through national leadership programmes such as Leading Better Care (LBC). Further online resources have been developed through LBC to assist people in understanding where national drivers align to the National Quality Strategy through to the practical integration of implementing different improvement approaches. Further information can be accessed on the LBC-hosted website, **www.nhsscotlandintegration.com**.

PUTTING INTEGRATED CARE PATHWAYS INTO PRACTICE

The importance of a robust development approach using local and national expertise cannot be overstated. This development model uses tried and tested improvement approaches, such as process mapping, supported by effective project management methodology. However, there are many challenges to overcome in getting ICPs into routine practice.

Some NHS Board areas have adopted the model of development whereby they spend many months authoring their ICP, consulting stakeholders, revising the ICP in line with feedback, consulting again, and eventually 'launching' the final ICP, ready for full implementation.

Experience in Scotland tells us that taking this 'big bang' approach can create a great deal of anxiety and resistance, as people can perceive that implementing the pathways will mean a great deal of 'extra work' and drastically-changed practice.

It needs to be acknowledged that consultation and involvement are crucial to success; however, it is essential that the ICP is tested out at various stages throughout the development process. This ensures that each element of the ICP can be tried and tested, prior to full implementation of the whole pathway. Adopting this approach is less onerous on teams, as they are only applying small changes over a period of time, and therefore risks are kept to a minimum.

ICPs often can be complex, multifaceted and contain numerous aspects of care that span a whole journey for an individual. Breaking the ICP down into manageable chunks, and getting different teams to try out small parts of the ICP during the development phases, allows the team to use this learning to influence the final ICP.

The Plan – Do – Study – Act (PDSA) model for improvement (developed by Dr. W. Edwards Deming) is one that supports ICP development and implementation perfectly. Teams will be more enthusiastic in trying out small changes and feeding back to the wider stakeholders. It is essential at this stage that no assumptions are made that the elements of the ICP being tried out automatically will produce the desired effect. It is important to keep an open mind and agree a willingness to change aspects of the ICP, in line with feedback from the team who are leading on the 'testing'. This is also another good reason why the PDSA model can be effective, as it reduces the likelihood of major changes to the overall ICP needing to be made once formal implementation has started. The gradual implementation of ICP using this model for improvement also helps to identify any training needs for staff prior to full implementation.

Throughout the testing phases, it is important that evaluation of the tests includes what has worked well, what has not worked, and what aspects require further development.

One of the issues that can arise is that the ICP lays out aspects of care that practitioners do not always feel confident or skilled in delivering. This in many ways seems surprising, as an effective ICP should be based on evidence-based good practice, and not dictate new ways of working that are unfamiliar. However, it is useful to acknowledge that often successful implementation may need investment of time and resources to ensure that those delivering the ICP have the required skills and tools to help them do so.

By using a phased implementation programme, any training issues can be identified early, thus ensuring that teams are equipped with the relevant skills and knowledge by the time the full ICP is rolled out. This might take the form of basic awareness-raising on particular aspects of care that are contained within the local ICP, or the delivery of formal and informal training programmes, customised to different stakeholder groups and individuals.

Training alone does not ensure that the ICP will be implemented effectively. The development of resources and information to support successful implementation of the ICP is also crucial. The testing phases can be used to identify where these resources or training materials might be required so they can be developed over time, ready to cascade as the ICPs are being fully implemented across the service.

CONCLUSION

The previous sections have provided some useful considerations in terms of the most practical ways to ensure successful implementation. It is important to emphasise that implementation does not end once the ICP has been rolled out. Sustainability of this model in the long term, in particular embedding ICP into routine practice, needs to be carefully considered.

As with many national and local strategies and improvement programmes, it is all too easy to become complacent and to compliment ourselves in having succeeded in our objectives to get something agreed and implemented. Often, this can be short-lived if effective infrastructures are not put in place to support long-term sustainability.

As mentioned earlier in the chapter, some NHS Boards invested finances to secure ICP project management to lead on the development of the local ICP. For many Boards, this was a short-term and ring-fenced investment, which is no longer in place. What has emerged over recent months is that without this dedicated resource, it is proving difficult to keep the momentum going and to ensure that the ICP agenda remains high profile in local governance and service improvement strategies.

By clearly identifying how ICPs underpin the overall improvement programme and by providing a platform for other work streams, these can help make the most effective use of skills, expertise and resources across a range of programmes, while also supporting them in the long term.

There are many lessons to be learned in relation to the approach taken in Scotland. It is anticipated that, over the coming years, the evidence emerging through further research and evaluations will continue to influence local and national mental health strategy.

REFERENCES

Clinical Standards Board for Scotland (2001). *Clinical Standards for Schizophrenia*, Edinburgh: Clinical Standards Board for Scotland.

Clinical Standards Board for Scotland (2004). *A Review of Schizophrenia Services in Scotland*, Edinburgh: Clinical Standards Board for Scotland.

NHS Quality Improvement Scotland (2007). *Standards for Integrated Care Pathways for Mental Health*, available from
http://library.nhsggc.org.uk/mediaAssets/dementiasp/
mentalhealth_standardsforICP_DEC07%5B1%5D.pdf.

NHS Quality Improvement Scotland (2004). *National Overview of Schizophrenic Services in Scotland*, Edinburgh: NHS Quality Improvement Scotland.

Scottish Executive Health Department (SEHD) (2006). *Delivering Mental Health*, Edinburgh: SEHD.

Scottish Government (2012). *Mental Health Strategy for Scotland 2012-2015*, Edinburgh: Scottish Executive Health Department.

19: EQUAL RECOGNITION BEFORE THE LAW: A CALL FOR A STATUTORY SOCIAL CARE ADVOCATE FOR VULNERABLE ADULTS IN INTEGRATING HEALTH AND SOCIAL CARE

Moira Jenkins

An unenforceable right or claim is a thing of little value to anyone (Bingham, 2010: 85).

Advocacy is concerned with getting one's needs, wants, opinions, and hopes taken seriously and acted upon. It allows people to participate more fully in society by expressing their own viewpoints, by participating in management and decision-making, and by availing of the rights to which they are entitled (Commission on the Status of People with Disabilities, 1996).

Advocacy enables the individual to access civil and human rights, therefore advocacy should be a right in itself – a necessary tool in participating in society as a full and equal citizen. Rights to services and a right to advocacy are not exclusive – one cannot exist without the other (Centre for Disability Studies, 2003: 37).

INTRODUCTION

Integration of care provides an opportunity to implement a coalescence of developments in recognition of legal capacity and the right to independent living in the community through the mechanism of advocacy. A legally-recognised and centrally-placed role of social care advocate to ensure the will and preferences of the person are central to care planning is missing from the proposed framework. Independent of all service providers and inspection mechanisms, the social care advocate could provide the catalyst and linchpin to facilitate the integration of health, social care and social work services in residential/community care practice. A legislative base is necessary to provide clarity for the vulnerable adult, their paid and unpaid carers and to allow future cohesive policy development on care in the community and care pathways. Various current initiatives, including the National Advocacy Service (NAS) and the proposed monitoring of professional home care by the Health Information and Quality Authority (HIQA), need to be consolidated in commenced legislation to ensure clarity on access to independent advocacy support for the vulnerable adult. Establishing a comprehensive social care advocacy support system may be exacting, but existing models of guardianship are no longer congruent with international human rights norms and must be replaced with supports for decision-making. Similarly, standard-setting for person-centred care in adult residential centres requires the resource of an independent advocate for those without appropriate supports – proposed moves to place the standards on a statutory basis in 2013 demands such a facility with legally-defined powers and duties. A social care advocate could both provide the support for exercising legal capacity demanded by the *Convention on the Rights for Persons with Disabilities* (United Nations (UN), 2006) and fulfil the stated promise of access to independent advocacy for those in residential care, whilst enabling the will and preferences of the individual to be asserted in integrated care planning.

WHY NOW?

This proposal is, in part, a response to the publication of the report of the Joint Committee on Justice, Defence and Equality (Oireachtas, 2012) on the hearings on the scheme of the *Mental Capacity Bill* on 1 May 2012. The report of the hearings coincided with the publication of *National Quality Standards for Safer Better Healthcare* (HIQA, 2012) on 26 June and the *National Quality Standards: Residential Services for People with Disabilities* (HIQA, 2009) and the *National Quality Standards for Residential Care Settings for Older People* (HIQA, 2011) (with the promise of a statutory basis for both in early 2013). All of these documents are premised on principles of dignity, autonomy and respect of/for the person. The Report and the published Standards explicitly recognise the central importance of advocacy in making rights real and thereby advancing equality. These developments occur against the background of a pressing human rights agenda of ratifying the *Convention on the Rights of Persons with Disabilities* (UN, 2006), in particular Article 12 on equal recognition before the law and Article 19 on the right to independent living, together with a promised Convention on our *Constitution* and moves to integrate health and social care services in Ireland. The proposal made here for a new statutory role of an independent professional social care advocate, with a core role of working with the vulnerable adult person in their care planning when beneficial in realising their constitutional and legal rights, could encompass these varied drivers.

It should be noted that, whilst the draft Scheme of Bill suggested by the Law Reform Commission (LRC) on Vulnerable Adults and the Law (LRC, 2006) only addressed adults who lack 'capacity' (on a now-questioned functional test) a wider application than that, or the definition of 'disability' in the *Disability Act, 2005*, is envisaged for access to a social care advocate. For the purpose of this proposal, the following definition of a vulnerable adult is borrowed from the UK policy document *No Secrets* (Department of Health (UK), 2000):

> ... a person over eighteen who is or maybe in need of community services by reason of mental or other disability, age or illness; and who is or maybe unable to take care of him or herself, or unable to protect him or herself against significant harm or exploitation.

The submissions to the Justice Committee on legal capacity (the 740-page Report of the Committee includes copies of the 70 submissions received and representations made at the hearings) and the referred-to ongoing debates on the far-reaching implications of Article 12 of the *Convention on the Rights of Persons with Disabilities* (UN, 2006) on equal recognition of all adult persons before the law have highlighted that concepts of 'guardianship', 'best interests', 'substitute' decision-making and 'mental' capacity are no longer fit for purpose with reference to adults. The need for an inclusive test of decision-making ability (legal capacity) that incorporates a right to appropriate support appears to be universally recognised. Therefore we need a range of decision-making arrangements to be regulated from the norm of independent decision-making (that includes with all supports necessary) to supported and facilitated decision-making where a person may be appointed with a status to express the known wishes of an individual with regulated relevant powers, duties and accountability. The pending (at time of writing) law reform developments in repealing archaic laws on 'lunacy' and plenary guardianship in the wards of court system could join with imminent legal capacity legislation to begin to advance what President Higgins has termed 'a culture of assisted citizenship' (2012a). The promise of these changes occur in a legal landscape where the three-pronged approach of the National Disability Strategy – *Disability Act, 2005* (needs assessment), *Citizens Information Act, 2007* (personal advocates) and *Education for Persons with Special Educational Needs Act, 2004* – has be, en largely unrealised. None of this legislation has been fully commenced, nor has it been repealed. An alarming attitude to the rule of law has emerged, whereby a Minister can announce that legislation will not be enforced in the foreseeable future by statement in the Dáil. On the non-appointment of the Director of Personal Advocacy Services under the 2007 Act, Mary Hanafin announced:

> ... having regard to the current budgetary circumstances, it will not be possible to proceed with this in 2009 ... the potential for a personal advocacy service is huge ... it is only on hold, however, until we get out of the current economic crisis. It was purely a budgetary decision not to go ahead at the moment, rather than a policy one (Oireachtas, 2009).

The on-going review of the National Disability Strategy must ensure implementation is monitored more rigorously in future.

As indicated above, instead of the statutory right to a personal advocate enacted in the *Citizen's Information Act, 2007*, albeit on exacting criteria, with attendant statutory powers to enter and make inquiries, obtain any necessary information about a person and attend and represent a person at any meeting where the interests of the person are being discussed, we now have the NAS.

Persuasive evidence in the form of independent evaluation of the benefits of independent advocacy has been produced (two examples from both community-based services and residential care being the report commissioned by the Citizens Information Board (CIB), *Evaluation of the Programme of Advocacy Services for People with Disabilities Final Report* in June 2010 (CIB, 2010), and *Evaluation of the National Advocacy Programme for Older People in Residential Care* (Pillinger, 2011). Despite the value of advocacy being acknowledged in the *National Standards for Residential Care* (HIQA, 2011), it remains, however, unclear how the obligations with regard to access to independent advocacy will be met. The issue of advocacy support for the vulnerable adult living in the community, particularly at times of transition to or from hospital or supported living accommodation, also should be anticipated in this context. Integrated care pathways (ICPs) demand a mechanism with the scope to address both and it is suggested that discussing advocacy support in relation to residential care or community independent living separately is short-sighted and a wasted opportunity.

There are other more aspirational reasons 'why now'. On 29 June 2012, President Michael D. Higgins launched the initial essays in the TASC project 'The Flourishing Society' in a speech entitled 'Towards an emancipatory discourse', noting that "the enormity of the task is clear. Irish society is being challenged to little less than to remould itself" (Higgins, 2012b). How we provide social care/support has become, and will remain, a core concern and challenge for all modern societies, including Ireland. It is worth recalling that, back in 1996, the Constitutional Review Group suggested that the criticised reference to the role of women and mothers in the home in Articles 41.2.1 and 41.2.2 be replaced with the following amendment:

> The State recognises that home and family life gives to society a support without which the community good cannot be achieved. The State shall endeavour to support persons caring for others within the home (Constitutional Review Group, 1996: 333-334).

It appears that a range of incremental yet incomplete reforms in social care law and policy in Ireland combine now with a number of human rights imperatives and system reviews to make this an opportune moment for a comprehensive initiative to integrate capacity supports into care planning and delivery. The policy formulations for residential care and, increasingly, domiciliary care have laudable ethos but the questions recur:

- Who will provide this independent advocacy?
- Who will ensure the will and preferences of the person are heard, particularly when in conflict with views of professionals and/or family?
- Who will assist the person to ascertain the extent to which their wishes for their life can be met within their home setting – whether in the community or in residential care?

It may not seem the time politically to suggest the setting-up of a new independent body but that is what is proposed by the *Report of the Taskforce to Establish the New Child and Family Support Agency* (Department of Children and Youth Affairs, 2012). In integrating social care and health care, and aiming to enable people to remain in the community or return to the community from residential care, it is argued that a body of advocacy professionals – independent from government, service providers and the HSE – also is required for the vulnerable adult.

If we wish to ratify the *Convention on the Rights of Persons with Disabilities* (UN, 2006) and regulate for standards in residential care for older people and/or people with disabilities in Ireland, we must create a comprehensive support network for exercising legal capacity – to not include that reform into the integration of care process is illogical.

WHERE WE ARE NOW

At the Social Care Ireland conference on 4 May 2012, *Taking Stock*, I attempted to outline what ought to be in place for people with disabilities, according to the enacted law, in a paper entitled 'Advocacy for People with Disabilities' (Jenkins, 2012). This chronicled the protracted and now-stalled progress towards a statutory entitlement to a personal advocate under the *Citizens Information Act, 2007* and the apparent replacement of that legislative promise with the NAS (see 'Speaking up for Advocacy' on **www.citizensinformation.ie** for contact details).

Whilst welcoming the independence of the NAS initiative, the paper echoed the concerns of others over the lack of statutory powers for the NAS advocate to access the person, to access necessary information and to representation at meetings (as provided for the personal advocate envisaged in section 5, *Citizens Information Act, 2007*, and the lack of criminal penalty for obstructing an advocate, also enshrined in the 2007 Act). It further queried how the 42 advocates currently employed by the NAS could meet the demands of the 32,000 people with a disability living in a residential home or hospital to their right to access independent advocacy as set out in the National Quality Standards – quite aside from meeting the similarly-stated rights of the people over 65 years of age living in the 607 residential homes in the State. The intersectionality of discrimination should be noted in the statistic that 36% of the 400,000 citizens with a disability are over 65 years of age (Central Statistics Office, 2008). The paper also discussed the results of the CIB's evaluation of the 2004-2010 pilot programme of representative advocacy in 46 community and voluntary projects around the country, referenced above, and the benefits ascertained from access to advocacy and the evidenced obstacles some advocates encountered.

That evaluation concluded that, in the absence of statutory powers, "isolated and vulnerable people with disabilities are dependent on the consideration of senior managers within service providing organisations to decide on their access to advocacy" (CIB, 2010: 20). This finding is echoed in the *United Nations Handbook for Parliamentarians on the Convention on the Rights of Persons with Disabilities*, where it is noted that "people in institutional settings are often denied support, even when it is available" (UN-DESA *et al.*, 2007: 91). A centrally-placed single Office of the Social Care Advocate, established by law, within the integrated care system, would allow both a public and professional awareness to develop and make real safeguards for vulnerable adults anticipated by, for example, changes in whistleblowing.

THE POTENTIAL OF A COHORT OF SOCIAL CARE PROFESSIONALS TO PROVIDE ADVOCACY IN INTEGRATED CARE

Writing on integrating social work and social care practice in 2005, Dr. Colm Doherty concluded:

> ... the re-active, *ad hoc* nature of policy-making in the personal social services contributes to a professional culture that is over-committed to short-term practice responses. The time has come to replace this 'stop-gap' practice with a new approach that will advance and promote both interprofessional collaboration and partnership between service providers and service users (O'Doherty, 2005: 249).

A legally-recognised social care advocate would need to be a professional, expert in both advocacy and social care – that is, someone adept at ascertaining the will and preferences of an individual and able to audit and broker supports that are, or may be, available to that person to enable the greatest possible independence in day-to-day living. A number of professional skills sets meet aspects of this job description – lawyers are very good at adhering to their clients' instructions; social workers at care planning; social care workers at assisting day-to-day living structures and arrangements; and primary health care nurses at community supports. Certainly, social care graduates are not the only degree students' equipped to take on the proposed role (and the range of backgrounds to the recently-appointed advocates to the NAS demonstrates the range of valid professional backgrounds) but it is worth noting the availability of the social care professional resource, particularly in light of the professional practice experience that must be completed to graduate.

CORU, established under the *Health and Social Care Professionals Act, 2005*, is about to finalise registration for social care professionals in the State. Social care graduates will be required to have completed at least 800 hours of supervised professional work placement with people across the care community, including those with disabilities, people in residential care, families and children, vulnerable older people, older people and the homeless. In discussing social care and social capital, Dr. O'Doherty described what the potential for social care is:

> Social care professionals acting as policy/practice pioneers can: activate the web of networks submerged in everyday life and enable service users to tie them into their own conditions of existence; act as connectors, catalysts and social relays between different communities and organisations (O'Doherty, 2006: 39).

It is suggested that the experience gained with working alongside people with a variety of needs, together with expertise in facilitating maximum independence in day-to-day living, is required for a social care advocate in integrated care planning and that social care professionals will be well placed to contribute.

WHAT CAN BE

Whilst the focus of this book is on integration of health and social care services, it is argued also that an even greater potential benefit exists in an enabling of access to public services by vulnerable adults, which could include legal services (particularly legal aid), the Family Mediation Service and child protection services, through the mechanism of the social care advocate. In addition to addressing the challenges posed by ratification of the *Convention on the Rights of Persons with Disabilities* (UN, 2006), and allowing the progression to a legislative base of the National Standards for Residential Care for Older People and People with Disabilities, the statutory establishment of an Office of the Social Care Advocate, together with the establishment of the HSE Integrated Services Programme, could allow for other synchronisation. Such an Office would not remove the need for the diverse self or voluntary and professional advocacy provision that exists or is being developed presently but would provide a vital complementary resource in accessing justice and equality for vulnerable adults and their carers – whether professional or voluntary. By ensuring access to independent social care advocacy at primary and community care conferences – particularly at transition points between the community and hospital/residential care and access to advocacy for adults in residential care – both people without networks of support and their carers would be able to address possible conflicts between the will and preferences of the individual and the views of their family or service provider. Such advocates would require statutory powers in line with those envisaged for personal advocates under the 2007 Act and the Office, crucially, must be independent and seen by all as independent from any State-funded service. The siting of the National Advocacy Service within the Citizens

Information Board is instructive, but other possibilities arise if the role is seen as having other dimensions beyond a core function of empowering the individual on care pathways, particularly at transition points across the health system (see Doocey and Reddy, 2010). It is contended that the potential for the role goes beyond the integration of health and social care and extends logically to a range of other potential advocacy roles currently provided in an *ad hoc* manner and not always with regulated professional supervision, including for example:

- The 'Person to Assist' arrangements in relation to child care proceedings provided currently by the Legal Aid Board (where the solicitor requires professional assistance to communicate effectively with her client. See *Legal Aid Board v. District Judge Patrick Brady and the Northern Area Health Board and Others*, March 2007, **www.ihrc.ie**). In time, the Office of the Social Care Advocate also could be used to provide a statutory provision of guardian *ad litem* for children/young adults in line with the Northern Ireland NIGALA system;

- The Office could facilitate the currently unregulated 'appropriate adult' under Part VI of the *Children Act, 2001* (relating to child suspects in Garda custody);

- The Care Representative role under section 21(1) of the *Nursing Home Support Scheme Act, 2009* (see the submission of the Social Work Department of the Mater University Hospital to the Justice Committee hearings (Oireachtas, 2012));

- Advocating with the older person in situations where HSE elder abuse officers may be involved, particularly if self-harm is the primary concern, and assisting the older person during *Domestic Violence Act, 1996* processes;

- Support for ex-offenders to reconnect with families and community on release, ideally through facilitation of peer-support networks, to reduce recidivism;

- Advocacy during review of 'voluntary' admissions under the *Mental Health Act, 2001* (also under review at time of writing).

If these allied roles in facilitating action on rights were accepted, then locating the Office within the Legal Aid Board, together with the Family Mediation Service, has some merit. Finally, however, this issue of advocacy support to ensure equality of treatment before the law is a human rights issue for us all and therefore, perhaps, the Office of the Social Care Advocate should be allied with, and sited with, the proposed merged Irish Human Rights Commission and Equality Authority. The idea of an Office of the Social Care Advocate has a number of precedent models (the Office of the Public Advocate in Victoria, Australia, is one example with a similar population catchment) but whilst, obviously and unashamedly, borrowing heavily from the powerful disability rights agenda and protection of the older person debate, the concept proposed is about realising rights for all – essentially effective and equal access to justice – and hence the criteria should be based on realising equality before the law not disability-defined (however attempted).

The above may appear overly ambitious and even naïve, but a grown-up, egalitarian legal system must be honest on what it is doing, as opposed to what it would like to be doing. There are harsh lessons to be taken from the history of non-implementation of the National Disability Strategy and we must attempt to provide to meet the stated aims of standards for residential care and community support, not just state them. Long on rhetoric and cruelly curtailed on arrival by not even reaching the statute book, it has ensured realisation of hard-fought-for reforms for people with disabilities. Non-commencement of statutes may survive scrutiny of constitutional lawyers on separation of powers grounds (see Morgan, 2001: 66-70), but non-implementation of legislation due to budgetary constraints by decree of a Minister made in the Dáil must be bad for the rule of law in Ireland and is dreadful for accessibility and accountability. An invidious non-choice has emerged – an *ad hoc* system where access to a service depends on the discretion of the provider and/or geographical location (for example, home supports) or non-implemented legislation that sits on the statute book and mocks the people who attended forums, discussion groups and meetings and thought they had achieved change.

Another false dawn in social care with regard to the new National Quality Standards for Residential Care and Health Care must be avoided. The Standards are long overdue and most welcome (backed by the steely scrutiny of HIQA and its willingness to publish inspection reports) and they share with other initiatives in the community the principles of dignity, autonomy, person-centredness and access to independent advocacy; but they lack the force of law presently. The promise that they will be legislated for in early 2013 also is welcome but vital references to access to independent advocacy in the Standards must be facilitated. Even if and when the National Standards for Residential Care for both persons with disabilities and older people are placed on a legislative base, a vital gap will remain between community and residential care planning. Arguably, even if the *Disability Act, 2005* was implemented, the definition is too narrow to address the needs of many who, for a temporary period, may have need for supported decision-making to exercise capacity or alternatively may have times when they can act independently. The time has come to integrate the various approaches to supporting people to exercise their legal capacity in a manner that promotes equality for all before the law and allows movement along a continuum of low to high support and back again as capacity or need grows. The planned system shift to integrated care could be the moment to realise the aim of advocacy to make rights real.

The preamble to the *Convention on the Rights of Persons with Disabilities* (UN, 2006) recognises that:

> ... disability is an evolving concept and that disability results from interaction between persons with impairments and attitudinal and environmental barriers that hinder their full and effective participation in society on an equal basis with others.

This chapter argues that we should shed the costly and time-consuming focus on assessment of needs and the categorisation of various disabilities and focus on promoting equality. It appears in tune with the spirit of the *Convention* that we remove the disability focus in social care advocacy provision and replace it with an equality focus.

In summary, the argument is for a separate Office of the Social Care Advocate that straddles the divide between community and residential care and provides skilled, accountable and independent advocacy for people vulnerable and without a network of support. It is envisaged that such provision would not only assist individuals and their families but also care staff in meeting their obligations to people to provide access to independent advocacy. The failure to acknowledge the intersectionality of discrimination over multiple grounds also would be mitigated by moving away from rigid definitions and replacing it with a focus on promoting equality.

The requirement for regulating the appointment, role, powers, supervision and accountability of advocates have been canvassed extensively and well already in various fora (see, for example: Bach, 2012; European Disability Forum, 2009). But in addition to these aspects, legislation is needed also to ensure safeguards in the form of facilitated/substitute decision-making are for the shortest time possible; to provide legal clarity and protection for staff acting in good faith (similar to section 5 of the UK *Mental Capacity Act, 2005*) and to provide for resolution of disputes between the advocate and the individual and others. It appears vital that care staff have recourse to external independent advocacy for those in their care when they perceive a failure to meet standards of care or afford dignity to the individual – in which regard the pending whistleblowing legislation, together with protected disclosures under the *Health Act*, is another crucial part of the change envisaged.

Often a person who requires support to have their will and preferences heard and acted upon will nominate a person with a demonstrated, trusting relationship with them for appointment as a supporter. Such a support person needs an authoritative appointment with clear duties to assert the known will and preferences of the individual and clear legal obligations on third parties to recognise the designated authority of the supporter. Failure to take reasonably practicable steps to ascertain the current will and preferences of an individual, including through a designated supporter and any documented direction (such as an advance care directive or power of attorney), should amount to professional negligence. Conversely, staff acting in good faith and with reasonable care in ascertaining and adhering to will and preferences should be clearly protected. Any formal supported decision-making (or facilitated decision-making) must be subject to regular review by a competent, impartial body with final appeal on a point of law to the Courts. The focus must be on restoring independent decision-making capacity to the individual as soon as possible.

The potential for the Office once established is great. The debate over whether there is a normative gap and hence a need for a United Nations *Convention on the Rights of Older People* will continue, although resisted by the European Union at present as duplication of the *Convention on the Rights of Persons with Disabilities*. We are living longer and we need to facilitate access to our community and domiciliary supports so people can remain in or return to their homes.

Other new departures in social care practice marry with the supports-for-capacity agenda and should be mentioned here, including individualised resource allocation systems (a system of individualised budgeting is recommended in the *Value for Money and Policy Review of Disability Services* (Department of Health and Children, 2012)). These new approaches require greater consideration in the near future in light of the closure of congregated settings. The Disability Federation of Ireland (DFI) welcomed the focus in the *Review* on the urgency of integrating people with disabilities into mainstream health and social services and "the importance of working across functional boundaries" (DFI, 2012: 176), but noted that there was limited guidance offered on how the HSE's Disability Services Programme could facilitate access to services across the health system and beyond. Establishing an Office of the Social Care Advocate would develop the structure required to progressively respond to emerging community needs and also provide a catalyst and co-ordination for further voluntary contributions by people to the wellbeing of all.

One final aspect to consider is with regard to 're-ablement'. In place in Northern Ireland and parts of the United Kingdom, re-ablement (see Social Care Institute of Excellence, 2012; Patient and Client Council, 2012) helps people to learn or adjust the skills necessary for daily living, following a period of illness or increased support needs, and thereby restoring or maintaining independent living. The emphasis is on intensive support over an average six-week period with a reduction in on-going support and thus it is distinct from traditional home care. The potential for this to enable people to gain confidence in their decision-making capacity is great. It could also be of benefit in family support and early intervention in child protection. Such recourse to an intensive, temporary social care support to 'get you sorted' and in touch with community supports seems a vital missing element in the plans for primary, community integrated care.

It is argued here that we should remove the criteria of 'disability' to secure a social care advocate and move towards a system of supports for people making legal decisions of some import on the basis that they are vulnerable and would benefit from assistance in realising their legal rights. The call now (O'Connor and Murphy, 2006) is for a social care practice that works in partnership with the service user. This aim accords with both the stated requirements of the disability rights campaign for supports for equal recognition before the law and, more generally, best practice in advocacy.

The *Convention on the Rights of Persons with Disabilities* (UN, 2006) has provided the catalyst for some overdue and fundamental debates on realising, rather than espousing, human rights. Concurrently, tragic failures in residential care have forced fundamental changes in ethos and accountability for some of the most vulnerable in society. Ultimately, the provision of independent advocacy as support to exercising legal rights is about equality – of treatment, opportunity, and outcome – and social justice. At the 30th Anniversary Conference of the Legal Aid Board, the Chairperson, Anne Colley, made the case for greater integration of public services to ensure access to justice (2010). She quoted Hazel Genn, in an address to the English Law Society in 2009, in identifying the fundamentals of access to justice: an awareness of rights, entitlements, obligations and responsibilities; an awareness of procedures for resolution; the ability effectively to access resolution systems/procedures; and the ability to effectively participate in the resolution process to achieve just outcomes. That seems an apt aim of a culture of assisted citizenship.

This proposal does not tackle the key obstacles of criteria for a social care advocate or attendant resources. Legislation is required to ensure that prioritising need is done in a transparent, fair and equitable manner. Nor does it address some of the most difficult cases, when some form of facilitated decision-making may be required – for example, where someone is suffering from psychosis. The idea of a social care advocate needs a cost-benefit analysis that would include the potential savings from such an innovation, but it is argued that the establishment of a stand-alone Office would increase community and professional awareness and allow an incremental, dynamic accumulation of expertise and credibility. Beyond initial investigation as to current wishes and situation, a practical facilitation of establishing structures to maintain independent living also would be within the training and experience of social care advocates and could be developed in time.

Overly ambitious or necessary, this is a response to a call for what we, as a society, can be and suggests what a social care advocate could contribute. Integrating health and social care in line with human rights imperatives requires the social care advocate.

REFERENCES

Bach, M. (2012). 'Personhood – The Right to Make Your Own Decisions and Have Them Respected by Others', *CDLP Summer School 2012*.

Bingham, T. (2010). *The Rule of Law*, London: Penguin.

Central Statistics Office (2008). *Statistical Yearbook of Ireland*, Cork: Central Statistics Office.

Centre for Disability Studies (2003). *Exploring Advocacy – Full Report*, available www.nda.ie, accessed 01.02.13.

Citizens Information Board (CIB) (2010). *Evaluation of the Programme of Advocacy Services for People with Disabilities in the Community and Voluntary Sector: Final Report*, Dublin: CIB.

Colley, A. (2010). 'Chairperson's Address', *30th Anniversary Conference of the Legal Aid Board*, 15 September, available www.legalaid.ie.

Commission on the Status of People with Disabilities (1996). *A Strategy for Equality: Report of the Commission on the Status of People with Disabilities*, Dublin: Stationery Office.

Commissioner for Human Rights (2012). *Who Gets to Decide? Right to Legal Capacity for Persons with Intellectual and Psychosocial Disabilities*, Strasbourg: Council of Europe Publishing, available at http://www.coe.int/t/commissioner/source/prems/IP_LegalCapacity_GBR.pdf.

Constitutional Review Group (1996). *Report of the Constitutional Review Group*, Dublin: Stationery Office.

Department of Children and Youth Affairs (2012). *Report of the Taskforce to Establish the New Child and Family Support Agency*, Dublin: Stationery Office.

Department of Health (UK) (2000). *No Secrets: Guidance on Developing and Implementing Multi-agency Policies and Procedures to Protect Vulnerable Adults from Abuse*, available www.dh.gov.uk/assetRoot/04/07/45/44/04074544.pdf.

Department of Health and Children (2012). *Value for Money and Policy Review of Disability Services in Ireland*, available http://www.dohc.ie, accessed 07.09.12.

Disability Federation of Ireland (2012). *Value for Money and Policy Review of the HSE's Disability Services Programme: DFI's Initial Analysis*, available www.disability-federation.ie, accessed 07.09.12.

Doocey, A. and Reddy, W. (2010). 'Integrated Care Pathways: The Touchstone of an Integrated Service Delivery Model for Ireland', *International Journal of Care Pathways*, March, 14(1): 27-29.

European Disability Forum (2009). *Equal Recognition before the Law and Equal Capacity to Act: Understanding and Implementing Article 12 of the UN CRPD*, Position Paper, Brussels: European Disability Forum.

Health Information and Quality Authority (HIQA) (2009). *National Quality Standards for Residential Care Settings for Older People in Ireland*, Dublin: HIQA.

Health Information and Quality Authority (HIQA) (2011). *National Quality Standards for Residential Care of People with Disabilities*, Dublin: HIQA.

Health Information and Quality Authority (HIQA) (2012). *National Standards for Safer Better Healthcare*, Dublin: HIQA.

Higgins, M.D. (2012a). 'Towards an Emancipatory Discourse', launch of the TASC Flourishing Society project, Áras an Uachtaráin, 29 June, available http://www.president.ie, accessed 09.07.2012.

Higgins, M.D. (2012b). Launch of the International Sumer School, Centre for Disability Law and Policy, NUI Galway.

Jenkins, M. (2012). 'Advocacy for People with Disabilities: Recent Legal, Policy and Service Developments in Social Care Advocacy for People with Disabilities: What is Available and What Remains to be Done to Enable Ratification of the CRPD', *Social Care Ireland Conference 2012, Taking Stock*, available www.socialcareireland.ie.

Judge, L. (2008). 'The Rights of Older People: International Law, Human Rights Mechanisms and the Case for New Normative Standards', *International Symposium on Ageing*, International Federation on Ageing (IFA) and HelpAge International, January.

Law Reform Commission (LRC) (2003). *Consultation Paper on the Law and the Elderly*, LRC CP 23-2003, Dublin: Stationery Office.

Law Reform Commission (LRC) (2005). *Consultation Paper on Vulnerable Adults and the Law: Capacity*, LRC CP 37-2005, Dublin: Stationery Office.

Law Reform Commission (LRC) (2006). *Report on Vulnerable Adults and the Law*, LRC 83-2006, Dublin: Stationery Office.

Law Reform Commission (LRC) (2011). *Report on Legal Aspects of Professional Home Care*, LRC 105-2011, Dublin: Stationery Office.

McCann James, C., de Róiste, Á. and McHugh, J. (2009). *Social Care Practice in Ireland: An Integrated Perspective*, Dublin: Gill and Macmillan.

McGreevy, R. (2012). 'The Capacity to Decide', *The Irish Times*, Health Matters, 24
     July, p.27.

Morgan, D.G.:(2001). *A Judgment Too Far? Judicial Activism and the Constitution,*
     Cork: Cork University Press.

National Children Office (2004). *Review of the Guardian* ad Litem *Service: Final
     Report from Capita Consulting Ireland (in association with the Nuffield Institute for
     Health)*, available http://www.childrendatabase.ie.

O'Connor, T. and Murphy, M. (eds.) (2006). *Social Care In Ireland: Theory, Policy and
     Practice*, Cork: CIT Press.

O'Doherty, C. (2005). 'Integrating Social Care and Social Work: Towards a Model
     of Best Practice' in Share, P. and McElwee, N. (eds.), *Applied Social Care: An
     Introduction for Irish Students*, Dublin: Gill and Macmillan.

O'Doherty, C. (2006). 'Social Care and Social Capital' in O'Connor, T. and Murphy,
     M. (eds.), *Social Care In Ireland: Theory, Policy and Practice*, Cork: CIT Press.

Oireachtas (2009). Dáil Debates, 30 April, Dublin: Stationery Office.

Oireachtas (2012). *Report of the Joint Committee on Justice, Defence and Equality on the
     Hearings on the Scheme of the Mental Capacity Bill, 1 May 2012*, Dublin:
     Stationery Office.

Patient and Client Council (2012). 'Care at Home: Older People's Experiences of
     Domiciliary Care', available www.patientclientcouncil.hscni.net.

Pillinger, J. (2011). *Evaluation of the National Advocacy Programme for Older People in
     Residential Care*, January 2011. Commissioned by the HSE/National Advocacy
     Programme Alliance, available http://www.hse.ie/eng/services/
     Publications/Your_Service,_Your_Say_Consumer_Affairs/AdvocacyResiden
     tialEvaluation.pdf.

Power, A. (2010). *Individualised Resource Allocation Systems: Models and Lessons for
     Ireland*, Policy Briefing No.2, Galway: Centre for Disability Law and Policy,
     NUI Galway.

Social Care Institute of Excellence (UK) (2012). 'Re-ablement: Emerging Practice
     Messages', available at www.scie.org, accessed 12.07.2012.

Third Age Ireland (2011). *Third Age National Advocacy Programme*, available
     http://www.thirdageireland.ie/what-we-do/41/national-advocacy-programme/.

Timonen, V. (2007). 'Home Care of Older People in Ireland: Main Issues and
     Challenges', *Home Care for Ageing Populations Conference*, 12 March 2007, Social
     Policy and Ageing Research Centre.

United Nations (2006). *Convention on the Rights of Persons with Disabilities*, available
     www.un.org/disabilties/convention.

United Nations Department of Economic and Social Affairs (UN-DESA), Office of
     the United Nations High Commissioner for Human Rights (OHCHR) and
     Interparliamentary Union (IPU) (2007). *From Exclusion to Equality: Realising the
     rights of persons with disabilities. A Handbook for Parliamentarians on the
     Convention on the Rights of Persons with Disability*, New York: United Nations.

Cases

*Legal Aid Board v. District Judge Patrick Brady and Northern Area Health Board and
     Others*, High Court No. 2005/474JR and 2006/653SS, available www.courts.ie.

20: INTEGRATED SUPPORTS FOR PEOPLE WITH DISABILITIES

Eithne Fitzgerald[16]

INTRODUCTION

In the field of medical care, the term 'integrated care' is used to describe a re-orientation of care around the needs of the individual. As the Health Service Executive (HSE) has put it:

> An integrated health and social care model develops services with the service user at the centre and services as close to home as is reasonably possible. Patients/clients in an integrated system are more likely to receive the type and quality of care they need, when they need it, in the most appropriate setting and from the most appropriate health professional (HSE, 2008).

People with Disabilities and the Integration of Supports

There is an analogous policy shift taking place in the area of disability supports. The *Disability Policy Review*, the report of an expert reference group published by the Department of Health and Children (DoHC), sets out proposals to re-orient disability services towards person-centred services, individualised programmes and personal budgets (DoHC, 2011). The policy emphasis is shifting away from segregated wrap-around services for people with disabilities towards a situation where people with disabilities:

- Access mainstream public services;
- Exercise choice and control;
- Live and participate in ordinary communities.

---

[16] The author wishes to thank Dharragh Hunt of the National Disability Authority for his assistance with this chapter.

Specialist Disability Services Are for a Minority

In 2009, specialist disability services funded through the HSE cost €1.5bn. However, most people with a disability live ordinary lives in the community, supported by family, friends and mainstream services, and it is only a minority who receive specialist disability services.

What the Statistics Show

In round figures, *Census 2006* showed 400,000 people with a disability (Central Statistics Office (CSO), 2007). The follow-up *National Disability Survey 2006* found that about 217,000 of these were at the more severe end of the spectrum, reporting that they either experienced a lot of difficulty or could not do everyday activities (CSO, 2008).

We can compare this with the number of people being served by HSE-funded specialist disability services. The Health Research Board's disability databases measure the number of people receiving, or on a waiting list for, specialist disability services and supports. For 2010, the numbers on its National Intellectual Disability database totalled about 26,500, while the estimated numbers getting or awaiting physical or sensory disability supports or equipment was 44,000.[17] This gives a total of 70,500 captured by specialist disability services. These figures suggest that only about one in three of those with more significant disabilities is being supported *via* specialist disability services.

SPECIALIST SERVICES TO PEOPLE WITH DISABILITIES

Specialist disability services in Ireland were largely developed by voluntary bodies, which include charitable organisations, religious orders, and organisations set up by parents and friends groups. Today, most of this activity is publicly-funded, alongside services delivered by the HSE itself.

How Services are Funded

There are two separate legal bases for funding voluntary organisations. Section 38 of the *Health Act, 2004* covers agencies delivering health or personal social services on behalf of the HSE. Most of the big disability service providers come under this heading. In 2009, there were 40 such

---

[17]   The Health Research Board estimates that its National Physical and Sensory Disability Database achieves about 66% coverage of this group, so the numbers recorded in 2010 of 29,000 would equate to an underlying 44,000.

service providers, which received over €5m (in fact, they averaged €26m) and accounted for 90% of funding to voluntary disability organisations.

Section 39 of the *Health Act, 2004* grant aids bodies providing services "similar to or ancillary to" HSE services. These are generally the smaller niche organisations, such as those serving people with a specific medical condition. Typically, these provide advice, support and advocacy for their members and, in some cases, some service provision. These organisations typically have income from fundraising, in addition to what they get from the HSE.

Voluntary providers receive block funding for services, which is not specifically calibrated to the levels of need of service users nor to achievement of quality standards. This funding model was criticised by the Comptroller and Auditor General in his 2005 Report (CAG, 2005). From 2010 on, formal service level agreements have become the norm.

The Provider Mix

The voluntary sector provides about 90% of specialist intellectual disability services and about 60% of specialist physical and sensory disability services. The HSE is also a significant service provider, while private for profit service provision is minimal.

Table 20.1: Disability Service Programme Expenditure by Service Type and Agency, 2009

Service area	%	HSE Share	Voluntary Agency Share
Residential	48	10%	90%
Adult Day Care	26	10%	90%
Multi-disciplinary teams	6	50%	50%
Personal Assistance Service	6	-	100%
Respite	4	5%	95%
National Rehabilitation Hospital and specialist services	3	20%	80%
Aids and appliances	3	80%	20%
Inappropriate Placements	3	50%	50%
Early intervention teams	1	30%	70%
Total	100	31%	69%

Source: DoHC. This excludes spending on allowances, now transferred to the Department of Social Protection.

About three-quarters of the disability services budget goes to provide residential or adult day services, principally serving people with intellectual disabilities. About 8,000 of the estimated 8,800 people in disability residential care have intellectual disabilities, as do 14,000 of the 25,000 people receiving adult day services.[18]

Wrap-around Services

The large disability service providers typically provide comprehensive wrap-around services. Their services may include education and training; transport; therapy support; day services; housing; and residential support. Many adults with disabilities may receive all their supports from one provider as an integrated package.

A review of disability services in six jurisdictions conducted by the National Disability Authority (NDA) in 2010 found that a similar wrap-around model was common in other developed countries until the 1990s (NDA, 2010a). While an advantage of this model can be that individuals receive seamless and joined-up services, disadvantages are that it can lead to segregated services and diminish choice.

A RIGHT TO LIVE IN AND BE PART OF THE COMMUNITY

Article 19 of the United Nations (UN) *Convention on the Rights of Persons with Disabilities* recognises:

> … the equal right of all persons with disabilities to live in the community, with choices equal to others, and shall take effective and appropriate measures to facilitate full enjoyment by persons with disabilities of this right and their full inclusion and participation in the community (UN, 2006).

However, many people with disabilities live lives that are removed from the mainstream community, and do not access mainstream services or community activities.

People in Residential Care

About half of those receiving disability residential care live in community group homes, while about half of those who live in disability residential care are living in centres of 10 or more people. As documented in the HSE report *Time to Move on from Congregated Settings* (2011a), these centres may

---

[18] National Intellectual Disability database 2010; National Physical and Sensory Disability database 2010; HSE (2012a).

be physically isolated; people may be living in dormitory accommodation; and there is strong international evidence of a poorer quality of life in residential centres compared to mainstream housing.

Article 19 of the *Convention on the Rights of Persons with Disabilities* states that persons with disabilities have the opportunity to choose their place of residence and where and with whom they live on an equal basis with others and are not obliged to live in a particular living arrangement (UN, 2006). The *Growing Older with an Intellectual Disability* report (Health Research Board, 2011) found that 68% of those living in community settings (mainly group homes) had no choice of where to live and 88% had no choice about who they lived with. The corresponding figures for those living in residential centres found over 90% without these choices.

Segregated Activities

The wrap-around service model is associated with group-based services that segregate people with disabilities from the general community.

As the *Disability Policy Review* states:

... this often involves service users attending a community setting as a group, on a special bus, often in a segregated manner (for example, a special hour for swimming or bowling). Those attending in the group usually have not selected that activity themselves. This is very different to an individual choosing to attend a swimming lesson, travelling to the swimming pool on public transport and taking the lesson with just a support person (not necessarily a health or social care professional) (DoHC, 2011: 10).

The consultation conducted for the *Disability Policy Review* showed a strong preference for people to live normal lives in normal places. As one mother put it:

"I don't want my daughter getting on a 'special' bus to a 'special' school and to be totally separated from the rest of the community... I want her to go to the same school as the other children and to have the same opportunities." (DoHC, 2011: 13-14).

Absence of Choice

The *Disability Policy Review* has criticised the absence of choice inherent in the wrap-around model of service (DoHC, 2011). In this model, the person is a passive recipient of a pre-determined service rather than an active determinant of an individually-tailored service that meets their needs and supports the achievement of their potential.

The *Growing Older with an Intellectual Disability* survey (Health Research Board, 2011) documented the degree to which those over 40 with an intellectual disability make everyday choices in their lives. What is striking is the absence of choice for those living in residential centres – 45% do not choose who they spend their free time with; 51% do not choose what they see on TV; and 64% do not choose when they go to bed.[19]

Different Elements of Service from Different Providers

Under current arrangements, where the service provider is also the landlord, people in residential care have no real option to switch services, as they would lose their home.

The consultation on the *Disability Policy Review* showed a strong preference that people would be free to get different elements of service from different providers (DoHC, 2011).

New Directions, the HSE's review of adult day services (HSE, 2012a), envisages moving away from group activities towards more individualised services where people would be supported to engage in mainstream community activities.

The proposal to move a share of the disability spend towards individualised budgets, as set out in the *Programme for Government 2011-2016*, would enable individuals and their families to choose how their funding was allocated across different providers and services (Fine Gael/Labour, 2011).

Therapy Supports

Half of public spending on provision of therapies to people with disabilities is *via* voluntary service providers. The traditional autonomy of voluntary service providers to decide their own model of service has resulted in an uneven geographical spread and uneven access to these therapy supports, depending on the local service provider or on which service someone attends. Access to therapy services, for example, may be easier for a child who is enrolled in a special school linked to a disability service provider, than for a child enrolled in a mainstream school, which is the preferred policy choice set out in the *Education for Persons with Special Education Need Act, 2004*.

As the D*isability Policy Review* noted:

> ... the almost exclusive location of many of the specialised therapy services (e.g. physiotherapy, occupation therapy, psychology etc.) within disability services means that these therapies are not routinely available outside of disability service settings. This drives demand for segregated services which are counter to policy objectives (DoHC, 2011).

---

[19]   Health Research Board, 2011: Table 8.1.

Recent initiatives and policy reviews have endorsed a change towards a single model of therapy support.

A REVIEW OF CHILDREN'S SERVICES

Following a HSE review entitled *Progressing Disability Services for Children and Young People* (HSE, 2011b), work has begun on reconfiguring existing therapy resources into geographically-based teams where HSE and voluntary therapy staff are pooled to serve each Integrated Services Area (typically a county).

The aims are:

- To provide one clear pathway to services for all children according to need;
- To ensure resources used to the greatest benefit for all children and families;
- To ensure health and education working together to support children to achieve their potential.

The new system envisages three levels of therapy provision:

- By the local primary care team (general practitioner, public health nurse, speech and language therapist, etc) when and where the child's needs can be met there;
- If the child's needs are more complex (whatever the nature of their disability) by early intervention and school age teams in each network area;
- The primary care and network teams should be supported as appropriate by specialist teams with a high level of expertise in particular fields.

The NDA's *Report on the Practice of Assessment of Need under Part 2 of the Disability Act, 2005* (NDA, 2011) found that areas with integrated early intervention teams were better equipped to meet the requirements of the *Disability Act, 2005* than areas with more fragmented provision. Also, parents of young children in areas where early intervention services were not integrated were found to have experienced more difficulty in accessing assessment and intervention.[20]

---

[20] This finding is based on interviews with 33 parents and on parents' subjective views of views of outcomes for their children, so must be treated with some caution.

OTHER REVIEWS TAKE A SIMILAR APPROACH

The HSE's *National Review of Autism Services Past, Present and Way Forward* (HSE, 2012b) has also recommended a similar approach:

> An integrated approach to meeting the health needs of people with disabilities is designed to ensure that generic health needs, which can be met at primary care level, are addressed by primary care teams and that only needs, where specialist knowledge, skill or expertise is required are referred to specialist services.

The *National Policy and Strategy for the Provision of Neurorehabilitation Services in Ireland 2011-2015* also set out a vertically-integrated model of service (HSE/DoHC, 2011).

The *Disability Policy Review* recommended that specialist disability supports be 'unbundled' or separated out into three distinct inputs that people with disabilities currently receive from specialist disability services funded by the health system:

- **Clinical inputs:** Addressing the health needs of an individual, providing specific treatments to cure/ease specific symptoms and disorders. These inputs are provided by medical and therapy professionals, usually in disability service settings in the current model;

- **Therapy inputs:** Aimed at increasing or sustaining functioning in various ways. These inputs are largely provided by therapy professionals and usually in disability service settings in the current model;

- **Personal social services:** Supporting people in activities of daily living (for example, self-care and accessing facilities in the community), with inputs from appropriate staff (such as personal assistants) (DoHC, 2011).

Furthermore, the *Review* recommended that there be equitable access to mainstream and specialist therapies and other health inputs for all people with disabilities within a specific catchment area/integrated service area.

The emerging policy is that the clinical and therapy interventions that people with disabilities require, in the future, will be structured into a model of vertically-integrated care, with primary care services as the initial access and referral points.

Findings from the NDA's *2011 National Survey of Public Attitudes to Disability in Ireland* highlighted difficulties that people with disabilities had in accessing general health services and community-based health services (NDA, 2011). It suggests that there is a need to ensure that primary care services are accessible to enable these services to function as an initial access and referral point to more specialised health and social services.

Second, a prerequisite to organising clinical and therapy supports into integrated care structures will be the 'unbundling' of clinical and therapy supports from personal social services and other ancillary services that disability services have historically delivered. The 'bundling' of clinical and therapy supports with personal social services may have driven demand for segregated disability services. However, experience from other jurisdictions shows that unbundling disability supports may result in people with disabilities finding it harder to access specialist therapy supports *via* mainstream primary care. Therefore, ensuring that adequate screening programmes and referral processes are in place will be required to ensure that people with disabilities do not get lost in the mainstream.

THE ROLE OF THE MAINSTREAM

If most people with disabilities, including those with significant disabilities, are living their lives without reference to specialist disability services, this underlines the importance of ensuring that mainstream services and supports are disability-friendly.

For those whose lives are largely lived within disability services – *circa* 9,000 people who live in residential care, and *circa* 25,000 adults who attend disability day services – the refocusing of those services towards a model to support people to live ordinary lives in ordinary places will put new demands on mainstream public services and on ordinary communities to rise to this challenge.

From a Health Model to an Equality Model

Disability policy was traditionally under the DoH, in keeping with a medical model of disability. An important break was when responsibility for disability policy was moved to the Department of Justice, Equality and Law Reform in 1993, signalling that advancing the inclusion of people with disabilities in Irish society was primarily an equality issue, not a medical issue.

The Report of the Commission on the Status of People with Disabilities (DoH, 1996), *Equal Citizens*, criticised the practice of segregated public services for people with disabilities.

Making Disability the Business of All Public Agencies

In June 2000, the then Government announced the policy that all public services would be obliged to include people with disabilities in their mainstream services ('mainstreaming'). This policy was given legal effect in the *Disability Act, 2005*.

The Act also required six Departments to prepare statutory plans on disability (Sectoral Plans), which were adopted by the Oireachtas in 2006, and were a core element of the National Disability Strategy. These plans set out a range of commitments covering employment and income support; housing and the built environment; transport; telecommunications; and the health service.

Challenges to Participation in Community Life

The NDA's *National Survey of Public Attitudes to Disability in Ireland* has documented some of the areas where people with disabilities said their participation has been restricted, and the degree to which this differs from the experience of others in the community (NDA, 2011).

Table 20.2: To What Extent Has Your Participation in the Following Areas been Restricted over the Past 12 Months?

Restrictions Experienced	Disabled %	Other %
Socialising (for example, meeting friends) ***	34	7
Employment or Job Seeking ***	31	11
Shopping ***	30	6
Sports or Physical Recreation ***	29	4
Community Life ***	26	2
Hospital Services ***	26	4
General Health Services ***	25	4
Community Based Health Services (for example, GPs, nurses, dentists) ***	25	3
Leisure /Cultural Activities ***	24	4
Mental Health Services ***	24	2
Living with Dignity ***	22	4
Education and Training ***	21	6
Family Life ***	21	4
Religion**	5	1
Base = 1,045 (2011); *Multiple responses possible; * $p<=0.05$; ** $p<=0.01$; *** p,=0.001		

Source: NDA, 2011.

THE NATIONAL DISABILITY STRATEGY

The National Disability Strategy, which is a whole-of-government approach to addressing the inclusion of people with disabilities, will be a key instrument to ensure there are systems, policies and actions in place to address the challenges to inclusion in the community.

As previous wrap-around services are unbundled in favour of a more individualised approach, the challenge will be for mainstream services to ensure they are genuinely inclusive for people with disabilities. Under the National Disability Strategy, the progressive achievement of public transport that is accessible to people with disabilities is one such example.

The co-ordination mechanisms under the National Disability Strategy are also critical. The policies of different Departments need to be mutually consistent, and not leave gaps, and set out clear protocols for interdepartmental co-ordination, which are translated down to local level.

Major Change in Disability Service Model

The *Disability Policy Review* (DoHC, 2011) was conducted by an expert reference group as part of a wider value-for-money and policy review. The vision set out in the *Review* is:

> To realise a society where people with disabilities are supported to participate fully in economic and social life and have access to a range of quality supports and services to enhance their quality of life and wellbeing.

The *Review* proposed two overarching goals:

- Full inclusion and self-determination for people with disabilities;
- The creation of a cost-effective, responsive and accountable system that will support the full inclusion and self-determination of people with disabilities.

Implication for Services and Supports for People with Disabilities

The *Disability Policy Review* (DoHC, 2011) summed up the contrast between the current model of disability services provision and the Expert Reference Group's new vision and, in particular, the contrast between the wrap-around nature of the current model of provision requirement for co-ordination between specialist, community and mainstream supports to deliver on the new vision of disability supports.

While the comprehensive wrap-around service from one provider often serves to isolate the person with a disability from being fully included in their local community and from mainstream provision, the advantage of such a model is the 'joined-up' nature of services. Thus, there is little need for co-ordination of services across sectors. The proposed model of a variety of support providers, both specialist and mainstream, and the separate provision of health and personal social supports will require a greater degree of liaison and co-ordination across sectors. This will include personal social services, such as transport and housing that come within the remit of other Government Departments.

Views of People with Disabilities on the New Approach

The NDA undertook research to establish how people with disabilities viewed the emerging new vision for disability supports emerging from this *Disability Policy Review* (DoHC, 2011). Specifically, focus groups representing people with disabilities, frontline staff, parents of children with disabilities and advocates were asked about their views on:

- Individualised supports;
- Mainstreaming (NDA, 2010a).

In relation to individualised supports, attitudes were generally positive, though somewhat sceptical about the capacity of the system to deliver such supports.

Many participants responded to the greater choice and control over funding, which they associated with an individualised funding mechanism. However, some of the participants also queried the capacity and willingness of the Government to deliver on this policy (NDA, 2011).

Similarly, participants were positive about mainstreaming when adequate supports were provided for those accessing mainstream services:

> [P]articipants were in favour of mainstreaming, provided appropriate supports were provided, which would enable people with disabilities access services they needed. (NDA, 2010a)

There appears, therefore, to be a consensus among policy-makers and people with disabilities that future disability supports and services should be based on:

- Individuals' choices and preferences;
- A greater use of mainstream and community services;
- A high-quality and transparently-funded support system.

TOWARDS INTEGRATED SUPPORTS

Integrated Care and Person-centred Approaches

The aim of integrated care appears to be what in the disability area are termed 'person-centred services'. In recent decades, a person-centred approach is seen as being key to driving changes within the disability service sector (NDA, 2010a).

The outcome of the person-centred planning process should be a plan of individualised supports – a combination of specialist, mainstream and informal supports co-ordinated to deliver the best outcome for a person, taking account of their abilities and aspirations (NDA, 2010b).[21] However, achieving co-ordination across specialist, mainstream and informal supports is a challenge (NDA, 2010b).[22] In the new model envisaged by the *Disability Policy Review*, it will be a key task to ensure the co-ordination of individualised services that may be provided by community, mainstream or specialised providers.

What changes in the organisation of the delivery across specialist, community and mainstream public services are required to develop a system of supports that are flexible, personalised and seamless from the point of view of the person with a disability?

Integration: A Challenge to Disability Supports Provision

While there is a consensus that integrated services should be flexible, personalised and seamless from the point of view of the person with a disability, there is much less consensus about how that can be achieved.

According to Kodner (2009), social service systems in many jurisdictions are now attempting to address key issues such as fragmented services, difficult-to-control costs and poor quality and access. Efforts to deal with these challenges increasingly are referred to as 'integration of care'.

The NDA's 2010 review of disability services in six jurisdictions (NDA, 2010c) did not find good examples of co-ordinated services and supports. So while streamlined, integrated, joined-up, transparent service system models, co-ordinated across departments and delivering mainstream services to people with disabilities are often proposed, they are not easily achieved. There are no ready models or frameworks to draw on.

---

[21] *See also* NDA, 2006.
[22] *See also* NDA, 2006.

Stewart *et al.* (2003) suggest the following are key preconditions to making progress towards more integrated care:

- Consistent and realistic national policy;
- Overcoming cultural suspicions and developing a practical understanding of how other organisations operate;
- Jointly identifying and accepting local unmet need;
- Addressing operational factors;
- Being open, flexible and take risks in the pursuit of clear goals, supported by strong management.

Housing Strategy for People with Disabilities

Disability service providers generally have owned and managed the homes in which people with disabilities who get residential support are living.

The *Housing Strategy for People for People with a Disability 2011-2016* (Department of the Environment, Community and Local Government, 2011) gives effect to the principle of mainstreaming, by placing responsibility for housing provision with local authorities, while the HSE would continue to fund associated care supports. Jointly launched by the Ministers with responsibilities for disability and housing, the *Strategy* has the following aim:

> To facilitate access, for people with disabilities, to the appropriate range of housing and related support services, delivered in an integrated and sustainable manner, which promotes equality of opportunity, individual choice and independent living.

The *Strategy* is very clear that the solution to providing housing in the community to people with disabilities can only be delivered by an integrated approach by national and local stakeholders. The actions identified in the *Strategy* include:

- New assessment and prioritisation criteria, including interagency protocols with the HSE;
- A requirement for strategic housing assessment to determine local need for housing supports for people with disabilities;
- Clarified roles and responsibilities and developing a joint working ethos for within agencies and organisations delivering services to people with disabilities;
- A commitment to developing a framework for interagency co-operation, with structured agreements, common goals and objectives;

- National protocols, to define funding responsibilities and to facilitate exchange of relevant information and advice to enhance service delivery.

CONCLUSION

The current model of specialist disability service provision, whereby a single provider wraps services around an individual, largely negated the need for integrated services and supports. However, it re-inforced segregation and risked causing social isolation. The new vision of supports for people with disabilities, as set out in the *Disability Policy Review* (DoHC, 2011), envisages more services being delivered in the community and by mainstream providers, and service delivery built around individuals' needs and preferences, to support people's capacity for independent living.

This vision of people with disabilities living independently, participating in mainstream community activities, and accessing mainstream public services is not something that any one provider can deliver. Responsibility for providing service to people with disabilities is likely in the years ahead to be shared across a greater number and range of providers. Whether this development results in a system of services and supports that is flexible, personalised and seamless from the point of view of the person with a disability will depend on whether the instruments – joint planning, joint needs assessment, service delivery protocols, key workers – and the ethos of integrated services and supports can be developed within and between specialist, community and mainstream service providers.

There are likely to be two major change processes shaping disability service provision over the coming years:

- Specialist disability services are likely to be unbundled;
- Greater levels of integration across specialist, community and mainstream providers are envisaged in the new vision of disability services.

At first sight, these processes may seem contradictory. However, the success of the unbundling of specialist disability services is dependent on the ability of specialist, community and mainstream providers to deliver integrated services. If specialist services are unbundled, but a significantly enhanced capacity to deliver integrated supports and services across specialist, community and mainstream providers is not achieved, people with disabilities will be faced with greater levels of service fragmentation.

The *Disability Act, 2005* provides for the position of Liaison Officer (known in the HSE as 'case managers'), whose task is to source the different services required to meet an individual's needs. Such a case manager or key worker role is a critical part of ensuring that the different pieces of the service jigsaw come together.

The National Disability Strategy Implementation Plan will be a critical element in ensuring that Departments, across the board, play their parts in making mainstream services responsive to the needs of people with disabilities, and in delivering a genuinely co-ordinated framework of services.

REFERENCES

Central Statistics Office (CSO) (2008). *National Disability Survey 2006*, Cork: CSO.

Central Statistics Office (CSO) (2007). *Census 2006*, Cork: CSO.

Comptroller and Auditor General (CAG) (2005). *Report of the Comptroller and Auditor General*, Dublin: Stationery Office.

Department of Health (DoH) (1996). *Equal Citizens: The Report of the Commission on the Status of People with Disabilities*, Dublin: Stationery Office.

Department of Health and Children (DoHC) (2011). *Report of the Disability Policy Review*, available http://www.dohc.ie/publications/pdf/ERG_Disability_Policy_Review_ Final.pdf?direct=1.

Department of the Environment, Community and Local Government (2011). *National Housing Strategy for People with a Disability 2011 – 2016*, available http://www.environ.ie/en/Publications/DevelopmentandHousing/Housing/FileDownLoad,28016,en.pdf.

Fine Gael/Labour (2011). *Towards Recovery, Programme for a National Government 2011-2016*, Dublin: Fine Gael/Labour.

Health Research Board (2011). *Growing Older with an Intellectual Disability*, Dublin: Health Research Board, available http://www.hrb.ie/uploads/media/Growing_Older_with_an_Intellectual_Disability_in_ Ireland_2011.pdf, Table 8.1.

Health Service Executive (HSE) (2008). *Corporate Plan 2008-2011*, available http://www.hse.ie/eng/services/Publications/corporate/Corporate_Plan_2 008_-_2011.pdf.

Health Service Executive (HSE) (2011a). *Time to Move On from Congregated Settings*, Dublin: HSE.

Health Service Executive (HSE) (2011b). *Progressing Disability Services for Children and Young People*, available http://www.hse.ie/eng/services/Publications/services/ Disability/multidisciplinarydisabilityserviceschildren.html.

Health Service Executive (HSE) (2012a). *New Directions: A Review of Adult Day Services*, Dublin: Stationery Office.

Health Service Executive (HSE) (2012b). *National Review of Autism Services Past, Present and Way Forward*, available http://www.hse.ie/eng/services/Publications/services/ Disability/autismreview2012.pdf.

Health Service Executive and Department of Health and Children (HSE/DOHC) (2011). *National Policy and Strategy for the Provision of Neurorehabilitation Services in Ireland 2011-2015*, available http://www.dohc.ie/publications/pdf/ NeuroRehab_Services1.pdf.

Kodner, D. (2009). 'All Together Now: A Conceptual Exploration of Integrated Care', *Healthcare Quarterly*, 13(Special): 6-15.

National Disability Authority (NDA) (2006). *Guidelines on Person-centred Planning in the Provision of Services for People with Disabilities in Ireland*, available http://www.nda.ie/cntmgmtnew.nsf/0/ 12AF395217EE3AC7802570C800430BB1/$File/main.pdf.

National Disability Authority (NDA) (2010a). *Individualised Supports and Mainstream Services Attitudes of People with Disabilities and Other Stakeholders to Policy Proposals by the Department of Health and Children*, available http://www.nda.ie/website/nda /cntmgmtnew.nsf/0/ E093380FB2F9DD5580257775003E0E6B/$File/Attitudes_of_people_with_disabili ties_and_other_stakeholders_to_policy_proposals_by_the_DoHC.pdf.

National Disability Authority (NDA) (2010b). *Advice Paper to the Value for Money and Policy Review of Disability Services Programme*, available http://www.nda.ie/ CntMgmtNew.nsf/DCC524B4546ADB3080256C700071B049/B6B630EA27AC 94CC8025787F003D54F0/$File/Value_For_Money.pdf.

National Disability Authority (NDA) (2010c). *Developing Services for People with Disabilities: A Synthesis Paper Summarising the Key Learning of Experiences in Selected Jurisdictions as at October 2010*, available http://www.nda.ie/CntMgmtNew.nsf/   . DCC524B4546ADB3080256C700071B049/FF7105D82D4C7E6D80257877005A8 745/$File/SynthesisReport.pdf.

National Disability Authority (NDA) (2011). *A National Survey of Public Attitudes to Disability in Ireland*, available http://www.nda.ie/CntMgmtNew.nsf/ DCC524B4546ADB3080256C700071B049/90F8D23334D786A880257987004FC F51/$File/Public_Attitudes_to_Disability_in_Irelandfinal.pdf.

National Disability Authority (NDA) (2011) *Report on the Practice of Assessment of Need under Part 2 of the Disability Act, 2005*, Dublin: NDA.

Stewart, A., Petch, A. and Curtice, L. (2003). 'Moving towards Integrated Working. in Health and Social Care in Scotland: From Maze to Matrix', *Journal of Interprofessional Care*, 17(4): 35-350, cited by Jarrett, D., Stevenson, T., Huby, G. and Stewart, A. (2009), 'Developing and Implementing Research as a Lever for Integration: The Impact of Service Context', *Journal of Integrated Care*, 38-48.

United Nations (2006). *Convention on the Rights of Persons with Disabilities*, New York: United Nations.

CONCLUSION

The international experience offers salutary conclusions for the development of integrated care in Ireland. The Northern Ireland (NI) experience, in particular, is significant. We have learned that perhaps NI is a UK leader in integrated care and is clearly ahead of the Republic of Ireland, which is still trying to get to grips with the organisational framework and delivery of integrated care.

In the context of the continuing failure to deliver primary care centres (PCCs) in Ireland as discussed by myself earlier (**Chapter 1**), and the belief by some that primary care teams (PCTs) can work while not all being housed under one roof, the NI experience clearly shows that this is unwise: "... locating professionals under the same roof and shared working space enables more comprehensive assessments of vulnerable adults and children to be undertaken".

My belief that a significant number of integrated care co-ordinators/managers will be needed in Ireland, if Integrated Service Areas and the Health Service Executive's (HSE) four-level model are to be implemented, is also supported by Campbell et al. in their chapter on Northern Ireland (**Chapter 2**): "... for example, Donnelly et al. (2004) found that a community-based team of health and social care professionals led by a community care manager (with access to consultant medical staff, if required) provided cost-effective rehabilitation in the homes of stroke patients, who in the absence of the service, would have had longer hospital stays and lower quality of life".

There are many chronic illnesses that will present very significant challenges for policy-makers and those in the health and social caring professions in the years ahead. One particular illness in this regard is diabetes. In the case of chronic illnesses such as diabetes, for McHugh and Perry in their chapter (**Chapter 6**): "The cracks in the delivery of health care are particularly precarious for those with complex chronic conditions who require planned, structured, multidisciplinary care that is integrated across professions and settings, including social and health care". Integrated care is urgently required to tackle these illnesses. The likely explosion of the incidence of diabetes in the coming years means that this is a 'model' disease for which an integrated care approach to dealing with other chronic illnesses can be based, according the authors. The need for this approach, with a high emphasis on modelling an integrated care approach to diabetes, also is found to be necessary in the chapter by Quinlan and Moran (**Chapter 9**).

The critical importance of implementing quality and effective management systems at the coalface of health and social care practice to deliver real integrated care is mentioned also by Hetherington *et.al.*, who welcome in **Chapter 8**: "… shared protocols, such as those developed by the HSE clinical care programmes and care pathways". The protocols themselves "promote continuity of care by defining roles and responsibilities for all team members/providers involved in the care process". It seems clear that dedicated and specialised field managers in health and social care will need to be educated and trained in integrated care, which is a specialism now in its own right. The specialist integrated care managers, of which there will need to be a significant number, will need to be involved in developing, implementing, monitoring and managing these protocols to ensure that all patients/clients are receiving the required standard of care and that there is continuity in the process, not gaps and blockages. **Chapter 3** by William Reddy clearly demonstrates the importance of established protocols: in this case, the importance of a discharge plan for each patient leaving hospital. But the implementation of this discharge plan and the building of the recommended services within primary and community care into a more comprehensive integrated care plan for the patient is a significant function. While teams will be involved in bringing forward the recommended inputs, a co-ordinator/manager still will be needed to bring all the necessary elements of care together and to manage its delivery in line with necessary protocols across the different levels of service delivery.

The management of integrated care in Ireland, at least in policy, seems to have learned from the Swedish use of 'chains of care' which are: "a Swedish concept of integration and collaboration in health care, which includes all the services provided for a specific group of patients within a defined geographical area", as discussed by Ahgren and Axelsson in **Chapter 5**. Teams of social workers and health professionals have collaborated at the local level in forming 'dementia teams' working within home care, the care of mental illness, addiction, care of refugees and other areas in Sweden. The results have been positive. However, a warning of the possible pitfalls for Ireland comes in the guise of professional disagreements: "there were many 'territorial' conflicts between the different organisations and professionals involved". A taste of this problem can be gleaned also from **Chapter 7** by Desmond and O'Connor on the implementation of the new NDRIC model for addiction services, where the enthusiasm of the policy-makers was not necessarily shared by all practitioners. This suggests that there is a clear need to develop and to roll out courses on interprofessional education, as called for in **Chapter 10** by McGrath. In this context, Jacob, in **Chapter 11**, argues that the profession of social work has a key role to play in the facilitation of interprofessional working: "As 'systems specialists', social workers in primary care have the opportunity to be the 'glue' that bonds primary and secondary services with the common aim of integrated care". Jacob provides an impressive array of information, particularly that from Siefert and Henk within the University of Michigan School of Social Work, on the strongly pivotal role of social workers in primary care, community care, health promotion, advocacy, disease prevention and a whole range of other areas, to strongly support her contention that social workers are uniquely placed as a profession to manage integrated care. That it might be better to have a 'social' profession as key in the management of integrated care is suggested from the Northern Ireland experience, where interprofessionalism has been rather too-greatly influenced by the biomedical model. Perhaps, however, fully- and newly-trained integrated care managers, drawing their knowledge holistically from both the biomedical and social models of health and social care, are the optimum solution for the effective management of integrated care.

It might be argued that, given the centrality of general practitioners (GPs) in primary care, GPs themselves need to have a significant role in the management of integrated care teams. Contrarily, one might argue that GPs spend years training to be clinicians and that integrated care management is not the role that GPs are trained for. The latter position seems obvious from **Chapter 9** by two Cork GPs, Quinlan and Moran, and also from **Chapter 12** by O'Riordan and Collins, representing the Irish College of General Practitioners. The authors argue for good management of primary care teams; but there are significant problems in this area at the moment, with only 54% of teams reporting full GP participation. The authors also highlight a quote from the Comptroller and Auditor General's *2011 Report* that: "There has not yet been a change at the level of control and management that would put PCTs at the centre of primary care delivery". O'Riordan and Collins highlight the success of GPs working closely with the local primary care manager and their interest in working as part of primary care teams: "GPs highly value managers who are pro-active, flexible, open communicators, showing a willingness to engage in a positive manner with them and thus encouraging participation and belief in the team concept. Naturally, this has led also to improved GP-HSE communications on all aspects of local service delivery". This allows us to make two conclusions: first, the centrality of management in integrated care is highlighted; second, there are only relatively few primary care managers nationally who have a very broad remit. The benefits of GPs' management experience would need to be replicated in a far larger number of specifically-trained integrated care managers to manage the integration between PCTs and other teams that operate in the community health and social care network, secondary care hospital teams, and at teams operating at the level of tertiary care. The management of discharge and appropriate integrated care plans need also to be managed, not alone across levels of care, but also with regard to a variety of integrated care groups: older people, mentally ill, stroke victims, cancer sufferers, diabetes patients, etc. Again, this requires highly-trained and specialised integrated care personnel to fulfil these highly demanding roles, which would also involve managing interprofessional working and any conflict that may arise from time to time.

However, irrespective of the primary profession of dedicated integrated care managers, an important lesson advanced by Fleming *et al.* on the Scottish experience in **Chapter 18** is that the development of integrated care pathways (ICPs) needs to happen on a phased basis and not all at once: "Experience in Scotland tells us that taking this 'big bang' approach can create a great deal of anxiety and resistance, as people can perceive that implementing the pathways will mean a great deal of 'extra work' and drastically-changed practice". Instead, the authors advise: " by using a phased implementation programme, any training issues can be identified early, thus ensuring that teams are equipped with the relevant skills and knowledge by the time the full ICP is rolled out". In Ireland, we don't have the ICPs in practice that we need for members of the general population or the various client/patient groups in need of them. As **Chapter 1** demonstrates, we have a new emphasis on integrated care in HSE policy and an integrated services model for the whole population. Other plans, such as *Vision for Change* for those with mental illness, fit this model, as does the hospital discharge plan. However, the micro application to practice of ICPs for the general population, those with diabetes, mental illness, disability, stroke, cancer and other challenges, have not been practically operationalised to date. This urgently needs to happen. In this context, returning to NI, Campbell *et al.* argue in **Chapter 3** that community and primary care partnership arrangements, linked as they need to be to hospital services, are key to delivering integrated care. The setting up of health and social care trusts to manage integrated care locally has shown to be successful in Northern Ireland, and to some extent also in Scotland, as illustrated in Chapter 18 by Fleming *et al.* Working on a study by Heenan and Birrell (2006), Campbell *et al.* state in relation to Northern Ireland: "… the problems caused by the separation of health and social care functions in the rest of the UK were viewed to be more easily resolved in the Northern Irish system because of the unified system of planning and delivery of services across this continuum". This was facilitated *inter alia* by the organisational management of health and social care trusts. They also found advantages in having programmes of care, which are already intrinsic to the Irish model (HSE), as pointed out in **Chapter 1**.

The issue of resources is critical as always in moving integrated care forward in Ireland. This includes human resources, physical infrastructure and requires a particular emphasis on strong communication systems. In order to facilitate the process, an incentivisation system for GPs, based on quality treatment outcomes for specific diseases such as diabetes and asthma, is needed according to Quinlan and Moran (**Chapter 9**), but also the Irish Medical Organisation authors (Hetherington *et al.*, **Chapter 8**). Regarding communication, Hetherington *et al.* note that: "Information and communications technology is widely considered a key tool for supporting/assisting integrated health care systems and the 'seamless' transfer of patients between clinical settings". This key need for strong communication systems has been highlighted also in the case of Northern Ireland by Campbell *et al.* (**Chapter 3**). The critical importance of strong communication systems is clear also from the Canadian experience, as shown by McAdam in **Chapter 13**.

On the issue of the much-lauded PCTs in Irish health policy, Hetherington *et al.* report in **Chapter 8** the poor functioning of PCTs currently, based on ICGP findings. In **Chapter 1**, the poor functioning of PCTs has been shown to be strongly influenced by the failure to provide most of the PCCs needed to house the teams in question, with a minimum of 300 still in the pipeline to be built/commissioned in the short- to medium term.

But the issue of resources presupposes a sustainable and quality funding stream for health in Ireland, which has always been a problem historically. The critical issue of how best to fund care and to provide Universal Health Insurance for the whole population is dealt with in **Chapter 4** by Thomas and Darker. The authors deal with highly complex arguments and ultimately point to the fact that there are pros and cons in both single-payer and multi-payer health insurance systems. However, on balance, it seems that a single-payer system (currently being rejected by the Irish government in favour of the more competitively-driven Dutch multi-payer model) offers the most balanced approach from a population health perspective, given that: "Single-payer systems usually are financed more progressively, and rely on existing taxation systems. Effectively, they distribute risks throughout one large risk pool and offer governments a high degree of control over the total expenditure on health. Multi-payer systems sacrifice this control for a greater ability to meet the diverse preferences of beneficiaries. However, this diversity tends to result in the segmentation of risk groups unless adequate safeguards against adverse selection are used".

Specific conclusions can be drawn also regarding integrated care delivery with specific service user groups. Starting with the care of older people, the Canadian experience of piloting integrated care based on home care family home teams, consisting of a variety of integrated health/social care professionals and using health information initiatives, in Québec and British Columbia, warns us of the dangers of not having a uniform and consistent delivery of services across the whole population (**Chapter 13**). Nonetheless, McAdam points to significant benefits for older people in receiving integrated care that can be delivered on a cost-neutral basis: "… there is Canadian evidence that supports increased investment in improving co-ordination of care for seniors because it has the potential to improve quality of care while not increasing system total costs". In addition, home care for the elderly in Canada offers an excellent example of innovation by way of its Home Care Assessment instrument: "Seven of the 10 provinces are using the Home Care Assessment instrument to collect uniform reliable data about home care clients. These data are used for care planning at the clinical level but they also allow policy-makers to group home care clients by risk level, map service plans against the supply of local services, and develop performance accountability measures". This would be a hugely advantageous system for the delivery of integrated elder care in Ireland.

Dementia is presenting itself as a significant population health problem for Ireland and is likely to increase over time. Research conducted by Suzanne Cahill (**Chapter 14**) has shown that there has been appalling neglect in the assessment and diagnosis of people with dementia, which has resulted in detrimental effects on the subsequent health of the individual. The case study on the failure of Marjorie Murphy by the health services highlights the fact that her deterioration into dementia, ultimately to the point where she was found wandering three miles from home, occurred over a period of up to 12 months whereby: "at no stage did she have a cognitive assessment undertaken, nor was any attempt made to discuss her discharge planning with Kevin or trial her at home". Prior to her case becoming apparent, Marjorie had spent four days on a trolley in A&E and was discharged with tranquillisers, having developed MRSA in hospital, and without a diagnosis of her condition been made. This should never happen again to older people like Marjorie, although it is probably happening as you read, due to the continuing failure in the area of home care, a key element of integrated care services. Irish health policy *inter alia* needs to remedy the fact that people with dementia in Ireland "fall between the cracks of disability services, services for older people and mental health services", according to Cahill. This is the antithesis to 'integrated care' and needs urgent attention. Cahill points out that, in Ireland, there are no dementia-specific teams or aged care teams in existence. What is needed are ICPs for dementia sufferers (currently non-existent in Ireland): "An integrated care pathway in dementia care ideally would mean community-based dementia teams, working in tandem with primary care teams and trained to conduct assessment and diagnostic services in peoples' homes and to help families come to terms with transitions into long-term care and into hospices. Flexible, around the clock, individualised services, underpinned by person-centred principles, would be organised around service users, in response to their individual needs". This is a clear conclusion and recommendation.

The neglect of older people in Ireland has been well-documented in this book by Des O'Neill in **Chapter 15**: one study from 2012 shows that over 80% of older people had "no support in place at the time of discharge" from hospital. Because of the failure of the system in general to adequately assess health and social care needs of older people once they leave hospital, over a quarter return to hospital in less than six weeks after discharge. This is "a telling argument for better assessment of, and provision for, care needs and their delivery in a better integrated manner". Going forward, a beacon on the horizon is the production of blueprints for the care of older people as part of the National Clinical Programme for Older People. This recognises "the complexity of care of older people" and uses a single assessment tool to assess their care needs. Ireland, however, is a latecomer to this process and trails behind many other countries such as the USA and most of Europe, in O'Neill's assessment. In addition, assessment tools are ineffective unless ICPs follow and resources are committed in training, infrastructure, communication and other areas.

The need for ICPs for older people as described by Cahill in **Chapter 14**, also is called for in this book by Irving *et al.*, who stress in **Chapter 16**, in line with similar conclusions already arrived at earlier, that specific training for those involved in these new roles will be required. They call for the government to honour its commitment to a National Dementia Strategy by 2013. The authors also call for a far greater service user involvement in the development of services and new roles of responsibility. In developing ICPs for dementia, several 'test sites' need to be piloted to cater for the full diversity of needs of dementia sufferers and carers. Measurement of the efficacy of these sites in terms of best practice and cost-effectiveness needs to be conducted in order to provide strong evidence to influence policy-makers. Otherwise, these sites will become "mere islands of good practice".

Astonishingly, ICPs for those with a mental illness, which at any given time can affect nearly one-third of Irish people, have been identified as far back as 2006 by way of *Vision for Change*, the government's accepted policy. **Chapter 1**, and more particularly that of Saunders (**Chapter 17**), makes this clear. The continuing failure to implement worked out pathways between PCTs and community mental health teams nationwide to any significant extent whatsoever has been recognised by Saunders. This doesn't bode well for the future development of ICPs for older people or those with disabilities. Saunders clearly speaks to the need to strengthen the advocacy role in society of service user groups and others in co-operation, a point that is also made by Irving *et al.* in **Chapter 16**. The use of human rights law, advocating that the government enforce the *Convention on the Rights of People with Disabilities*, is eloquently described by Moira Jenkins in **Chapter 19**. This could be a useful strategy in pressurising policy-makers to deliver integrated care for 'vulnerable adults'. In that event, the statutory recognition and provision of a new role of 'social care advocate' is intrinsic to the integration of health and social care services for the vulnerable adult, as Jenkins concludes. She offers the very useful observation that: "The idea of an Office for the Social Care Advocate has a number of precedent models (the Office of the Public Advocate in Victoria, Australia is one example)". Clearly, there is a need for overt political pressure to mobilise for the development and delivery of ICPs for disabled people, mentally ill, older people and others. The work of advocacy organisations such as the Mental Health Coalition, the Alzheimer Society of Ireland and others cannot be overstated in this regard.

The role of the National Disability Authority has provided a wealth of valuable research to aid the development of better services for the disabled community and has pointed the way forward for disability policy in recent years. **Chapter 20** by Fitzgerald decries the current failure to allow many disabled people in Ireland the human right to live in a community of their choice, as set out under Article 19 of the UN *Convention on the Rights of Persons with Disabilities*. There is a clear need to move a large number of those with disabilities out of institutional residential care and to allow them to live in their own community. The current 'absence of choice' is an abuse of human rights. Integrated care services, particularly those in primary care and within community health and social care networks, are needed to foster this de-institutionalisation. For Fitzgerald, the role of the Liaison Officer, established under the *Disability Act, 2005*, is pivotal in order to act as a 'case manager' to co-ordinate integrated services for those with a disability and whereby "the different pieces of the jigsaw come together".

These conclusions are the ones that 'jump off the page' from the various chapters in this book. However, there are myriads of other conclusions contained within the chapters themselves that require more detailed examination. I would encourage anybody with a deep interest in integrated care to dig deeper and to examine more closely the in-depth and highly analytical discussions within each chapter. The text has been divided into sections, based on their specific interest. Nonetheless, there is a significant cross-fertilisation and cross-validation of themes, conclusions and findings across the various chapters, only a flavour of which is derived from reading my conclusions above. If you have a passion for understanding integrated care, I can state without reservation that reading this book in its totality will prove a very worthwhile and rewarding experience.

INDEX

3 Es, 49

A&E, 24, 183, 236, 276, 356 – *see also* Emergency Departments
academic institution(s), 310
access, 61, 69, 70, 73, 80, 82, 84, 114, 137, 214, 256, 257, 329
accountability, 78, 134, 217, 319, 326, 329
accountable care, 144
activities of daily living (ADLs), 237, 238, 247, 256, 257, 260, 340
acute care, 63, 83, 99, 223, 241, 248
acute coronary syndrome, 23
acute facilities, management of, 84
acute hospital care, 84, 248
acute hospital(s), 8, 10, 11, 12, 13, 14, 16, 21, 22, 24, 41, 62, 139
Acute Medicine Programme, 256, 258
acute re-actionary service(s), 105
acute secondary care hospital(s), 21
acute service(s), 194
acute stomach pain, 161
acutely ill patient(s), 207
addiction, 3, 4, 35, 37, 95, 120, 122, 123, 126, 127, 132, 188
addiction care, 351
addiction counsellor(s), 124, 127, 128, 134, 135, 352
addiction service(s), 119, 122-123, 127, 132-133
Adelaide Hospital Society (AHS), 70, 74, 75, 79, 82, 84
administration, 49, 75, 199
administration, personnel/staff, 27, 181, 297
administrator(s), 13, 48, 126, 161, 196, 208, 232
admission(s), 11, 13, 15, 52, 53, 61-62, 144, 152, 180, 183, 201, 267, 272
adolescent(s), 38
adult care, 51, 52
advance care directive(s), 247, 328
adverse selection, 77, 355

advocacy, 135, 150, 153, 162, 194, 195, 201, 241, 251, 317-330, 352, 357 – *see also* case advocacy
aetiologies, 266
Afghanistan, 120
Age Action Ireland, 11, 241
age-attuned care, 258
age-attuned education and training, 255
aged care, 246
aged care assessment team(s), 248, 356
ageing demographic(s), 20
ageing population(s), 182, 207, 266
ageist practice(s), 256
Aging at Home Strategy (Ontario) (Canada), 230
Alberta (AB) (Canada), 225, 233
Alberta Health and Wellness (Canada), 233
Alberta Health Services (Canada), 233
Alberta Medical Association (Canada), 233
alcohol, 120, 121
alcohol abuse/misuse, 17, 121, 160
alcohol and drug treatment service(s), 123
allied health professional(s), 105, 143, 184, 185, 189, 196, 197, 214, 251
alternate level of care (ALC), 228
Alzheimer Society of Ireland (ASI), 241, 243, 357
Alzheimer's disease, 237, 238, 265, 291
ambulance service(s), 16, 22, 160
ambulatory health, 223
American Association of Colleges of Nursing, 174
American Association of Colleges of Osteopathic Medicine, 174
American Association of Colleges of Pharmacy, 174
American Dental Education Association, 174
Amnesty International, 40
An Bord Altranais, *see* Bord Altranais, An
anaesthetic, 37
ancillary service(s), 143, 194, 213

ABOUT OAK TREE PRESS

Oak Tree Press develops and delivers information, advice and resources for entrepreneurs and managers. It is Ireland's leading business book publisher, with an unrivalled reputation for quality titles across business, management, HR, law, marketing and enterprise topics. NuBooks is its recently-launched imprint, publishing short, focused ebooks for busy entrepreneurs and managers.

In addition, Oak Tree Press occupies a unique position in start-up and small business support in Ireland through its standard-setting titles, as well training courses, mentoring and advisory services.

Oak Tree Press is comfortable across a range of communication media – print, web and training, focusing always on the effective communication of business information.

Oak Tree Press, 19 Rutland Street, Cork, Ireland.
T: + 353 21 4313855 F: + 353 21 4313496.
E: info@oaktreepress.com W: www.oaktreepress.com.